An Illustrated Dictionary of Dermatologic Syndromes

An Illustrated Dictionary of Dermatologic Syndromes

Susan Bayliss Mallory MD
Associate Professor of Dermatology
Washington University School of Medicine
St. Louis, Missouri.

with

Susana Leal-Khouri MD
Washington University School of Medicine
St. Louis, Missouri.

With a foreword by
Walter B. Shelley

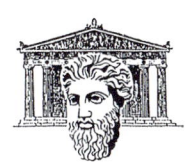

The Parthenon Publishing Group
International Publishers in Medicine, Science & Technology

NEW YORK　　　　　　　　　　　　　　　　　　　LONDON

Published in North America by
The Parthenon Publishing Group Inc.
One Blue Hill Plaza, PO Box 1564
Pearl River
New York 10965, USA

Published in the UK and Europe by
The Parthenon Publishing Group Limited
25 Blades Court
London SW15 2NU, UK

Copyright © 1994 The Parthenon Publishing Group Inc.

Library of Congress Cataloging-in-Publication Data
Mallory, Susan B.
  An Illustrated Dictionary of Dermatologic Syndromes /
Susan Bayliss Mallory with Susana Leal-Khouri.
       p. cm.
  Includes bibliographic references.
  ISBN 1-85070-458-9
  1. Cutaneous manifestations of general diseases—Dictionaries.
  2. Syndromes—Dictionaries. I. Leal-Khouri, Susana. II.Title.
       [DNLM: 1. Skin Diseases—dictionaries. 2. Skin Diseases—atlases.
  3. Skin Manifestations—dictionaries. 4. Skin Manifestations—atlases.
  WR 13 M2551 1994]
  RL100.M35 1994
  616.5'003—dc20
  DNLM/DLC   94–15125
  for Library of Congress   CIP

British Library Cataloguing in Publication Data
Mallory, Susan B.
  Illustrated Dictionary of Dermatologic Syndromes
  I. Title II. Leal-Khouri, Susana
  616.5075

  ISBN 1-85070-458-9

No part of this book may be reproduced, stored in a retrieval system, or transmitted in any form or by any means, electronic, mechanical, photocopying, recording or otherwise, without prior permission from the publishers.

Color reproduction by Colorplan, Leeds, UK
Printed and bound in Spain by T.G. Hostench, S.A.

CONTENTS

Foreword vii

Introduction ix

Acknowledgements x

General References xi

Dictionary 1

Appendix: Classification by Syndrome Manifestation 243

FOREWORD

You now hold in your hand a magnificent collection of syndromes that will greatly enhance your diagnostic ability. You simply have to turn the pages to discover old classics, half-forgotten syndromes and the best of the new world syndromy.

This compilation of over 700 syndromes can provide endless variations on the skin diseases you see in your practice. For instance, the ichthyosis section has 24 variations, the epidermolysis bullosa section has 27 different types, and there are 49 aberrations of the nail plate.

Here are some of the new enticing syndromes you will meet: the happy puppet syndrome, the prune belly syndrome, Sly syndrome, Sweet syndrome and the lip-tip syndrome. They are all there. The rich heritage of both pediatric and dermatologic knowledge awaits you in this book. If you can recognize the kinky hair syndrome or the wildlife syndromes (LAMB, LEOPARD and Robin) they may just appear in your office!

All of these syndromes are displayed in a clear format of lovely color photographs and lists which are very easy to read. References, current to 1993, sit in adjoining blue boxes for easy access. When only a few parts of a syndrome come to mind, you can go to the Appendix where you will be directed to each syndrome containing your fragment of information. For instance, if your patient has annular erythematous plaques, the Appendix will introduce you to 17 possible diseases.

Here is an *aide-mémoire* for the finer points of clinical diagnosis. What's more, it's a great book for browsing. Here is your 'symphony' of syndromes. Let its music fill the halls of your office every day.

Walter B. Shelley, MD, PhD, MACP
Professor of Dermatology,
Medical College of Ohio,
Toledo, Ohio
July 1994

INTRODUCTION

An Illustrated Dictionary of Dermatologic Syndromes contains pertinent points about dermatologic syndromes and their associations. It is designed for use by dermatology residents, pediatric residents, and medical students as well as dermatologists, pediatricians, and primary care practitioners.

As both a dermatology and pediatric resident, I often found it difficult to remember the many syndromes which dominate our specialties. I tried many different ways to bring order to the chaos but found that what I really needed to achieve this was an accessible compendium of the pertinent entities of syndromes, to jog my memory when it failed. Therefore, in this dictionary, I have put together a list of some of the most familiar (and some not so familiar) syndromes that have mainly cutaneous and/or physical findings. Its purpose is to help physicians become familiar with a wide variety of syndromes and to serve as a reference for identification when an individual case arises. This is not an exhaustive list of syndromes and some of the syndromes included may not seem to 'fit the mold' of well-known syndromes. Some were chosen because a proper name was attached to the disorder and others were chosen because they had multiple names associated with various parts of the disease – for example, syphilis and Hutchinson's triad.

It would be useful to define a few terms here. The term *syndrome* simply means findings which run together. Most syndromes consist of one or more major anomalies together with a varying number of minor abnormalities. It is the pattern of anomalies which is important in identifying a syndrome, not necessarily the individual parts.

Deformations are anomalies which are caused by mechanical pressure on the fetus, such as compression of the nose or the ear and also positional club foot in a breech presentation. *Disruptions* are caused by some outside agent causing actual destruction of the tissue, leading to cell death. Amniotic bands with resulting amputations or constrictions are examples. A *malformation* is an intrinsic change in a tissue or body structure. The causes of malformations are largely unknown, but errors in migration, differentiation, and proliferation may be involved.

The perpetual learning experience is what makes medicine so interesting – learning does not end when formal education stops. Each patient teaches us a lesson. Seeing actual cases imprints knowledge upon the memory, but reiteration and placement of this knowledge into its context is essential for a well-rounded perspective. We need to be patient ourselves, and listen to them.

In this book I have tried to include recent key references so that interested physicians can investigate specific syndromes in greater detail. My hope is that you will use this book to learn these syndromes!

Susan Bayliss Mallory, MD
Associate Professor of Dermatology (Medicine),
Washington University School of
Medicine in St Louis,
Missouri.
July 1993

ACKNOWLEDGEMENTS

Immense thanks are given to many people, but especially to the following, without whom I would not have been able to write this book – my ever-patient, loving husband, George B. Mallory, Jr, MD; my children, Elizabeth and Meredith, who so kindly gave me time to write; the residents who inspired me to begin this endeavor: Dow Stough, MD, David Jackson, MD, Francine Brunyeel-Rapp, MD, Marty Okun, MD and Laura Grady, MD; my faithful and hard-working secretaries: Sherry Eagle, Pat Elrod, and Tina Brown; my parents, Dr and Mrs Milward W. Bayliss, who inspired me to go into medicine; and my godparents, Major General and Mrs Elbert DeCoursey, who continually asked me what I was doing to stimulate my mind!

Lastly, I would like to thank Jere D. Guin, MD and Arthur Z. Eisen, MD for inspiring me to achieve high goals and who have been tremendously supportive throughout this endeavor. Nancy Esterly, MD and Larry Solomon, MD have encouraged me far more than they ever realized, and S. Bruce Dowton, MB, BS helped with the manuscript. I thank God for giving me the desire to learn and keep on learning.

Susan Bayliss Mallory

The following figures have been reproduced from the sources listed below by kind permission of the publishers and, where relevant, the authors.

Figure 43 *Genetic Disorders of the Skin* by JC Alper. With kind permission of Mosby-Year Book, Inc. and JC Alper MD.

Figure 45 Champlin TL, Mallory SB: J Arkansas Med Soc 1989; 86:115–117.

Figures 57 & 58 Moore DJ, Mallory SB: Pediatr Dermatol 1989; 6:251–253. With kind permission of Blackwell Scientific Publications, Inc.

Figure 78 Mallory SB: Pediatr Clin N Amer 1991; 38:745–759. With kind permission of W. B. Saunders Company.

Figure 87 Ring DS, Mallory SB: Pediatr Dermatol 1992; 9:80–82. With kind permission of Blackwell Scientific Publications, Inc.

Figure 89 Cleveland M, Mallory SB: J Am Acad Dermatol 1993; 29:788–789. With kind permission of Mosby-Year Book, Inc.

Figure 109 Snell JA, Mallory SB: Pediatr Dermatol 1990; 7:77–78. With kind permission of Blackwell Scientific Publications, Inc.

Figure 113 Mallory SB, Stough SB: Dermatol Clin 1987; 5:221–230. Courtesy of Leonard Swinyer MD.

Figure 141 Mallory SB, Wiener E, Nordlund JJ: Pediatr Dermatol 1986; 3:119–124. With kind permission of Blackwell Scientific Publications, Inc.

GENERAL REFERENCES

1. Fitzpatrick, T.B., Eisen A.Z., Wolff K., Freedberg I.M., and Austen K.F. (eds.) (1993) *Dermatology in General Medicine,* 4th edn. (New York: McGraw-Hill, Inc.)

2. Schachner L.A. and Hansen R.C. (eds.) (1988) *Pediatric Dermatology,* 1st edn. (New York: Churchill Livingstone)

3. Moschella S.L. and Hurley H.J. (eds.) (1985) *Dermatology,* 2nd edn. (Philadelphia: W.B. Saunders Company)

4. Rook A., Wilkinson D.S., Ebling F.J.G., Champion R.H. and Burton J.L. (eds.) (1992) *Textbook of Dermatology,* 5th edn. (Oxford: Blackwell Scientific Publications)

5. Rook A. and Dawber R. (1982). *Diseases of the Hair and Scalp.* (Oxford: Blackwell Scientific Publications)

6. Buyse M.L. (ed.) (1990) *Birth Defects Encyclopedia.* Center for Birth Defects Information Services, Inc., Dover, MA, USA (Blackwell Scientific Publications, Inc.)

7. Jones K.L. (1988). *Smith's Recognizable Patterns of Human Malformation,* 4th edn. (Philadelphia: W.B. Saunders Company)

8. Wiedemann H.R., Kunze J., Grosse F-R. and Dibbern H. (1992). *Atlas of Clinical Syndromes. A Visual Aid to Diagnosis.* (St Louis: Mosby-Year Book, Inc.)

9. Hall J.G. (ed.) (1992). *Medical Genetics I.* Pediatr. Clin. N. Amer., **39** (February)

10. Alper J.C. (1991). *Genetic Disorders of the Skin.* (St Louis: Mosby-Year Book, Inc.)

11. Beighton P. (ed.) (1993). *McKusick's Heritable Disorders of Connective Tissue,* 5th edn. (St Louis: Mosby-Year Book, Inc.)

12. Magalini S.I., Magalini S.C. and deFrancisci G. (1990). *Dictionary of Medical Syndromes.* (Philadelphia: J.B. Lippincott Company)

13. Scriver C.R., Beaudet A.L., Sly W.S., *et al.* (eds.) (1989). *The Metabolic Basis of Inherited Disease,* 6th edn. (New York: McGraw-Hill, Inc.)

A

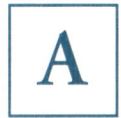

AARSKOG SYNDROME,
FACIODIGITOGENITAL DYSPLASIA

Manifestations and Major Findings
digital deformities
- short, broad hands and feet
- syndactyly
- hyperextensible proximal interphalangeal joints
- clinodactyly
- short thumb
- short fingers due to hypoplasia of the digital phalanges

shawl scrotum
small stature
pectus excavatum

Characteristic Facies
broad, prominent forehead
hypertelorism
ptosis
short, broad nose
anteverted nostrils
long philtrum

References
Berry C, Cree J, Mann T: Aarskog's syndrome. Arch Dis Child 1980; 55:706–710.
Nielsen KB: Aarskog syndrome in a Danish family: an illustration of the need for dysmorphology in paediatrics. Clin Genet 1988; 33:315–317.
Porteous MEM, Goudie DR: Aarskog Syndrome. J Med Genet 1991; 28:44–47.
Teebi AS, Naguib KK, Al-Awadi SA, Al-Saleh QA: New autosomal recessive faciodigitogenital syndrome. J Med Genet 1988; 25:400–406.

ACHONDROPLASIA

Manifestations and Major Findings
short-limbed dwarfism
limb shortening (especially marked in humerus and femur)
trunk almost normal in size
short, trident hand
large head compared to body
caudal narrowing of spinal canal
increased lumbar lordosis
bell-shaped or flat thorax
genu varus
hearing loss (occasional)
normal mental development
delayed motor development in infancy and early childhood

Characteristic Facies
hypoplasia of mid-face
frontal bossing
depressed nasal bridge
prognathism

autosomal dominant

References
Clark RN: Congenital dysplasias and dwarfism. Pediatr Rev 1990; 12:149–159.
Hecht JT, Francomano CA, Horton WA, Annegers JF: Mortality in achondroplasia. Am J Hum Genet 1987; 41:454–464.
Horton WA, Rotter JI, Rimoin DL, Scott CI, et al.: Standard growth curves for achondroplasia. J Pediatr 1978; 93:435–438.
Thompson JN, Schaefer GB, et al.: Achondroplasia and parental age. N Engl J Med 1986; 314:521–522.

ACATALASEMIA see TAKAHARA SYNDROME

ACQUIRED IMMUNODEFICIENCY SYNDROME (AIDS)

Manifestations and Major Findings
infection with a human immunodeficiency virus – HIV-1, HIV-2, human T cell lymphoma virus (HTLV-III), AIDS-related virus (ARV), lymphadenopathy-associated virus (LAV)
decreased T-helper lymphocytes
AIDS-related complex (ARC)
lymphadenopathy syndrome (LAS)
ARC and LAS are defined as a constellation of symptoms in persons with an increased risk of developing AIDS. Signs include: lymphadenopathy, weight loss, fever, chronic diarrhea, and oral thrush. Kaposi sarcoma and opportunistic infections are not present.

DRUG ERUPTIONS
trimethroprim–sulfamethoxazole (TMP–SMX)-induced morbilliform rash
zidovudine hyperpigmentation
multiple drug sensitivity (especially with antibiotics)

OPPORTUNISTIC INFECTIONS
mycobacteria
candidiasis of esophagus, trachea, bronchi, or lungs
cytomegalovirus
cryptococcosis
coccidioidomycosis
histoplasmosis
toxoplasmosis
Pneumocystis carinii pneumonia
herpes simplex
herpes zoster
recurrent bacterial infections (*Haemophilus, Streptococcus, Salmonella*)
syphilis

MALIGNANCIES
lymphoma
squamous cell carcinoma and adenocarcinomas of the mouth, pharynx, and rectum

INCREASED-RISK GROUPS
homosexuals
intravenous drug abusers
hemophiliacs
multiple blood transfusion recipients
prostitutes
sexual partners of infected individuals
infants of infected mothers

Cutaneous Manifestations
Kaposi sarcoma
seborrheic dermatitis
papulopruritic eruption
eosinophilic folliculitis
herpes zoster
herpes simplex
candidiasis
oral hairy leukoplakia (secondary to Epstein–Barr virus)
tinea corporis and tinea cruris
molluscum contagiosum
verruca vulgaris
condyloma acuminatum
bacillary angiomatosis
psoriasis
Reiter syndrome
granuloma annulare
prurigo-like lesions
gingivitis

References
Cockerell CJ: Immunodeficiency virus infection and the skin. Arch Intern Med 1991; 151:1295–1303.
Coldiron BM, Bergstresser PR: Prevalence and clinical spectrum of skin disease in patients infected with human immunodeficiency virus. Arch Dermatol 1989; 125:357–361.
Dover JS, Johnson RA: Cutaneous manifestations of human immunodeficiency virus infection. Arch Dermatol 1991; 127:1383–1391.
Gallo RC, Montanier L: AIDS in 1988; Sci Am 1988; 259:41–48.
Greene WC: The molecular biology of human immunodeficiency virus type 1 infection. N Engl J Med 1991; 324:308–317.
Pizzo PA, Eddy J, Faloon J: Acquired immune deficiency syndrome in children. Am J Med 1988; 85 (Suppl 2A):195–202.
Prose NS: Mucocutaneous disease in pediatric human immunodeficiency virus infection. Pediatr Clin N Am 1991; 38:977–990.
Strako BF, Whitaker DL, Morrison SH, Oleske JM, Grant-Kels JM: Cutaneous manifestations of the acquired immunodeficiency syndrome in children. J Am Acad Dermatol 1988; 18:1089–1102.

ACROCEPHALOSYNDACTYLY
see APERT SYNDROME

ACRODERMATITIS CONTINUA OF HALLOPEAU, ACROPUSTULOSIS, ACRODERMATITIS PERSTANS

Manifestations and Major Findings
chronic pustular eruption (sterile) involving fingertips and toes (may evolve into generalized pustular psoriasis)
nail folds and nail bed involvement leads to nail dystrophy
slowly progressive

References
Mahowald ML, Parrish RM: Severe osteolytic arthritis mutilans in pustular psoriasis. Arch Dermatol 1982; 118:434–437.
O'Keefe E, Braverman IM, Cohen I: Annulus migrans. Arch Dermatol 1973; 107:240–244.

ACRODERMATITIS ENTEROPATHICA

Manifestations and Major Findings
zinc deficiency
- acral and peri-orificial erosive dermatitis (Fig. 1)
psoriasiform plaques over bony prominences
diarrhea
alopecia

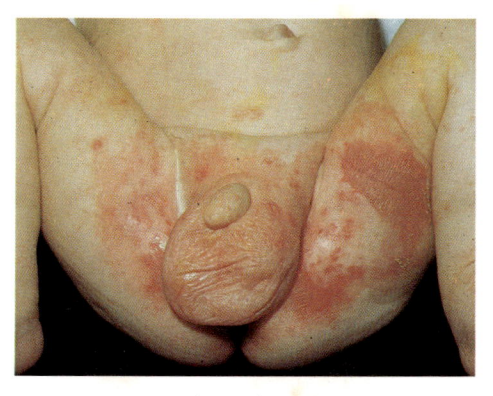

- *Figure 1 Erosive diaper dermatitis in acrodermatitis enteropathica.*

Other Findings
glossitis
growth failure
personality changes
photophobia, conjunctivitis, blepharitis
poor wound healing
paronychia, nail dystrophy
immune dysfunction
secondary infections with bacteria and *Candida albicans*
Acrodermatitis enteropathica usually begins 4–6 weeks after weaning from breast milk, or earlier in bottle-fed infants.

autosomal recessive or acquired

References
Fraker PJ, Jardieu P, Cook J: Zinc deficiency and immune function. Arch Dermatol 1987; 123:1699–1701.
Glover MT, Atherton DJ: Transient zinc deficiency in two full-term breast-fed siblings associated with low maternal breast milk zinc concentration. Pediatr Dermatol 1988; 5:10–13.
Lee MG, Hong KT, Kim JJ: Transient symptomatic zinc deficiency in a full-term breast-fed infant. J Am Acad Dermatol 1990; 23:375–379.
Miller SJ: Nutritional deficiency and the skin. J Am Acad Dermatol 1989; 21:1–30.

ACRODYNIA see PINK DISEASE

ACROGERIA see GOTTRON SYNDROME

ACROKERATOELASTOIDOSIS OF COSTA

Manifestations and Major Findings
- small, firm, translucent, round papules (pearl-like) on dorsal aspects of fingers, and margins of palms and soles (Fig. 2)
histology shows fragmented and decreased elastic fibers with homogenization of collagen
hyperhidrosis
onset in childhood or adolescence
sun exposure or chronic trauma may induce this condition in adulthood

autosomal dominant or acquired

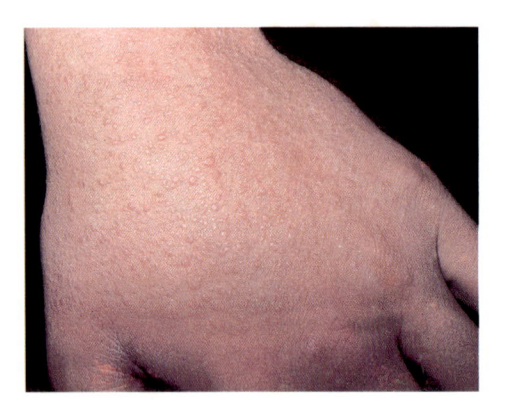

Figure 2 Small, firm, translucent, 'pearl-like' papules in acrokeratoelastoidosis of Costa.

References
Costa OG: Acrokeratoelastoidosis. Arch Dermatol 1954; 70:228–231.
Highet AS, Rook A, Anderson JR: Acrokeratoelastoidosis. Br J Dermatol 1982; 106:337–344.
Korc A, Hansen RC, Lynch PJ: Acrokeratoelastoidosis of Costa in North America. J Am Acad Dermatol 1985; 12:832–836.
Saruk M, Taylor MR, Rudolph RI, Parhizgar B, Wood MG: Acrokeratoelastoidosis. Cutis 1983; 32:248–251.

ACROKERATOSIS PARANEOPLASTICA
see BAZEX SYNDROME

ACROKERATOSIS VERRUCIFORMIS OF HOPF

Manifestations and Major Findings
verrucous, skin-colored or reddish brown, flat papules
predominantly affects the dorsa of hands and feet but may appear on forearms, knees, and elbows
punctate keratosis on palms and nails
histology shows papillomatosis, hyperkeratosis, acanthosis, and thickened granular cell layer, and no dyskeratotic cells
early onset – may be present at birth
Differential diagnosis includes: Darier disease, epidermodysplasia verruciformis, and verruca plana.

autosomal dominant

References
Panja RK: Acrokeratosis verruciformis (Hopf) – a clinical entity? Br J Dermatol 1977; 6:643–652.
Schueller WA: Acrokeratosis verruciformis of Hopf. Arch Dermatol 1972; 106:81–83.

ACROPIGMENTATION SYMMETRICA OF DOHI, SYMMETRICAL DYSCHROMATOSIS OF THE EXTREMITIES, DYSCHROMATOSIS SYMMETRICA HEREDITARIA

Manifestations and Major Findings
mottled, hyperpigmented and hypopigmented macules, without atrophy, on dorsum of hands and feet
pigmentation coalesces to form stellate patches
more common in Japan

autosomal dominant or recessive

References
Fulk CS: Primary disorders of hyperpigmentation. J Am Acad Dermatol 1984; 10:1–16.
Gonzalez JR, Botet MV: Acromelanosis. J Am Acad Dermatol 1980; 2:128–131.
Nishigori C, Miyachi Y, Takebe H, Imamura S: A case of xeroderma pigmentosum with clinical appearance of dyschromatosis symmetrica hereditaria. Pediatr Dermatol 1986; 3:410–413.

ACTINIC PURPURA
see BATEMAN PURPURA

ACUTE FEBRILE NEUTROPHILIC DERMATOSIS *see* SWEET SYNDROME

ADAM COMPLEX
see AMNIOTIC BAND SYNDROME

ADAMS–OLIVER SYNDROME
see also APLASIA CUTIS CONGENITA

Manifestations and Major Findings
aplasia cutis congenita (scalp) with or without underlying bone defects
terminal transverse limb defects
persistent cutis marmorata
digital deformities
– short fingers and toes
– small or absent nails

autosomal dominant (variable expression)

References
Bork K, Pfeifle J: Multifocal aplasia cutis congenita, distal limb hemimelia, and cutis marmorata telangiectatica in a patient with Adams–Oliver syndrome. Br J Dermatol 1992; 127:160–163.
Fryns JP: Congenital scalp defects with distal limb reduction anomalies. J Med Genet 1987; 24:493–496.
Küster W, Lenz W, Kääriäinen H, Majewski F: Congenital scalp defects with distal limb anomalies (Adams–Oliver syndrome): report of ten cases and review of the literature. Am J Med Genet 1988; 31:99–115.

ADDISON DISEASE, ADRENAL INSUFFICIENCY SYNDROME, ADRENOCORTICAL INSUFFICIENCY

Manifestations and Major Findings
hypocorticism due to insufficiency of the adrenal glands (primary insufficiency) or to hypopituitarism
- bronze-like pigmentation of the skin (Fig. 3) and mucous membranes, concentrated in areas of light exposure, flexures, areolae, scrotum, labia, palmar creases, scars, and nevi
linea alba darkens, becoming linea nigra
loss of pubic, axillary, and scalp hair
longitudinal pigmented bands in nails
calcification of ear cartilage
xerosis
muscular asthenia
hypotension
abdominal pain and diarrhea

Other disorders associated with Addison disease include: vitiligo, pernicious anemia, thyroiditis, diabetes mellitus, alopecia areata, chronic mucocutaneous candidiasis, chronic active hepatitis.

References
Feingold KR, Elias PM: Endocrine–skin interactions. J Am Acad Dermatol 1988; 19:1–20.
Kung AWC, Pun KK, Lam K, Wang C, Leung CY: Addisonian crisis as presenting feature in malignancies. Cancer 1990; 65:177–179.
Sadeghi-Nejad A, Senior B: Adrenomyeloneuropathy presenting as Addison's disease in childhood. N Engl J Med 1990; 322:13–16.

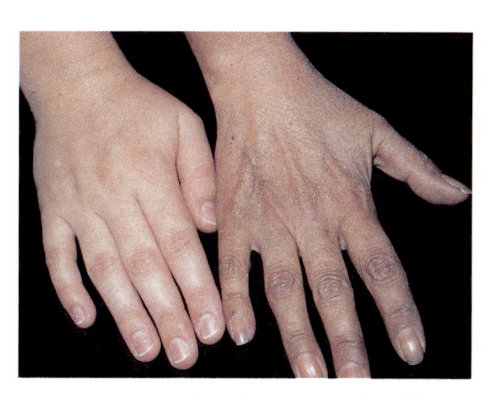

- *Figure 3 Bronze-like pigmentation of the skin in Addison disease. Normal skin color is on the left.*

ADIPOSIS DOLOROSA
see DERCUM DISEASE

ADRENAL INSUFFICIENCY SYNDROME
see ADDISON DISEASE

ADRENOGENITAL SYNDROME
see CONGENITAL ADRENAL HYPERPLASIA

AEC SYNDROME
see ANKYLOBLEPHARON–ECTODERMAL DYSPLASIA–CLEFTING SYNDROME

AGAMMAGLOBULINEMIA OF BRUTON

Manifestations and Major Findings
congenital absence of immunoglobulins
markedly reduced B cell counts
recurrent pyogenic infections – predominantly of middle ear, sinuses, lungs, skin
increased prevalence of atopic eczema

X-linked recessive, occurs in males

> **References**
> Bruton OC: Agammaglobulinemias. Pediatrics 1952; 9:722–727.
> Lederman HM, Winkelstein JA: X-linked agammaglobulinemia: an analysis of 96 patients. Medicine 1985; 64:145–156.

AIDS see ACQUIRED IMMUNODEFICIENCY SYNDROME

ALAGILLE SYNDROME,
WATSON–ALAGILLE SYNDROME, ARTERIOHEPATIC DYSPLASIA

Manifestations and Major Findings
congenital hypoplasia of intrahepatic bile ducts with chronic cholestasis
splenomegaly
jaundice
pruritus
xanthomas (which may resolve)
porphyria cutanea tarda-like photosensitivity
vascular malformations
cardiovascular anomalies
peripheral pulmonary artery hypoplasia or stenosis
defects of vertebral arches (butterfly-like arch defects)
growth retardation
mental retardation
hypogonadism
bone abnormalities
ocular anomalies
high-pitched voice

Characteristic Facies
prominent forehead
hypertelorism (slight)
deeply set eyes
saddle nose or accentuated, straight nasal bridge
sharp-pointed chin

autosomal dominant (variable penetrance)

> **References**
> Alagille D, Estrada A, Hadchouel M, Gautier M, et al.: Syndromic paucity of interlobular bile ducts (Alagille syndrome or arteriohepatic dysplasia): review of 80 cases. J Pediatr 1987; 110:195–200.
> Alagille D, Odièvre M, Gautier M, Dommergues JP: Hepatic ductular hypoplasia associated with characteristic facies, vertebral malformations, retarded physical, mental, and sexual development, and cardiac murmur. J Pediatr 1975; 86:63–71.
> Camacho-Martínez F, Moreno-Gimenez JC, Sánchez-Pedreño P: Xanthomatous biliary cirrhosis in Alagille's syndrome. J Am Acad Dermatol 1988; 18:746–747.
> Sokol RJ, Heubi JE, Balistreri WF: Intrahepatic "cholestasis facies": is it specific for Alagille syndrome? J Pediatr 1983; 103:205–208.
> Weston CFM, Burton JL: Xanthomas in the Watson–Alagille syndrome. J Am Acad Dermatol 1987; 16:1117–1121.
> Zhang F, Deleuze J-F, Aurias A, Dutrillaux A-M, Hugon R-N, Alagille D, Thomas G, Hadchouel M: Interstitial deletion of the short arm of chromosome 20 in arteriohepatic dysplasia (Alagille syndrome). J Pediatr 1990; 116:73–77.

ALBINISM, OCULOCUTANEOUS ALBINISM

Manifestations and Major Findings
disorder of melanin synthesis in hair, skin, and eyes
melanocyte number is normal
melanin synthesis is abnormal
hypopigmentation or depigmentation at birth
photophobia
decreased visual acuity
nystagmus

commonly inherited as autosomal recessive (except dominant albinoidism)

Types of Albinism and Distinguishing Features

1 tyrosinase-negative albinism
- snow-white hair (Fig. 4)
- pink-white skin (Fig. 4)

gray-blue/pink irides that transilluminate
severe nystagmus
markedly decreased visual acuity
susceptibility to skin neoplasia
negative dopa reaction of hair bulbs
melanosome stages I and II, no III or IV
inability to synthesize tyrosinase

2 tyrosinase-positive albinism
some melanin in hair, skin, and eyes
yellow or red hair, darkens with age
pink to cream colored skin
blue, yellow, or brown eyes
nystagmus
photophobia
poor visual acuity
susceptibility to skin neoplasia
positive dopa reaction of hair bulbs
melanosome stages I, II, and some III present
most common type in Americans, American Indians, and Chinese

3 yellow mutant albinism
skin white at birth, tans slightly when exposed to sun
yellow, red, or brown hair
mild nystagmus
mild photophobia
poor visual acuity
blue eyes, darkening with age
pigmented nevi
most prevalent in Amish families in USA
melanosome stages I and II present, and III with uneven pigment, resembling pheomelanosomes

4 Hermansky–Pudlak syndrome
(see Hermansky–Pudlak syndrome)

5 Chédiak–Higashi syndrome
(see Chédiak–Higashi syndrome)

6 brown oculocutaneous albinism
found in New Guineans and Nigerians
cream to light tan skin
hazel to light brown eyes
medium brown hair
with or without nystagmus
with or without photophobia
melanosome stages I–III present, some lightly pigmented IV

7 rufous oculocutaneous albinism
most common in African Americans and New Guineans
mahogany red-brown skin and hair
red-brown irides
mild nystagmus
mild photophobia
melanosome stages unknown

8 platinum oculocutaneous albinism
pink skin
gray to blue irides
poor visual acuity
susceptibility to skin neoplasia
melanosome stages I, II, and few III present

9 black locks–albinism–deafness
not a true albinism because there are no melanocytes in white hair and skin
snow-white hair in patches, and black locks of hair
white skin except for brown macules
gray to blue irides
deafness
nystagmus
photophobia
poor visual acuity
normal melanocytes in pigmented hair and skin
melanosomes normal, stages I–IV
absent melanocytes in areas of leukoderma

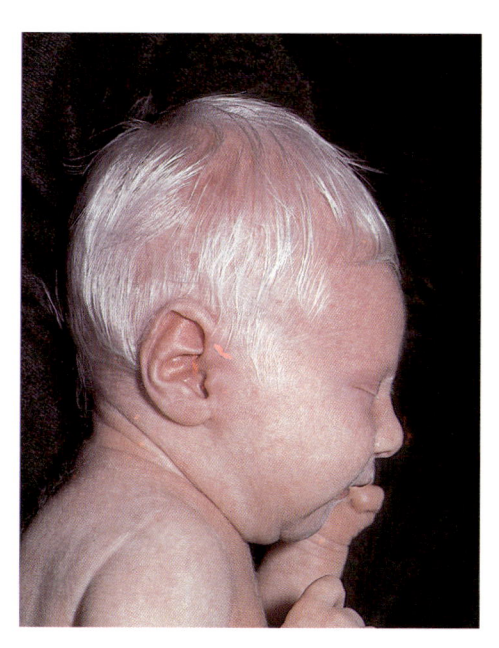

- *Figure 4* Snow-white hair and pink-white skin as features of tyrosine-negative albinism.

▷ ▷ ▷

▷ ▷ ▷
10 Cross syndrome
(see Cross syndrome)

11 Griscelli syndrome (see also Griscelli syndrome)
melanocytes lack normal dendrites
defect most likely due to transfer block of melanosomes to keratinocytes

12 dominant albinism
pale skin and hair
blue eyes
no eye abnormalities, nystagmus, or photophobia
melanosome stages I–III
autosomal dominant

> **References**
> Bolognia JL, Pawelek JM: Biology of hypopigmentation. J Am Acad Dermatol 1988; 19:217–255.
> Eady RAJ, Gunner DB, Garner A, Rodeck CH: Prenatal diagnosis of oculocutaneous albinism by electron microscopy of fetal skin. J Invest Dermatol 1983; 80:210–212.
> Gershoni-Baruch R, Benderly A, Brandes JM, Gilhar A: Dopa reaction test in hair bulbs of fetuses and its application to the prenatal diagnosis of albinism. J Am Acad Dermatol 1991; 24:220–222.
> O'Donnell FE, Hambrick GW, Green R, Iliff WJ, Stone DL: X-linked ocular albinism. Arch Ophthalmol 1976; 94:1883–1892.
> Spritz RA, Strunk KM, Giebel LB, King RA: Detection of mutations in the tyrosinase gene in a patient with type IA oculocutaneous albinism. N Engl J Med 1990; 322:1724–1728.
> Witkop CJ, Hill CW, Desnick S, Thies JK, et al.: Ophthalmologic, biochemical, platelet, and ultrastructural defects in the various types of oculocutaneous albinism. J Invest Dermatol 1973; 60:443–456.

ALBRIGHT HEREDITARY OSTEODYSTROPHY, ALBRIGHT SYNDROME, McCUNE–ALBRIGHT SYNDROME, POLYOSTOTIC FIBROUS DYSPLASIA, SEABRIGHT BANTAM SYNDROME

Manifestations and Major Findings
• osteoma cutis (Fig.5)
short stature
round facies
ptosis

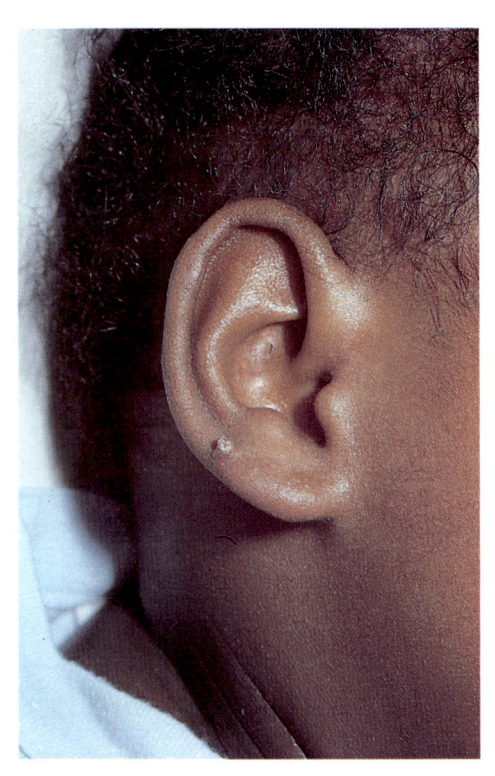

• *Figure 5* Osteoma cutis of the ear in Albright hereditary osteodystrophy.

skeletal abnormalities
– short metacarpals and metatarsals of digits (especially 4th and 5th)
– short distal phalanges
– • dimpling sign over knuckles (Fig. 6) when fist is clenched
– thumb sign – short distal phalanx
short broad nails
basal ganglia calcification
mental retardation
tetany due to hypocalcemia
cataracts
Albright hereditary osteodystrophy is associated with pseudohypoparathyroidism or pseudopseudohypoparathyroidism.

autosomal dominant with variable expression, or X-linked dominant

> **References**
> Fitch N: Albright's hereditary osteodystrophy: a review. Am J Med Genet 1982; 11:11–29.
> ▷ ▷ ▷

▷ ▷ ▷
Patten JL, Johns DR, Valle D, Eil C, Gruppuso PA, Steel G, Smallwood PM, Levine MA: Mutation in the gene encoding the stimulatory G protein of adenylate cyclase in Albright's hereditary osteodystrophy. N Engl J Med 1990; 322:1412–1419.
Prendiville JS, Lucky AW, Mallory SB, Mughal Z, et al.: Osteoma cutis as a presenting sign of pseudohypoparathyroidism. Pediatr Dermatol 1992; 9:11–18.
Spiegel AM: Albright's hereditary osteodystrophy and defective G proteins. N Engl J Med 1990; 322: 1461–1462.
Tsang RC, Venkataraman P, Ho M, Steichen JJ, Whitsett J, et. al.: The development of pseudopseudohypoparathyroidism. Am J Dis Child 1984; 138:654–658.

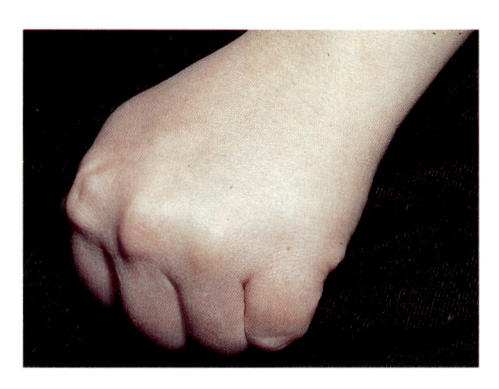

• *Figure 6 Dimpling of the fifth knuckle; a feature of Albright hereditary osteodystrophy.*

ALBRIGHT SYNDROME
see ALBRIGHT HEREDITARY OSTEODYSTROPHY OR McCUNE–ALBRIGHT SYNDROME

ALKAPTONURIA,
ALCAPTONURIA, OCHRONOSIS, HOMOGENTISIC ACID OXIDASE DEFICIENCY

Manifestations and Major Findings
dusky, blue-black or gray discoloration of sclerae, pinnae, face, cartilage, and nails, caused by homogentisic acid accumulation in tissues
dark sweat
thickened pinnae; later calcified and dark black cerumen
deafness
arthropathy – mainly lumbar spine, knees, shoulders, and hips and beginning in the fourth decade
calcific aortic disease
porous black renal stones
prostatic concretions
urine turns dark upon standing or alkalinization
normal life span

autosomal recessive

References
Albers SE, Brozena SJ, Glass LF, Fenske NA: Alkaptonuria and ochronosis: case report and review. J Am Acad Dermatol 1992; 27:609–614.
Lee EB: Metabolic diseases and the skin. Pediatr Clin N Am 1983; 30:597–608.

ALLERGIC GRANULOMATOSIS SYNDROME *see* CHURG–STRAUSS SYNDROME

ALLEZANDRINI SYNDROME

Manifestations and Major Findings
unilateral degenerative retinitis
ipsilateral facial vitiligo
poliosis of eyebrows and eyelashes
deafness
affects young adults or adolescents

References
Hoffman MD, Dudley C: Suspected Alezzandrini's syndrome in a diabetic patient with unilateral retinal detachment and ipsilateral vitiligo and poliosis. J Am Acad Dermatol 1992; 26:496–497.
Lorincz AL: Disturbance of melanin pigmentation. In: Moschella SL, Hurley JH, eds. Dermatology; vol 2. Philadelphia: WB Saunders, 1985:1297.

ALPORT SYNDROME, HEREDITARY NEPHRITIS WITH DEAFNESS AND OCULAR ABNORMALITIES

Manifestations and Major Findings
deafness
cataracts, myopia, keratoconus, and nystagmus

macrothrombocytopathy and thrombocytopenia
easily bruised and prone to bleeding
visceral leiomyomas (esophageal, genital, tracheal)
growth delay

X-linked dominant or autosomal dominant

> **References**
> Cochat P, Guibaud P, Torres RG, Roussel B, et al.: Diffuse leiomyomatosis in Alport syndrome. J Pediatr 1988; 113:339–343.

AMNIOTIC BAND SYNDROME,
CONSTRICTION BAND SYNDROME, ADAM COMPLEX (AMNIOTIC DEFORMITY, ADHESIONS, MUTILATIONS), AMNIOTIC BAND SEQUENCE, STREETER ANOMALY

Manifestations and Major Findings
congenital deformities caused by fetal entanglement in strands of ruptured amniotic sac, or arrested development manifested at birth
sporadic occurrence
no two fetuses identically affected

LIMB DEFECTS
constrictive bands
amputation
syndactyly
talipes equinovarus
distal lymphedema

CRANIOFACIAL DEFECTS
encephalocele
anencephaly
facial clefting (often unusual clefting)
microphthalmia
incomplete calcification of the cranium

VISCERAL ANOMALIES
abdominal or thoracic wall defects
gastroschisis
omphalocele
pelvic bone and vertebral anomalies

> **References**
> Bamforth JS: Amniotic band sequence: Streeter's hypothesis reexamined. Am J Med Genet 1992; 44:280–287.
> Garza A, Cordero JF, Mulinare J: Epidemiology of the early amnion rupture spectrum of defects. Am J Dis Child 1988; 142:541–544.
> Higgenbottom MC, Jones KL, Hall BD, Smith DW: The amniotic band disruption complex: timing of amniotic rupture and variable spectra of consequent defects. J Pediatr 1979; 95:544–549.
> Keller H, Neuhäuser G, Durkin-Stamm MV, Kaveggia EG, et al.: "ADAM" complex (Amniotic Deformity, Adhesions, Mutilations) – a pattern of craniofacial and limb defects. Am J Med Genet 1978; 2:81–98.
> Ray M, Hendrick SJ, Raimer SS, Blackwell SJ: Amniotic band syndrome. Intern J Dermatol 1988; 27:312–314.

ANDROGEN INSENSITIVITY SYNDROME *see* TESTICULAR FEMINIZATION

ANETODERMA *see* JADASSOHN–PELLIZZARI ANETODERMA AND SCHWENINGER–BUZZI ANETODERMA

ANGELMAN SYNDROME,
HAPPY PUPPET SYNDROME

Manifestations and Major Findings
ataxic jerky movements of the extremities
stiff gait
unprovoked paroxysms of laughter
no speech development
unusual position of the arms
mental retardation
seizures common
ocular anomalies – choroidal pigment deficiency, optic pallor or atrophy, blue irides
generalized hypopigmentation

Characteristic Facies
microcephaly
pale-blue eyes
maxillary hypoplasia
large mouth
tongue protrusion

prognathism

chromosome 15 abnormality

> **References**
> Clayton-Smith J: Angelman's syndrome. Arch Dis Child 1992; 67:889–891.
> King RA, Wiesner GL, Townsend DW, et al.: Hypopigmentation in Angelman syndrome. Am J Med Genet 1993; 46:40–44.
> Knoll JHM, Nicholls RD, Magenis RE, Graham JM, et al.: Angelman and Prader–Willi syndromes share a common chromosome 15 deletion but differ in parental origin of the deletion. Am J Med Genet 1989; 32:285–290.
> Smeets DFCM, Hamel BCJ, Nelen MR, Smeets HJM: Prader–Willi syndrome and Angelman syndrome in cousins from a family with a translocation between chromosomes 6 and 15. N Engl J Med 1992; 326:807–811.

ANGIOEDEMA see HEREDITARY ANGIOEDEMA

ANGIOKERATOMAS

Clinical Characteristics
asymptomatic, firm, dark red to black papules or plaques
vascular malformations
histology shows dilated capillaries in the dermal papillae with overlying hyperkeratosis and acanthosis

Types of Angiokeratomas and their Features

1 solitary papular angiokeratoma
usually on an extremity
often preceded by trauma
nonhereditary

2 angiokeratoma circumscriptum
- large, solitary, hyperkeratotic, hemangiomatous, verrucous plaques (Fig. 7)
usually present at birth
occurs in bands, streaks, or linear arrangements
usually on an extremity

3 angiokeratoma of Mibelli
cold injury as a provocative factor

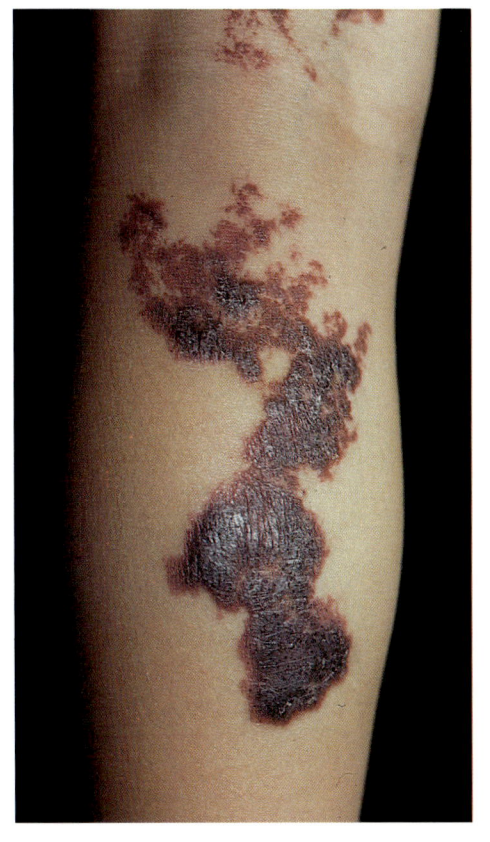

• *Figure 7 Angiokeratoma circumscriptum; large, solitary, hyperkeratotic, hemangiomatous, verrucous plaque on the lower leg.*

usually occurs in adolescent females
minute bright red macules which slowly increase in size and become warty on the digits
familial predisposition

4 angiokeratoma of the scrotum (Fordyce)
common in middle-aged males
- 3–5mm multiple lesions on the scrotum (Fig. 8)

5 angiokeratoma corporis diffusum (see also Fabry disease)
lysosomal hydrolase α-galactosidase A deficiency
ceramide trihexoside accumulates in blood vessels
angiokeratomas (0.5–2mm) mainly on thighs, buttocks, lower back, penis, and scrotum, although lesions may be seen on the trunk or buccal mucosa
hypertension

▷ ▷ ▷

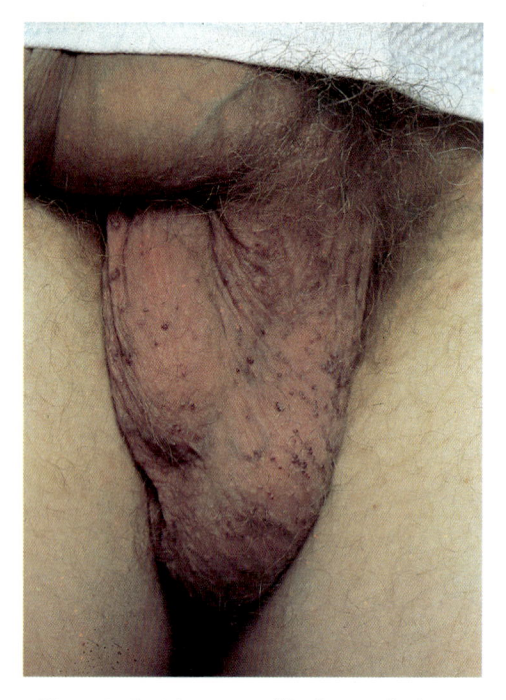

• **Figure 8** Angiokeratoma of Fordyce; multiple lesions on the scrotum.

▷ ▷ ▷
ocular findings:
– corneal linear opacities
– dilated and tortuous blood vessels
– edema of eyelids
neurological findings:
– transient cerebrovascular accidents
– severe episodic paresthesias
febrile episodes
renal failure (most common cause of death)
electron microscopy shows concentrically lamellated inclusions
X-linked recessive

6 fucosidosis (see also fucosidosis)
lysosomal enzyme α-L-fucosidase deficiency
multiple angiokeratomas on the trunk and upper legs, beginning in early childhood
mental retardation
weakness
spasticity

References
Imperial R, Helwig EB: Angiokeratoma, a clinicopathological study. Arch Dermatol 1967; 95:166–175. ▷ ▷ ▷

▷ ▷ ▷
Marsden J, Allen R: Widespread angiokeratomas without evidence of metabolic disease. Arch Dermatol 1987; 123:1125–1127.
Somasundaram V, Premalatha S, Rao NR, Razack EMA, et al.: Hemangiectatic hypertrophy with angiokeratoma circumscriptum. Intern J Dermatol 1988; 27:45–46.

ANGIOLYMPHOID HYPERPLASIA WITH EOSINOPHILIA

Manifestations and Major Findings
vascular, purple-red or translucent nodule, or clustered nodules
primarily on the head and neck
histopathology shows benign local hyperplasia of blood vessels with lymphocytes and eosinophils
elevated serum IgE and peripheral eosinophilia
most common in young adults
female predominance
spontaneous regression common

References
Botet MV, Sanchez JL: Angiolymphoid hyperplasia with eosinophilia: report of a case and a review of the literature. J Dermatol Surg Oncol 1978; 4:931–936.
Kung ITM, Gibson JB, Bannatyne PM: Kimura's disease: a clinico-pathological study of 21 cases and its distinction from angiolymphoid hyperplasia with eosinophilia. Pathol 1984; 16:39–44.
Nelson DA, Jarratt M: Angiolymphoid hyperplasia with eosinophilia. Pediatr Dermatol 1984; 1:210–214.
Olsen TG, Helwig EB: Angiolymphoid hyperplasia with eosinophilia. J Am Acad Dermatol 1985; 12:781–796.
vonden Driesch P, Gruschwitz M, Schell H, Sterry W: Distribution of adhesion molecules, IgE, and CD23 in a case of angiolymphoid hyperplasia with eosinophilia. J Am Acad Dermatol 1992; 26:799–804.

ANKYLOBLEPHARON– ECTODERMAL DYSPLASIA– CLEFTING SYNDROME, AEC SYNDROME, ECTODERMAL DYSPLASIA (HAY–WELLS SYNDROME)

Manifestations and Major Findings
ankyloblepharon (partial fusion of eyelids)

ectodermal dysplasia
- absent or rudimentary nails
- sparse, wiry hair
- pointed, widely spaced teeth
- hypohidrosis
clefting – facial (lip and/or palate)
widespread erosions at birth
dry, scaly skin
deformed ears
hyperthermia at birth
normal mentation

OCCASIONAL ABNORMALITIES OR ASSOCIATIONS
ear deformities
deafness
syndactyly
supernumerary nipples
microphthalmia
lacrimal duct atresia
ptosis
congenital heart defects

autosomal dominant

> **References**
> Hay RJ, Wells RS: The syndrome of ankyloblepharon, ectodermal defects and cleft lip and palate: an autosomal dominant condition. Br J Dermatol 1976; 94:277–289.
> Shwayder TA, Lane AT, Miller ME: Hay–Wells syndrome. Pediatr Dermatol 1986; 3:399–402.
> Spiegel J, Colton A: AEC syndrome: ankyloblepharon, ectodermal dysplasia and cleft lip and palate. Report of two cases. J Am Acad Dermatol 1985; 12:810–815.

ANTIPHOSPHOLIPID ANTIBODY SYNDROME, ANTICARDIOLIPIN SYNDROME, LUPUS ANTICOAGULANT SYNDROME

Manifestations and Major Findings
systemic lupus erythematosus
multiple spontaneous thromboses
recurrent spontaneous abortions
thrombocytopenia
nonthrombotic or thrombotic neurologic disorders
livedo reticularis
repeated digital gangrene
purpura
leg ulcers
atrophie blanche
pulmonary hypertension
valvular heart disease
labile hypertension

> **References**
> Grob JJ, Bonerandi JJ: Thrombotic skin disease as a marker of the anticardiolipin syndrome. J Am Acad Dermatol 1989; 20:1063–1069.
> O'Neill A, Gatenby PA, McGaw B, Painter DM, McKenzie PR: Widespread cutaneous necrosis associated with cardiolipin antibodies. J Am Acad Dermatol 1990; 22:356–359.
> Smith KJ, Skelton HG, James WD, Angritt P, et al: Cutaneous histopathologic findings in 'Antiphospholipid Syndrome'. Arch Dermatol 1990; 126:1176–1183.
> Sontheimer RD: The anticardiolipin syndrome. Arch Dermatol 1987; 123:590–595.

α-1-ANTITRYPSIN DEFICIENCY

Manifestations and Major Findings
chronic obstructive lung disease
low α-1-antitrypsin (proteinase inhibitor) level in serum

SEVERE DEFICIENCY
proteinase inhibitor pi ZZ phenotype (usually) associated with:
  emphysema in third decade
  panniculitis – painful, severe
  hepatitis
  cirrhosis
  hepatoma
  cutaneous vasculitis
  angioedema/urticaria

PARTIAL DEFICIENCY
proteinase inhibitor pi MZ phenotype (usually) associated with:
  severe psoriasis
  angioedema

autosomal recessive (normal phenotype is Pi MM)

References
Edmonds BK, Hodge JA, Rietschel RL: Alpha-1-antitrypsin deficiency-associated panniculitis: case report and review of the literature. Pediatr Dermatol 1991; 8:296–299.
Hendrick SJ, Silverman AK, Solomon AR, Headington JT: Alpha-1-antitrypsin deficiency associated with panniculitis. J Am Acad Dermatol 1988; 18:684–692.
Heng MCY, Moy RL, Lieberman J: α-1-Antitrypsin deficiency in severe psoriasis. Br J Dermatol 1985; 112:129–133.
Ibarguen E, Gross CR, Savik SK, Sharp HL: Liver disease in alpha-1-antitrypsin deficiency: prognostic indicators. J Pediatr 1990; 117:864–870.
Lipkin G, Galdston M, Kueppers F: α-1-antitrypsin deficiency genes: contributory defect in a subset of psoriatics? J Am Acad Dermatol 1984; 11:615–619.
Smith KC, Pittelkow MR, Su WPD: Panniculitis associated with severe alpha-1-antitrypsin deficiency. Arch Dermatol 1987; 123:1655–1661.
Snider GL: Pulmonary disease in alpha-1-antitrypsin deficiency. Ann Intern Med 1989; 111:957–959.

APERT SYNDROME,
ACROCEPHALOSYNDACTYLY TYPE I,
VOGT CEPHALODACTYLY

Manifestations and Major Findings
craniosynostosis (turribrachycephaly)
syndactyly of fingers and toes, symmetrical and extensive (including osseous fusion)

Characteristic Facies
broad, flat face
malar hypoplasia
hypertelorism with prominent eyes
parrot-beak type nose

OTHER FINDINGS
mental retardation common
moderate to severe acne, often on the extremities
cardiac anomalies
– pulmonary stenosis
– overriding aorta
– ventricular septal defect

autosomal dominant

References
McNaughton PZ, Rodman OG: Apert's syndrome. Cutis 1980; 25:538–540.
Robison D, Wilms NA: Successful treatment of the acne of Apert syndrome with isotretinoin. J Am Acad Dermatol 1989; 21:315–316.
Solomon LM, Fretzin D, Pruzansky S: Pilosebaceous abnormalities in Apert's syndrome. Arch Dermatol 1970; 102:381–385.
Steffan C: Acneiform eruption in Apert's syndrome. Arch Dermatol 1982; 118:206–208.

APLASIA CUTIS CONGENITA (ACC)

Categories of ACC, Areas Involved, and Features

1 • **scalp ACC (Fig. 9) without multiple anomalies**
midline scalp affected
associated abnormalities: cleft lip and palate; tracheoesophageal fistula; omphalocele; mental retardation; polycystic kidney; others
autosomal dominant or sporadic inheritance

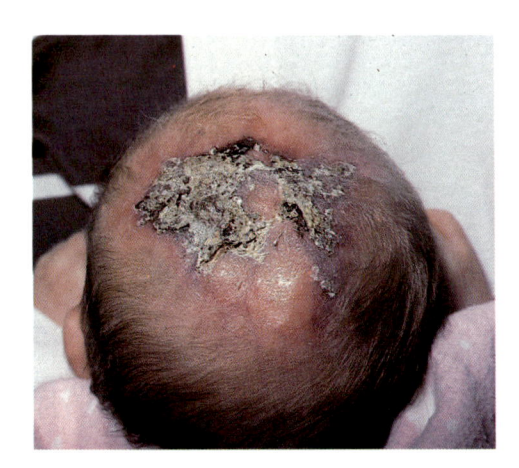

• *Figure 9 A large plaque of aplasia cutis congenita of the scalp.*

2 **scalp ACC with associated limb abnormalities (see Adams–Oliver syndrome)**
midline scalp affected
associated abnormalities: limbs reduced; syndactyly; clubfoot; encephalocele; nail absence or dystrophy; persistent cutis marmorata
autosomal dominant

Dermatologic Syndromes

3 scalp ACC with associated epidermal or sebaceous nevi
  scalp affected, may be asymmetric
  associated abnormalities: epidermal or sebaceous nevi (usually of scalp); corneal opacities; scleral dermoids; eyelid colobomas; mental retardation; seizures
  sporadic inheritance

4 ACC overlying embryologic malformations
  any site affected
  associated abnormalities: meningomyeloceles; spinal dysraphia; cranial stenosis; leptomeningeal angiomatosis; gastroschisis
  inheritance depends upon underlying condition

5 ACC with associated fetus papyraceus or placental infarcts
  multiple symmetric areas affected, often stellate or linear
  associated abnormalities: delivery of dead twin or triplet; single umbilical artery; developmental delay; spastic paralysis; clubbed hands and feet; amniotic bands
  sporadic inheritance

6 ACC associated with epidermolysis bullosa (EB)
  extremities, trunk, or head affected
  associated abnormalities: blistering of skin and/or mucous membranes; deformed nails; pyloric or duodenal atresia; abnormal ears and nose; ureteral stenosis; renal anomalies; amniotic bands
  inheritance depends upon type of EB (usually junctional or dystrophic)

7 ACC localized to extremities without blistering
  pretibial areas, dorsa of hands and feet, extensor areas of wrists affected
  associated abnormalities: none
  autosomal dominant or recessive

8 ACC caused by teratogens or intrauterine infections
  scalp affected (with methimazole for hyperthyroidism) and any area (with infection)
  associated abnormalities: imperforate anus (with methimazole); other signs of intrauterine infection (with varicella or herpes simplex infection)
  not inherited

9 ACC-associated malformation syndromes
  scalp or any location affected
  associated abnormalities: trisomy 13; 4p syndrome; ectodermal dysplasias; focal dermal hypoplasia; amniotic band syndrome
  inheritance depends upon syndrome

References
Frieden IJ: Aplasia cutis congenita: A clinical review and proposal for classification. J Am Acad Dermatol 1986; 14:646–660.
Levin DL, Nolan KS, Esterly NB: Congenital absence of skin. J Am Acad Dermatol 1980; 2:203–206.
Sybert VP: Aplasia cutis congenita: A report of 12 new families and review of the literature. Pediatr Dermatol 1985; 3:1–14.

ARGINOSUCCINIC ACIDURIA,
ARGINOSUCCINASE DEFICIENCY

Types of Arginosuccinic Aciduria and Features

1 neonatal
  poor feeding
  lethargy
  seizures
  death

2 subacute type
  feeding difficulties
  failure to thrive
  seizures
  developmental delay
  hepatomegaly

3 late-onset type
  neurologic abnormalities (irritability, seizures, ataxia)
  vomiting episodes
  mental retardation
  • trichorrhexis nodosa (Fig. 10)
  dull, brittle hair
  autosomal recessive

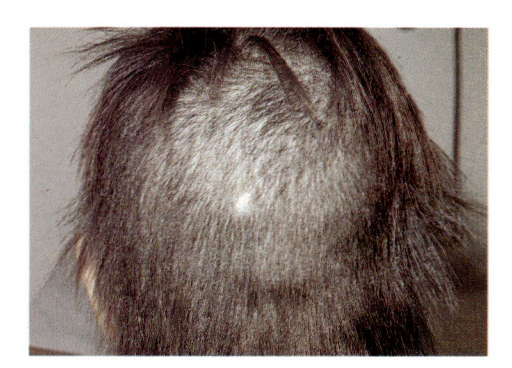

• *Figure 10 Hair displaying tricchorhexis nodosa in late-onset type arginosuccinic aciduria.*

ASCHER SYNDROME

Manifestations and Major Findings
thickened puffy eyelids
progressive enlargement of upper lip caused by hypertrophy and inflammation of labial glands
enlarged thyroid
endocrine abnormalities
– acromegaly
– dysmenorrhea

References
Held JL, Schneiderman P: A review of blepharochalasis and other causes of the lax, wrinkled eyelid. Cutis 1990; 45:91–94.
Mathew MS, Srinivasan R, Goyal JL, Ratnakar C, et al.: Ascher's syndrome: an unusual case with entropion. Int J Dermatol 1992; 31:710–712.
Navas J, Rodriquez-Pichardo A, Camacho F: Ascher syndrome: A case study. Pediatr Dermatol 1991; 8:122–123.

ATAXIA TELANGIECTASIA, LOUIS–BAR SYNDROME

Manifestations and Major Findings
progressive cerebellar ataxia (begins at about 2 years of age)
• oculocutaneous telangiectasias (Fig. 11) (begins about 2–6 years of age)
bulbar conjunctiva, ears, and flexor folds of the extremities
nystagmus
strabismus
blepharitis
progressive mental deterioration
frequent sinopulmonary infections

References
Lee EB: Metabolic diseases and the skin. Pediatr Clin N Am 1983; 30:597–608.
Porter PS: Genetic disorders of hair growth. J Invest Dermatol 1973; 60:493–502.
Price VH: Office diagnosis of structural hair anomalies. Cutis 1975; 15:231–239.

defective ce
– lymphope
– anergic skin testing
– hypoplastic thymus
humoral immunity abnormal – IgA, IgE, IgG-2, IgM all decreased
breaks and rearrangements of chromosomes, particularly 7 and 14
fibroblasts hypersensitive to killing by X-ray and certain chemicals, but not hypermutable
insulin-resistant diabetes
hypogonadism in males
ovarian agenesis
delayed or absent development of secondary sexual characteristics
growth retardation
hepatic dysfunction
usually fatal in second decade

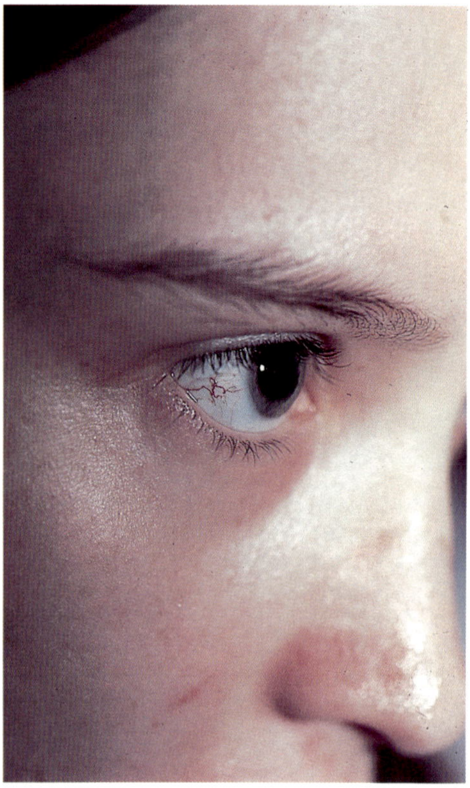

• **Figure 11** *Oculocutaneous telangiectasias of the conjunctiva in ataxia telangiectasia.*

elevated α-fetoprotein in the blood
high incidence of neoplastic disorders (lymphoma, leukemia, breast carcinomas, etc.) in patients and carriers

Cutaneous Manifestations
acanthosis nigricans
• granulomatous sterile plaques (Fig. 12)
vitiligo
premature graying of hair
hypo- or hyperpigmentation
atrophy
chronic skin infections

autosomal recessive, chromosome 11q 22–23

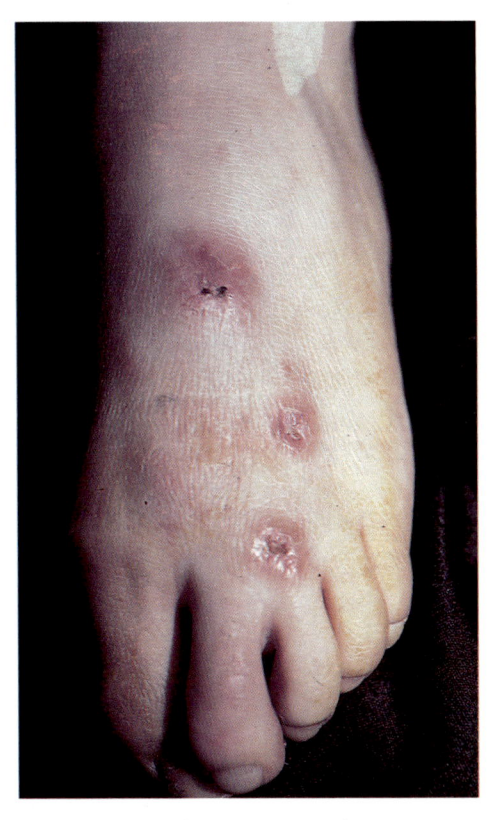

• *Figure 12 Sterile cutaneous granulomas in ataxia telangiectasia.*

References
Boder E, Sedgwick RP: Ataxia telangiectasia. A familial syndrome of progressive cerebellar ataxia, oculocutaneous telangiectasia and frequent pulmonary infection. Pediatrics 1958; 21:526–554.
Carbonari M, Cherchi M, Paganelli R, Giannini G, et al.: Relative increase of T cells expressing the gamma/delta rather than the alpha/beta receptor in ataxia-telangiectasia. N Engl J Med 1990; 322:73–76.
Cohen LE, Tanner DJ, Schaefer HG, Levis WR: Common and uncommon cutaneous findings in patients with ataxia telangiectasia. J Am Acad Dermatol 1984; 10:431–438.
Paller AS, Massey RB, Curtis MA, Pelachyk JM, et. al.: Cutaneous granulomatous lesions in patients with ataxia telangiectasia. J Pediatr 1991; 119:917–922.
Swift M, Morrell D, Massey RB, Chase CL: Incidence of cancer in 161 families affected by ataxia-telangiectasia. N Engl J Med 1991; 325:1831–1836.
Waldmann TA, Misiti J, Nelson DL, Kraemer KH: Ataxia-telangiectasia a multisystem hereditary disease with immunodeficiency, impaired organ maturation, x-ray hypersensitivity, and a high incidence of neoplasia. Ann Intern Med 1983; 99:367–379.

ATROPHODERMA OF PASINI AND PIERINI *see* PASINI AND PIERINI ATROPHODERMA

ATYPICAL MOLE SYNDROME
see DYSPLASTIC NEVUS SYNDROME

AURICULOTEMPORAL SYNDROME, FREY SYNDROME

Manifestations and Major Findings
pain, • vasodilatation, and/or hyperhidrosis of the cheek (Fig. 13) while eating (usually unilateral)
usually occurs after damage to the parotid area (autonomic fibers to sweat glands and salivary glands damaged), or begins in childhood spontaneously

References
Beck SA, Burks AW, Woody RC: Auriculotemporal syndrome seen clinically as food allergy. Pediatr 1989; 83:601–603.   ▷ ▷ ▷

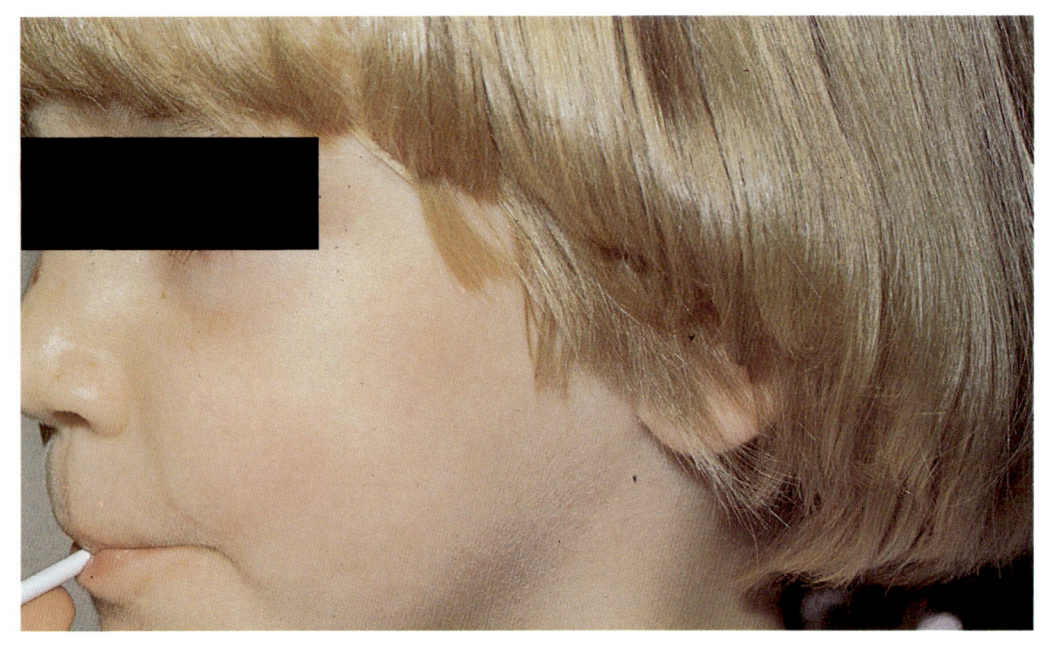

• *Figure 13* Vasodilation and flushing of the cheek during eating seen in auriculotemporal syndrome.

▷ ▷ ▷
Glaister DH, Hearnshaw JR, Heffron PF, Peck AW: The mechanism of post-parotidectomy gustatory sweating (the auriculotemporal syndrome). Br Med J 1958; 2:942–946.
Harper KE, Spielvogel RL: Frey's syndrome. Int J Dermatol 1986; 25:524–526.
Sato K, Kang WH, Saga K, Sato KT: Biology of sweat glands and their disorders. II. Disorders of sweat gland function. J Am Acad Dermatol 1989; 20:713–726.
Sato K, Ohtsuyama M, Samman G: Eccrine sweat gland disorders. J Am Acad Dermatol 1991; 24:1010–1014.

AUTOERYTHROCYTE SENSITIZATION SYNDROME,
GARDNER–DIAMOND SYNDROME, PAINFUL BRUISING SYNDROME

Manifestations and Major Findings
recurrent painful ecchymoses, most commonly on extremities
prodromal stinging or burning in the area prior to a lesion developing
psychiatric symptoms
systemic complaints
– severe headaches
– diplopia
– abdominal pain
– nausea
– muscle pain
uncertain etiology – may be factitious or an allergic sensitivity reaction
predominantly affects adult women (95%)

References
Berman DA, Roenigk HH, Green D: Autoerythrocyte sensitization syndrome (psychogenic purpura). J Am Acad Dermatol 1992; 27:829–832.
Campbell AN, Freedman MH, McClure PD: Autoerythrocyte sensitization. J Pediatr 1983; 103:157–160.
Hanna WT, Fitzpatrick R, Krauss S, Machado E, Dunn CDR: Psychogenic purpura (autoerythrocyte sensitization). South Med J 1981; 74:538–542.
Meister MM, Bodner AC: Autoerythrocyte sensitization – a psychogenic purpura? Cutis 1977; 19:221–224.
Settle JC: Autoerythrocyte sensitization successfully treated with antidepressants. J Am Med Assoc 1983; 250:1749–1750.
Stefanini M, Baumgart ET: Purpura factitia, an analysis of criteria for its differentiation from autoerythrocyte sensitization purpura. Arch Dermatol 1972; 106:238–241.

B

BADS SYNDROME *see* ALBINISM

BALANITIS OF ZOON *see* ZOON BALANITIS

BANNAYAN–ZONANA SYNDROME,
BANNAYAN SYNDROME, MACROCEPHALY WITH MULTIPLE LIPOMATA AND HEMANGIOMAS *see also* RILEY–SMITH SYNDROME *and* RUVALCABA–MYHRE–SMITH SYNDROME

Manifestations and Major Findings
macrocephaly
multiple cutaneous and visceral vascular malformations
pseudopapilledema
lymphangiomas
lipomas (often multiple)
normal development or mental retardation
intracranial tumors (meningioma)
high palate
hyperextensibility of the joints
pectus excavatum
amblyopia
strabismus

Characteristic Facies
frontal bossing
down-slanting palpebral fissures

autosomal dominant with variable expression

References
Dvir M, Beer S, Aladjem M: Heredofamilial syndrome of mesodermal hamartomas, macrocephaly, and pseudopapilledema. Pediatrics 1988; 81:287–290.

Higginbottom MC, Schultz P: The Bannayan syndrome: an autosomal dominant disorder consisting of macrocephaly, lipomas, hemangiomas, and the risk for intracranial tumors. Pediatrics 1982; 69:632–634.
Klein JA, Barr RJ: Bannayan–Zonana Syndrome associated with lymphangiomyomatous lesions. Pediatr Dermatol 1990; 7:48–53.
Miles JH, Zonana J, McFarlane J, Aleck KA, Bawle E: Macrocephaly with hamartomas: Bannayan–Zonana syndrome. Am J Med Genet 1984; 19:225–234.
Zonana J, Rimoin DL, Davis DC: Macrocephaly with multiple lipomas and hemangiomas. J Pediatr 1976; 89:600–603.

BANNWARTH SYNDROME,
LYMPHOCYTIC MENINGORADICULITIS, GARIN–BUJADOUX–BANNWARTH SYNDROME

Manifestations and Major Findings
neurological manifestation of an arthropod-transmitted borreliosis – either *Borrelia burgdorferi* or closely related species
characterized by pain with sensory and motor disturbances in peripheral nerves (especially facial nerve)
headache
fever
stiff neck
somnolence
memory deficits
inability to concentrate
cranial neuritis
facial palsy
erythema chronicum migrans
described mainly in Europe

BARAITSER SYNDROME

Manifestations and Major Findings
premature aging
short stature
multiple pigmented nevi
low birth weight
mental retardation

Characteristic Facies
small chin
lack of facial fat
broad forehead
prominent ear lobes

OTHER FINDINGS
hypospadias
high-pitched voice
fine hair
hepatomegaly
low serum IgG
diabetes mellitus

> **References**
> Baraitser M, Insley J, Winter RM: A recognisable short stature syndrome with premature aging and pigmented nevi. J Med Genet 1988; 25:53–56.

BARDET–BIEDL SYNDROME

Manifestations and Major Findings
mental retardation
severe retinal dystrophy causing blindness
polydactyly, syndactyly, or brachydactyly
obesity (especially truncal)
hypogenitalism
structural or functional renal abnormalities
diabetes mellitus

autosomal recessive

> **References**
> Cramer B, Green J, Harnett J, Johnson GJ, et al.: Sonographic and urographic correlation in Bardet–Biedl syndrome (formerly Laurence–Moon–Biedl syndrome). Urol Radiol 1988; 10:176–180.
> Green JS, Parfrey PS, Harnett JD, Farid NR, et al.: The cardinal manifestations of Bardet–Biedl syndrome, a form of Laurence–Moon–Biedl syndrome. N Engl J Med 1989; 321:1002–1009.

BARE LYMPHOCYTE SYNDROME

Manifestations and Major Findings
absence of HLA class I and/or II antigens on peripheral mononuclear cells
absence of β-2-microglobulin on lymphocytes
sinobronchial disease
diarrhea
combined immunodeficiency with infections – particularly *Candida*, *Pneumocystis carinii*, and viral infections
erythematous pustular eczematous plaques and nodules
ichthyosis vulgaris
skin lesions with histology similar to necrobiosis lipoidica

autosomal recessive

> **References**
> Touraine J-L: The bare lymphocyte syndrome: report on the registry. Lancet 1981; 1:319–320.
> Touraine J-L, Betuel H, Souillet G, Jeune M: Combined immunodeficiency disease associated with absence of cell-surface HLA-A and -B antigens. J Pediatr 1978; 93:47–51.
> Watanabe S, Iwata M, Maeda H, Ishibashi Y: Immunohistochemical studies of major histocompatibility antigens in a case of the Bare Lymphocyte Syndrome without immunodeficiency. J Am Acad Dermatol 1987; 17:895–902.

BARTONELLOSIS see CARRION DISEASE

BART SYNDROME

Manifestations and Major Findings
congenital localized absence of the skin
epidermolysis bullosa (simplex, junctional, or dystrophic)
trauma induced blisters, with or without scarring
oral mucosal lesions
shedding or dystrophy of the nails
rapid healing of erosions
usual spontaneous resolution by 12 months of age

> **References**
> Bart BJ, Gorlin RJ, Anderson VE, Lynch FW: Congenital localized absence of skin and associated abnormalities resembling epidermolysis bullosa. Arch Dermatol 1966; 93:296–304.
> Butler DF, Berger TG, James WD, Smith TL, Stanley JR, et al.: Bart's syndrome: microscopic, ultrastructural, and immunofluorescent mapping features. Pediatr Dermatol 1986; 3:113–118.
> Fisher GB, Greer KE, Cooper PH: Congenital self-healing (transient) mechanobullous dermatosis. Arch Dermatol 1988; 124:240–243.
> Kanzler MH, Smoller B, Woodley DT: Congenital localized absence of the skin as a manifestation of epidermolysis bullosa. Arch Dermatol 1992; 128:1087–1090.

BASAL CELL NEVUS SYNDROME,
NEVOID BASAL CELL CARCINOMA SYNDROME, GORLIN SYNDROME

Manifestations and Major Findings
multiple basal cell carcinomas at an early age
- palmoplantar pits (Fig. 14)

multiple jaw cysts (odontogenic keratocysts) with malignant potential
- hypertelorism (Fig. 15)

medulloblastomas
ovarian fibromas, carcinomas, calcified cysts
milia
lipomas
epidermal cysts of skin
mental retardation
calcification of the falx cerebri
agenesis of the corpus callosum
- frontal bossing (Fig. 15)

elevated mutant circulating T lymphocytes
fibroblasts defective in repair from ionizing radiation damage
radiotherapy should be avoided

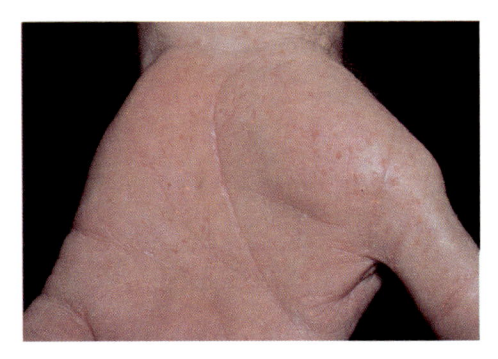

• *Figure 14 Palmar pits in basal cell nevus syndrome.*

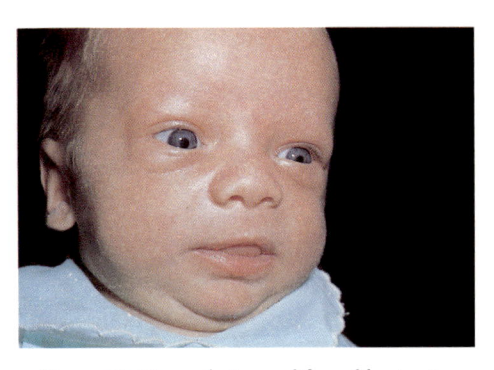

• *Figure 15 Hypertelorism and frontal bossing in a baby with basal cell nevus syndrome.*

SKELETAL ABNORMALITIES
spina bifida occulta
rib anomalies (splayed, bifid, fused, missing, etc.)
scoliosis
short fourth metacarpals
mandibular prognathism
vertebral anomalies
pectus excavatum

autosomal dominant

> **References**
> Applegate A, Goldberg LH, Ley RD, Anathaswamy HN: Hypersensitivity of skin fibroblasts from basal cell nevus syndrome patients to killing by Ultraviolet B but not ultraviolet C radiation. Cancer Res 1990; 50:637–641.
> Bale AE, Bale SJ, Murli H, Ivett J, Mulvihill JJ, et al.: Sister chromatid exchange and chromosome fragility in the nevoid basal cell carcinoma syndrome. Cancer Genet Cytogenet 1989; 42:273–279.
> Goldberg LH, Hsu SH, Alcalay J: Effectiveness of isotretinoin in preventing the appearance of basal cell carcinomas in basal cell nevus syndrome. J Am Acad Dermatol 1989; 21:144–145.
> Gorlin RJ: Nevoid basal-cell carcinoma syndrome. Medicine 1987; 66:98–113.
> Gutierrez MM, Mora RG: Nevoid basal cell carcinoma syndrome. J Am Acad Dermatol 1986; 15:1023–1030.
> Newton JA, Black AK, Arlett CF, Cole J: Radiobiological studies in the naevoid basal cell carcinoma syndrome. Br J Dermatol 1990; 123:573–580.

BASAN TYPE ECTODERMAL DYSPLASIA

Manifestations and Major Findings
hypohidrosis
hypotrichosis – body, scalp, eyebrows, eyelashes
very fine dermal ridges over the hands and feet
single palmar flexion creases
dysplastic nails
tooth loss early, secondary to decay

MINOR FINDINGS
xerosis (dry skin)
dry mucous membranes

Characteristic Facies
thin nasal alae
long philtrum
thin upper lips

autosomal dominant

BATEMAN PURPURA, ACTINIC PURPURA, SENILE PURPURA

Manifestations and Major Findings
purpura seen on sun-damaged skin of the elderly – usually on hands and forearms due to diminished strength of blood vessel walls, damaged collagen, and trauma

> **References**
> Lever WF, Schaumburg-Lever G: Histopathology of the Skin. 7th edition. J.B. Lippincott, Philadelphia, 1990, p.185.

BATTEN DISEASE, NEURONAL CEROID LIPOFUSCINOSIS

Manifestations and Major Findings
onset from 2 years of age to adulthood
hereditary neurodegenerative disease
seizures
myoclonus
optic atrophy
progressive blindness
mental and motor regression
elevated urinary sediment of dolichols
skin biopsy shows osmiophilic material accumulated in lysosomes, visible with lipid stains

> **References**
> Berkovic SF, Andermann F, Carpenter S, et al.: Progressive myoclonus epilepsies: specific causes and diagnosis. N Engl J Med 1986; 315:296–305.
> Carpenter S: Skin biopsy for diagnosis of hereditary neurologic metabolic disease. Arch Dermatol 1987; 123:1618–1621.
> Carpenter S, Karpati G, Andermann F, Jacob JC, et al.: The ultrastructural characteristics of the abnormal cytosomes in Batten–Kufs' disease. Brain 1977; 100:137–156.

BATTERED CHILD SYNDROME, CHILD ABUSE

Characteristic Findings
lesions caused by nonaccidental trauma
- bruising (Fig. 16) – linear, often on back or buttocks

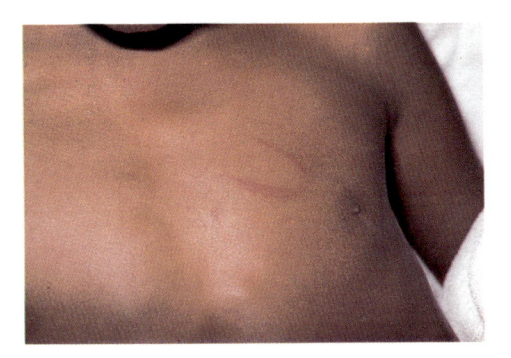

Figure 16 Cord-mark bruising; a typical finding in battered child syndrome.

bite marks
burns due to cigarettes, scalding, ropes, heaters, or hot grids
head injuries
multiple fractures
sexual abuse – sexually transmitted disease in a prepubertal child
internal injuries – hematomas or rupture of viscera

FEATURES SUGGESTIVE OF BATTERED CHILD SYNDROME
delay in seeking medical advice
details vague or inconsistent
history not compatible with observed injury
lack of concern by caregiver
child's acknowledgement of inflicted injury
child's disposition to complete compliance or marked reluctance
hostility of caregiver to medical personnel

References
Committee on Child Abuse and Neglect, American Academy of Pediatrics. Guidelines for the evaluation of sexual abuse of children. Pediatrics 1991; 87:254–260.
Raimer BG, Raimer SS, Hebeler JR: Cutaneous signs of child abuse. J Am Acad Dermatol 1981; 5:203–212.
Reece RM, Grodin MA: Recognition of nonaccidental injury. Pediatr Clin N Am 1985; 32:41–59.
Schachner L, Hankin DE: Assessing child abuse in childhood condyloma accuminatum. J Am Acad Dermatol 1985; 12:157–160.

BAZEX SYNDROME, ACROKERATOSIS PARANEOPLASTICA

Manifestations and Major Findings
violaceous psoriasiform lesions on external ears, fingers, feet, cheeks, elbows, and knees
squamous cell carcinoma in pulmonary or upper gastrointestinal tract, often with metastases to cervical lymph nodes
alopecia
palmoplantar keratoderma
nails with subungual hyperkeratosis, onycholysis, paronychia
more common in middle-aged white males

References
Gregory B, Ho VC: Cutaneous manifestations of gastrointestinal disorders. Part I. J Am Acad Dermatol 1992; 26:153–166.
Grimwood RE, Lekan C: Acrokeratosis paraneoplastica with esophageal squamous cell carcinoma (letter). J Am Acad Dermatol 1987; 17:685–686.
Martin RW, Cornitius TG, Naylor MF, Neldner KH: Bazex's syndrome in a woman with pulmonary adenocarcinoma. Arch Dermatol 1989; 125:847–848.
Pecora AL, Landsman L, Imgrund SP, Lambert WC: Acrokeratosis paraneoplastica (Bazex' syndrome). Arch Dermatol 1983; 119:820–826.
Richard M, Giroux J-M: Acrokeratosis paraneoplastica (Bazex' syndrome). J Am Acad Dermatol 1987; 16:178–183.
Witkowski JA, Parish LC: Bazex' Syndrome: paraneoplastic acrokeratosis. J Am Med Assoc 1982; 248:2883–2884.

BAZEX SYNDROME, FOLLICULAR ATROPHODERMA AND BASAL CELL CARCINOMA SYNDROME, BAZEX–DUPRÉ–CHRISTOL SYNDROME

Manifestations and Major Findings
follicular atrophoderma on the dorsum of hands and feet, face, and extensor surfaces from birth
multiple basal cell carcinomas from adolescence
generalized hypohidrosis or localized anhidrosis
hypotrichosis
pili torti (twisted hair shafts) or trichorrhexis nodosa
skeletal defects
milia

comedones
punctate keratoderma
scrotal tongue

autosomal dominant or X-linked

References
Tüzün Y, Mat MC, Serdaroglu S, Kotogyan A: Follicular atrophoderma with scrotal tongue. Pediatr Dermatol 1987; 4:328–331.
Viksnins P, Berlin A: Follicular atrophoderma and basal cell carcinomas. The Bazex syndrome. Arch Dermatol 1977; 113:948–951.

BAZIN DISEASE, ERYTHEMA INDURATUM, NODULAR VASCULITIS

Manifestations and Major Findings
persistent or recurrent painful nodules (panniculitis) mainly on the calves
irregular and shallow ulcers with a bluish edge
perniotic circulation in lower legs
more common in women than men
past or active focus of tuberculosis
may represent a hypersensitivity reaction to *Mycobacterium tuberculosis*

References
Kuramoto Y, Aiba S, Tagami H: Erythema induratum of Bazin as a type of tuberculid. J Am Acad Dermatol 1990; 22:612–616.
Ollert MW, Thomas P, Korting HC, Schraut W, et al.: Erythema induratum of Bazin. Arch Dermatol 1993; 129:469–473.
Rademaker M, Lowe DG, Munro DD: Erythema induratum (Bazin's disease). J Am Acad Dermatol 1989; 21:740–745.

BEAN SYNDROME see BLUE RUBBER BLEB NEVUS SYNDROME

BECKER MELANOSIS, BECKER NEVUS

Manifestations and Major Findings
- unilateral hyperpigmented macular patch with hypertrichosis (Fig. 17)
hypertrichosis usually appears after hyperpigmentation

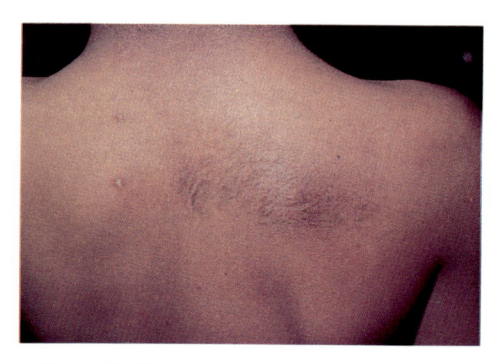

• *Figure 17* Becker melanosis presents as a hyperpigmented macular patch with hypertrichosis, typically over the shoulder.

no nevus cells found on biopsy
most common location on shoulder or back
becomes prominent in second to third decade
usually affects males
associated with pilar smooth muscle hamartoma

References
Fulk CS: Primary disorders of hyperpigmentation. J Am Acad Dermatol 1984; 10:1–16.
Glinick SE, Alper JC, Bogaars H, et al.: Becker's melanosis: associated abnormalities. J Am Acad Dermatol 1983; 9:509–514.
Moore JA, Schosser RH: Becker's melanosis and hypoplasia of the breast and pectoralis major muscle. Pediatr Dermatol 1985; 3:34–37.
Person JR, Longcope C: Becker's nevus: an androgen-mediated hyperplasia with increased androgen receptors. J Am Acad Dermatol 1984; 10:235–238.

BECKWITH–WIEDEMANN SYNDROME, EXOMPHALOS–MACROGLOSSIA–GIGANTISM (EMG) SYNDROME

Manifestations and Major Findings
(may be variable)
macroglossia
visceromegaly (liver, spleen, adrenals, pancreas, kidney, etc.)
omphalocele
anomalies of intestinal rotation
fetus is large for gestational age
asymmetry/hemihypertrophy
ear lobe creases
punched-out depressions on posterior pinna

neonatal hypoglycemia, hypocalcemia, and
  polycythemia
nevus flammeus of central forehead and eyelids
thick subcutaneous tissue
polyhydramnios
predisposition to Wilms tumor,
  hepatoblastoma, and other tumors
mild mental retardation
zosteriform dermatosis at birth

> **References**
> Chesney RW, Kaufman R, Stapleton FB, et al.:
> Association of medullary sponge kidney and
> medullary dysplasia in Beckwith–Wiedemann
> syndrome. J Pediatr 1989; 115:761–764.

BEHÇET SYNDROME

Manifestations and Major Findings
multisystem disorder with a classic triad of oral
  ulcers, genital ulcers, and ocular inflammation
- intermittent painful aphthous ulcerations of
  the mouth (Fig. 18)
painful recurrent ulceration of the genitals
central nervous system symptoms
  – meningoencephalitis
  – cerebral infarcts
pulmonary involvement
cardiac involvement
vascular involvement
  – aneurysms
  – arterial occlusions
  – venous occlusions
  – varices
  – thrombophlebitis
gastrointestinal ulcerations
renal involvement
immunologic abnormalities
  – suppressor T cell dysfunction
  – changes in serum complement
  – circulating immune complexes
arthralgias/arthritis
associated with HLA-B5, -Bw51, -B27,
  and -B12
more common in middle-aged males
more common in the Middle East, China, and
  Japan

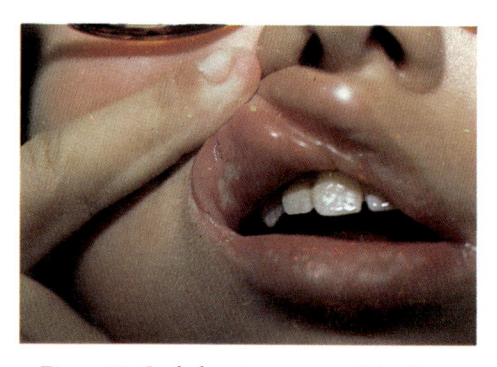

- *Figure 18* Oral ulcerations are one of the classic triad of findings in Behçet syndrome.

OCULAR ABNORMALITIES
iridocyclitis
keratitis
retinal vasculitis
optic neuritis
uveitis
hypopyon

Cutaneous Manifestations
erythema nodosum-like lesions
pathergy-sterile pustules at sites of injections
leukocytoclastic vasculitis

> **References**
> Arbesfeld SJ, Kurban AK: Behçet's disease. New
> perspectives on an enigmatic syndrome. J Am Acad
> Dermatol 1988; 19:767–779.
> Gilhar A, Winterstein G, Turani H, Landau J,
> Etzioni A: Skin hyperreactivity response (pathergy) in
> Behçet's disease. J Am Acad Dermatol 1989;
> 21:547–552.
> **International Study Group for Behçet's disease.**
> Criteria for diagnosis of Behçet's disease. Lancet
> 1990; 335:1078–1080.
> Jorizzo JL, Solomon AR, Zanolli MD, Leshin B:
> Neutrophilic vascular reactions. J Am Acad Dermatol
> 1988; 19:983–1005.
> Lee SH, Chung KY, Lee WS, Lee S: Behçet's
> syndrome associated with bullous necrotizing
> vasculitis. J Am Acad Dermatol 1989; 21:327–330.
> O'Duffy JD: Behçet's syndrome. N Engl J Med 1990;
> 322:326–328.
> Yazici H, Pazarli H, Barnes CG, Tüzün Y, et al.: A
> controlled trial of azathioprine in Behçet's syndrome.
> N Engl J Med 1990; 322:281–285.

BENIGN FAMILIAL PEMPHIGUS
see HAILEY–HAILEY DISEASE

BERLIN SYNDROME, ECTODERMAL DYSPLASIA (BERLIN TYPE)

Cutaneous Manifestations
mottled dyschromia – more prominent on the extremities
poikiloderma over the elbows, knees, and fingers
palmar and plantar hyperkeratosis
sparse eyebrows and pubic hair
normal scalp hair
telangiectasias of the lips
thick lips
normal nails
normal sweating

OTHER FINDINGS
short stature
flat, saddle-shaped nose
dental abnormalities
– missing teeth
– delayed dentition
sexual underdevelopment
mental retardation

autosomal recessive

> **References**
> Berlin C: Congenital generalized melanoleucoderma associated with hypodontia, hypotrichosis, stunted growth, and mental retardation occurring in 2 brothers and 2 sisters. Dermatologica 1961; 123:227–243.
> Fulk CS: Primary disorders of hyperpigmentation. J Am Acad Dermatol 1984; 10:1–16.
> Pinheiro M, Pereira LC, Freire-Maia N: A previously undescribed condition: tricho-odonto-onycho-dermal syndrome. A review of the tricho-odonto-onychial subgroup of ectodermal dysplasias. Br J Dermatol 1981; 105:371–382.

BESNIER–BOECK–SCHAUMANN SYNDROME see SARCOIDOSIS

BIDS SYNDROME
see TRICHOTHIODYSTROPHY

BIOTIN DEFICIENCY AND BIOTIN-RESPONSIVE DISORDERS

Biotin is a water-soluble vitamin belonging to the B complex.

Types of Biotin-Related Disorders and Features

1 holocarboxylase deficiency/multiple synthetase carboxylase deficiency (neonatal onset)
neurologic abnormalities – seizures, hypotonia
recurrent vomiting
life-threatening acidosis and ketosis
biotin-responsive (in large doses)
cutaneous findings:
– candidal infections
– alopecia universalis
– erythroderma with scaling
autosomal recessive

2 biotinidase deficiency/multiple carboxylase deficiency (juvenile onset)
infantile onset
developmental delay
neurologic abnormalities:
– ataxia
– seizures
– hypotonia
– nerve deafness
– optic nerve atrophy
life-threatening acidosis and ketosis
cutaneous findings – skin lesions resembling acrodermatitis enteropathica
patchy or diffuse alopecia
abnormal T cell responses to *Candida*
keratoconjunctivitis
autosomal recessive

3 dietary disorder
too many raw eggs in diet (contains avidin which binds to biotin) or total parenteral nutrition lacking in biotin
skin lesions resembling acrodermatitis enteropathica

References
Nyhan WL: Inborn errors of biotin metabolism. Arch Dermatol 1987; 123:1696–1698a.
Sweetman L, Surh L, Baker H, Peterson RM, Nyhan WL: Clinical and metabolic abnormalities in a boy with dietary deficiency of biotin. Pediatrics 1981; 68:553–558.
Thoene J, Baker H, Yoshino M, Sweetman L: Biotin-responsive carboxylase deficiency associated with subnormal plasma and urinary biotin. N Engl J Med 1981; 304:817–820.
Wolf B, Grier RE, Allen RJ, Goodman SI, et al.: Phenotypic variation in biotinidase deficiency. J Pediatr 1983; 103:233–237.
Wolf B, Heard GS: Screening for biotinidase deficiency in newborns:worldwide experience. Pediatrics 1990; 85:512–517.
Wolf B, Hsia YE, Sweetman L, Feldman G, et al.: Multiple carboxylase deficiency: clinical and biochemical improvement following neonatal biotin treatment. Pediatrics 1981; 68:113–118.

BIRT–HOGG–DUBÉ SYNDROME,
BIRT SYNDROME, HORSTEIN–KNICKENBERG SYNDROME

Manifestations and Major Findings
fibrofolliculomas (multiple) in generalized distribution
trichodiscomas
acrochordons
intestinal polyposis
hidradenomas
carcinoma of the thyroid gland or gastrointestinal tract

autosomal dominant

References
Birt AR, Hogg GR, Dubé WJ: Hereditary multiple fibrofolliculomas with trichodiscomas and acrochordons. Arch Dermatol 1977; 113:1674–1677.
Rongioletti F, Hazini R, Gianotti G, Rebora A: Fibrofolliculomas, trichodiscomas, and acrochordons (Birt–Hogg–Dubé) associated with intestinal polyposis. Clin Exp Dermatol 1989; 14:72–74.
Ubogy-Rainey Z, James WD, Lupton GP, Rodman OG: Fibrofolliculomas, trichodiscomas, and acrochordons: the Birt–Hogg–Dubé syndrome. J Am Acad Dermatol 1987; 16:452–457.

BJÖRNSTAD SYNDROME

Manifestations and Major Findings
pili torti (twisted hair shafts)
sensorineural deafness
hypogonadism (rare)

autosomal recessive

References
Price VH: Disorders of the hair in children. Pediatr Clin N Am 1978; 25:305–320.
Reed WB, Stone VM, Boder E, Ziprkowski L: Hereditary syndromes with auditory and dermatological manifestations. Arch Dermatol 1967; 95:456–461.
Scott MJ, Bronson DM, Esterly NB: Björnstad syndrome and pili torti. Pediatr Dermatol 1983; 1:45–50.

B–K MOLE SYNDROME
see DYSPLASTIC NEVUS SYNDROME

BLACK LOCKS–ALBINISM–DEAFNESS (BADS) SYNDROME
see ALBINISM

BLASCHKO LINES

Manifestations and Major Findings
pattern of lines on the body that follow a 'V' configuration over the spine and anterior neck, an 'S' shape on the lateral and anterior trunk, and frequently form whorls; on limbs they have a more perpendicular direction
on the scalp, lines arranged in a spiral pattern from the frontal and temple area, converging on the vertex

Diseases which follow Blaschko Lines

1 nevoid skin diseases
- linear epidermal nevus (Fig. 19)
- linear sebaceous nevus (Fig. 20)
nevus comedonicus
Becker melanosis
nevoid telangiectasia
nevus angiolipomatosis   ▷ ▷ ▷

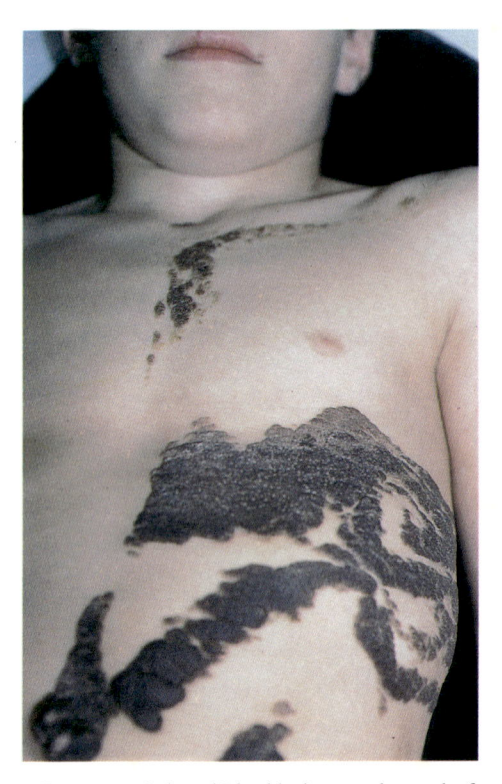

Figure 19 S-shaped Blaschko lines on the trunk of a patient with linear epidermal nevus.

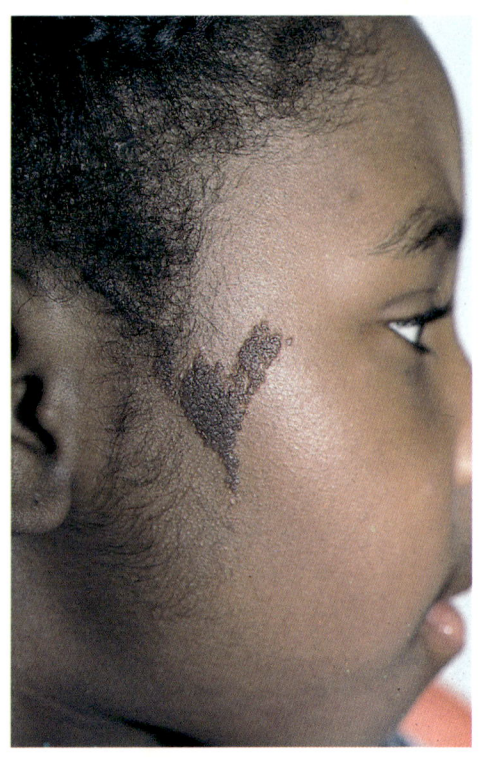

Figure 20 V-shaped Blaschko line on the face of a patient with linear sebaceous nevus.

▷ ▷ ▷
2 acquired skin diseases
linear scleroderma
lichen striatus
linear porokeratosis

3 X-linked genodermatoses
incontinentia pigmenti
focal dermal hypoplasia
chondrodysplasia punctata (Conradi disease)
hypohidrotic ectodermal dysplasia
Menkes syndrome

References
Happle R: Lethal genes surviving by mosaicism: a possible explanation for sporadic birth defects involving the skin. J Am Acad Dermatol 1987; 16:899–906.
Jackson R: Epidermal nevi and the epidermal nevus syndrome. J Am Acad Dermatol 1990; 22:320.
Kalter DC, Griffiths WA, Atherton DJ: Linear and whorled nevoid hypermelanosis. J Am Acad Dermatol 1988; 19:1037–1044.

BLOCH–SULZBERGER SYNDROME
see INCONTINENTIA PIGMENTI

BLOOM SYNDROME, CONGENITAL TELANGIECTATIC ERYTHEMA AND STUNTED GROWTH

Manifestations and Major Findings
short stature (prenatal onset)
telangiectatic facial erythema (butterfly distribution)
malar hypoplasia
photosensitivity (not true poikiloderma)
hypogonadism
high-pitched voice
high incidence of malignancy – especially leukemias, lymphomas, and gastrointestinal tract cancer
increased susceptibility to infections

OTHER FINDINGS
café au lait macules
acanthosis nigricans
hypogonadism
testicular atrophy
clinodactyly
syndactyly
abnormal immunity
– low immunoglobulins (particularly IgA and IgM)
– lymphocyte defects
chromosome breaks and rearrangements, quadriradial figures, sister chromatid exchanges
normal mentation or mild mental retardation
predominantly affects males

autosomal recessive

> **References**
> **Bloom D:** The syndrome of congenital telangiectatic erythema and stunted growth. J Pediatr 1966; 68:103–113.
> **German J, Bloom D, Passarge E:** Bloom's syndrome XI. Progress report for 1983. Clin Genet 1984; 25:166–174.
> **Van Kerckhove CW, Ceuppens JL, Vanderschueren-Lodeweyckx M, Eggermont E, et al.:** Bloom's syndrome. Clinical features and immunologic abnormalities of four patients. Am J Dis Child 1988; 142:1089–1093.

BLUE RUBBER BLEB NEVUS SYNDROME, BEAN SYNDROME

Manifestations and Major Findings
- bluish, compressible, rubbery venous channels of the skin (Fig. 21) and mucous membranes
skin lesions usually asymptomatic, but may be tender or painful (especially at night)
few or numerous vascular lesions which tend to increase in size and number with age

OTHER FINDINGS
gastrointestinal tract vascular malformations
supralesional sweating
bleeding from intestinal vascular malformations, leading to anemia
onset at birth or early childhood

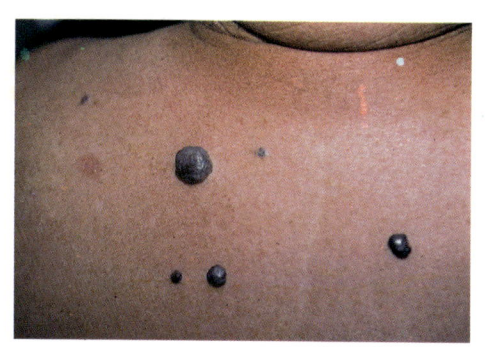

• *Figure 21 Typical skin lesions in blue rubber bleb syndrome with blue color and spongy feel.*

liver, spleen, and central nervous system may have vascular malformations

autosomal dominant

> **References**
> **Gregory B, Ho VC:** Cutaneous manifestations of gastrointestinal disorders. Part II. J Am Acad Dermatol 1992; 26:371–383.
> **Morris SJ, Kaplan SR, Ballan K, Tedesco FJ:** Blue rubber-bleb nevus syndrome. J Am Med Assoc 1978; 239:1887.
> **Morris L, Lynch PM, Gleason WA, Schauder C, et al.:** Blue rubber bleb nevus syndrome: laser photocoagulation of colonic hemangiomas in a child with microcytic anemia. Pediatr Dermatol 1992; 9:91–94.
> **Munkvad M:** Blue rubber bleb nevus syndrome. Dermatologica 1983; 167:307–309.
> **Oranje AP:** Blue rubber bleb nevus syndrome. Pediatr Dermatol 1986; 3:304–310.
> **Sandhu KS, Cohen H, Radin R, Buck FS:** Blue rubber bleb nevus syndrome presenting with recurrences. Dig Dis Sci 1987; 32:214–219.

BOCKHART IMPETIGO, FOLLICULAR IMPETIGO

Manifestations and Major Findings
infection of the follicular ostium with *Staphylococcus aureus*
scalp and limbs most commonly affected
lesions are individual, dome-shaped, yellow pustules which heal within 7–10 days

BOGORAD SYNDROME
see CROCODILE TEARS SYNDROME

BONNET–DECHAUME–BLANC SYNDROME see WYBURN–MASON SYNDROME

BONNEVIE–ULLRICH SYNDROME see TURNER SYNDROME

BÖÖK SYNDROME

Manifestations and Major Findings
hyperhidrosis of the palms and soles
premature canities (graying of the hair)
hypodontia (premolar aplasia)
malocclusion

autosomal dominant

> **References**
> Böök JA: Clinical and genetical studies of hypodontia. Am J Hum Genet 1950; 2:240–263.

BOURNEVILLE DISEASE
see TUBEROUS SCLEROSIS

BOWEL BYPASS SYNDROME, BOWEL-ASSOCIATED DERMATOSIS–ARTHRITIS SYNDROME

Manifestations and Major Findings
pustular vasculitis associated with jejunoileal bypass procedure, inflammatory bowel disease, or blind loop after bowel surgery
lesions usually occur in crops on upper body
pathergy (sterile pustules at the site of trauma)
fever
persistent diarrhea
myalgias
malaise
polyarthritis
bacterial overgrowth in bypassed bowel segment

> **References**
> Gregory B, Ho VC: Cutaneous manifestations of gastrointestinal disorders. Part II. J Am Acad Dermatol 1992; 26:371–383.
> Jorizzo JL, Solomon AR, Zanolli MD, Leshin B: Neutrophilic vascular reactions. J Am Acad Dermatol 1988; 19:983–1005.

BOWEN DISEASE

Manifestations and Major Findings
squamous cell carcinoma *in situ*
- persistent, progressive, red, scaly plaque on the skin (Fig. 22)

associated with chronic sun damage, arsenic exposure, radiation therapy, or possibly *Papillomavirus*

> **References**
> Callen JP: Bowen's disease and internal malignant disease. Arch Dermatol 1988; 124:675–676.
> Chuang T-Y, Reizner GT: Bowen's disease and internal malignancy. J Am Acad Dermatol 1988; 19:47–51.
> Kossard S, Rosen R: Cutaneous Bowen's disease. An analysis of 1001 cases according to age, sex, and site. J Am Acad Dermatol 1992; 27:406–410.
> Reymann F, Ravnborg L, Schou G, Engholm G, et al.: Bowen's disease and internal malignant diseases. Arch Dermatol 1988; 124:677–679.

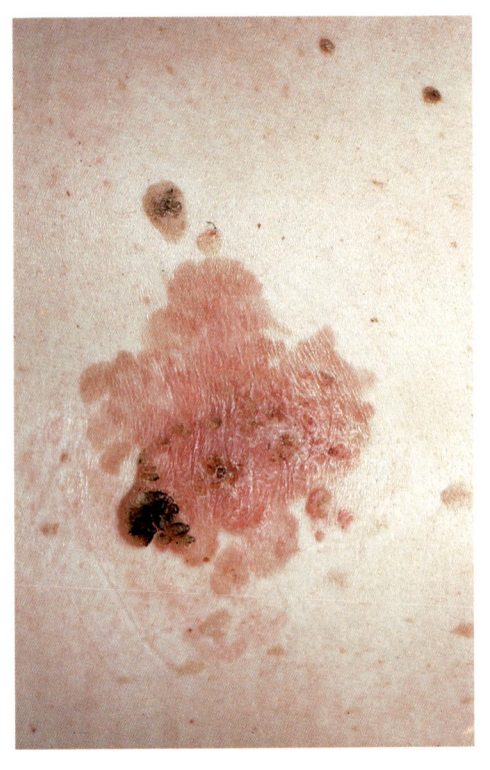

- *Figure 22* Red, scaly plaque seen in Bowen disease.

BRANCHIO-OCULOFACIAL SYNDROME

Manifestations and Major Findings
cleft lip or prominent vertical ridges on the upper lip resembling a poorly repaired cleft lip
branchial cleft with a sinus
hemangiomatous or atrophic skin lesions in the postauricular area
lacrimal duct obstruction
broad, flat nose

OTHER FINDINGS
subcutaneous scalp cysts
premature graying of hair (canities)
prognathic jaw
frontal bossing
microphthalmia
epicanthal folds
coloboma
lacrimal anomalies
cataracts
myopia
malformed ears
conductive hearing loss
lip pits
growth deficiency
hand anomalies

autosomal dominant or sporadic inheritance

References
Barr RJ, Santa Cruz DJ, Pearl RM: Dermal thymus. Arch Dermatol 1989; 125:1681–1684.
Lee WK, Root AW, Fenske N: Bilateral branchial cleft sinuses associated with intrauterine and postnatal growth retardation, premature aging, and unusual facial appearance: a new syndrome with dominant transmission. Am J Med Genet 1982; 11:345–352.

BRAZILIAN PEMPHIGUS FOLIACEUS *see* FOGO SELVAGEM

BRILL–ZINSSER DISEASE, RECRUDESCENT TYPHUS, SPORADIC TYPHUS

Manifestations and Major Findings
Rickettsia prowazekii as causative organism
transmitted by human body louse (*Pediculus hominis* var. *corporis*)
recurrent epidemic typhus which persists in tissues following primary typhus infection
fever and rash less prominent (may be absent) than with epidemic typhus
interepidemic reservoir of typhus

References
Burnett JW: Rickettsioses: a review for the dermatologist. J Am Acad Dermatol 1980; 2:359-373.

BRONZE BABY SYNDROME

Manifestations and Major Findings
complication of phototherapy for neonatal hyperbilirubinemia
grayish-brown skin (generalized)
hyperbilirubinemia (elevated direct bilirubin)
brown serum and urine
probably induced by photooxidation product of bilirubin, and biliverdin pigments
hepatic dysfunction
hyperporphyrinemia
usually resolves within 4–8 weeks

References
Ashley JR, Littler CM, Burgdorf WHC, Brann BS: Bronze baby syndrome. J Am Acad Dermatol 1985; 12:325–328.
Purcell SM, Wians FH, Ackerman NB, Davis BM: Hyperbiliverdinemia in the bronze baby syndrome. J Am Acad Dermatol 1987; 16:172–177.

BROOKE SYNDROME, EPITHELIOMA ADENOIDES CYSTICUM OF BROOKE, MULTIPLE TRICHOEPITHELIOMAS

Manifestations and Major Findings
multiple trichoepitheliomas, symmetrical over nasolabial folds, nose, forehead, upper lip, and ears, appearing in childhood or early teens, and enlarging slowly
lesions usually skin colored, yellow, pink, or bluish

autosomal dominant

References
Anderson DE, Howell JB: Epithelioma adenoides cysticum: genetic update. Br J Dermatol 1976; 95:225–232.
Berberian BJ, Sulica VI, Kao GF: Familial multiple eccrine spiradenomas with cylindromatous features associated with epithelioma adenoides cysticum of Brooke. Cutis 1990; 46:46–50.
Brichta RF, Feldman BD: Multiple flesh-colored facial papules. Diagnostic Challenges 1991; 1:25–26.
Brooke JD, Fitzpatrick JE, Golitz LE: Papillary mesenchymal bodies: a histologic finding useful in differentiating trichoepitheliomas from basal cell carcinomas. J Am Acad Dermatol 1989; 21:523–528.
Goldblum OM: Multiple nodules on the face. Diagnostic Challenges 1991; 1:21–24.
Wheeland RG, Bailin PL, Kronberg E: Carbon dioxide (CO2) laser vaporization for the treatment of multiple trichoepithelioma. J Dermatol Surg Oncol 1984; 10:470–475.

BRUNSTING–PERRY SYNDROME,
CICATRICIAL PEMPHIGOID OF THE BRUNSTING–PERRY TYPE, LOCALIZED CHRONIC PEMPHIGOID

Manifestations and Major Findings
chronic, localized bullous pemphigoid of the head and neck
atrophic scarring of the affected areas with severe burning and itching in affected areas
more common in middle-aged or older men
no mucosal involvement

References
Brunsting LA, Perry HO: Benign pemphigoid? Arch Dermatol 1957; 75:489-501.
Leenutaphong V, von Kries R, Plewig G: Localized cicatricial pemphigoid (Brunsting–Perry): electron microscopic study. J Am Acad Dermatol 1989; 21:1089–1093.
Monihan JM, Nguyen TH, Guill MA: Brunsting–Perry pemphigoid simulating basal cell carcinoma. J Am Acad Dermatol 1989; 21:331–334.

BRUSHFIELD–WYATT SYNDROME

Manifestations and Major Findings
unilateral nevus flammeus
cerebral vascular malformation
visual hemianopia
contralateral hemiplegia
mental retardation

BRUTON AGAMMAGLOBULINEMIA
see AGAMMAGLOBULINEMIA OF BRUTON

BUERGER DISEASE, THROMBOANGIITIS OBLITERANS

Manifestations and Major Findings
painful peripheral arterial and venous thrombosis without atherosclerosis or inflammation
most common in male smokers aged 20–45 years
Raynaud phenomenon of the hands
- superficial migratory thrombophlebitis (Fig. 23)

neuropathy in the affected limb
erythema nodosum
can lead to digital gangrene and amputations

References
Giblin WJ, James WD, Benson PM: Buerger's disease. Int J Dermatol 1989; 28:638–642.
Samlaska, CP, James WD: Superficial thrombophlebitis II. J Am Acad Dermatol 1990; 23:1–18.
Scully RE, ed.: Case records of the Massachusetts General Hospital. N Engl J Med 1989; 320:1068–1076.

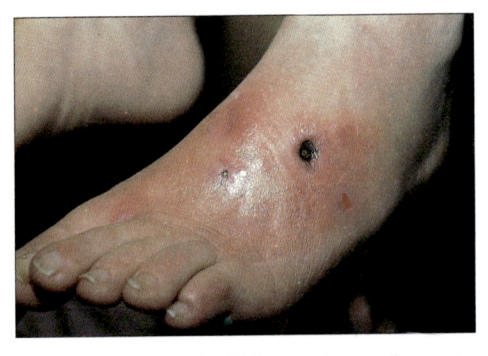

- *Figure 23 Thrombophlebitis with central necrosis of the foot in Buerger disease.*

BÜRGER–GRÜTZ SYNDROME
see HYPERLIPIDEMIAS, TYPE I

BURULI ULCER

Manifestations and Major Findings
ulcerating nodule caused by *Mycobacterium ulcerans*
leads to edema, necrotizing panniculitis, and crippling contractures
usually painless ulcer
named after a region of Uganda

> **References**
> Muelder K: Wounds that will not heal: the Buruli ulcer. Int J Dermatol 1992; 31:25–26.
> Muelder K, Nourou A: Buruli ulcer in Benin. Lancet 1990; 336:1109–1111.

BUSCHKE–FISCHER DISEASE,
KERATODERMA PALMOPLANTARIS PAPULOSA,
HEREDITARY PUNCTATE KERATODERMA

Manifestations and Major Findings
punctate keratoses with a central depression distributed irregularly over the palms and soles
onset between 10–45 years of age
nail abnormalities with longitudinal fissures and onychogryphosis

autosomal dominant

> **References**
> Rachid A, Freire-Maia N, Pinheiro M: Brief report: Autosomal dominant painful plantar callosities. Am J Med Genet 1987; 26:185–187.

BUSCHKE–LÖWENSTEIN TUMOR

Manifestations and Major Findings
low-grade, well differentiated squamous cell carcinoma (verrucous carcinoma) of the anogenital area
giant condyloma acuminatum – slow growing, painful
tends to ulcerate
associated most frequently with human papilloma virus types 6 and 11

> **References**
> Schwartz RA: Buschke–Löwenstein tumor: verrucous carcinoma of the penis. J Am Acad Dermatol 1990; 23:723–727.
> Schwartz RA, Nychay SG, Lyons M, Sciales CW, Lambert WC: Buschke–Löwenstein tumor: verrucous carcinoma of the anogenitalia. Cutis 1991; 47:263–266.
> Sherman RN, Fung HK, Flynn KJ: Verrucous carcinoma (Buschke–Löwenstein tumor). Int J Dermatol 1991; 30:730–733.
> Zemtsov A, Koss W, Dixon L, Tyring S, et al.: Anal verrucous carcinoma associated with human papilloma virus type 2: magnetic resonance imaging and flow cytometry evaluation. Arch Dermatol 1992; 128:564–565.

BUSCHKE–OLLENDORFF SYNDROME, DERMATOFIBROSIS LENTICULARIS DISSEMINATA

Manifestations and Major Findings
multiple small asymptomatic cutaneous connective tissue nevi, mainly on the lower trunk and extremities
connective tissue nevi are composed of abnormal elastic fibers and abnormally distributed collagen
osteopoikilosis (asymptomatic opacified sclerotic circumscribed lesions in long bones)
onset of lesions usually before puberty (may be present at birth)

autosomal dominant with variable expression

> **References**
> Sears JK, Stone MS, Argenyi Z: Papular elastorrhexis: a variant of connective tissue nevus. J Am Acad Dermatol 1988; 19:409–414.
> Trattner A, David M, Rothem A, et al.: Buschke–Ollendorff syndrome of the scalp: histologic and ultrastructural findings. J Am Acad Dermatol 1991; 24:822–824.
> Uitto J, Santa Cruz DJ, Starcher BC, Whyte MP, et al.: Biochemical and ultrastructural demonstration of elastin accumulation in the skin lesions of the Buschke–Ollendorff syndrome. J Invest Dermatol 1981; 76:284–287.
> Uitto J, Shamban A: Heritable skin diseases with molecular defects in collagen or elastin. Dermatol Clin 1987; 5:63–84.

C

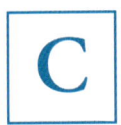

CANCER FAMILY SYNDROME

Manifestations and Major Findings
three or more first degree relatives with malignant neoplasms
early onset of colorectal cancer in the absence of polyposis coli
associated with multiple other primary cancers

References
Buckley C, Thomas V, Crow J, Houlston R, et al.: Cancer family syndrome associated with multiple malignant melanomas and a malignant fibrous histiocytoma. Br J Dermatol 1992; 126:83–85.
Lynch HT, Fusaro RM, Roberts L, Voorhees GJ, Lynch JF: Muir–Torre syndrome in several members of a family with a variant of the Cancer Family Syndrome. Br J Dermatol 1985; 113:295–301.

CANNON DISEASE, FAMILIAL WHITE FOLDED DYSPLASIA OF THE MUCOUS MEMBRANE, WHITE SPONGE NEVUS

Manifestations and Major Findings
white spongy appearing lesions of mucous membranes (oral, vaginal, anal)
buccal mucosa always involved

autosomal dominant

References
Jorgenson RJ, Levin LS: White sponge nevus. Arch Dermatol 1981; 117:73–76.

CANTU SYNDROME

Manifestations and Major Findings
small (1–2 mm) brownish macules that become confluent to form irregular patches on the face, dorsal surfaces of forearms, and feet
hyperkeratotic palms and soles
begins in early adolescence
progressive until adulthood, then stable

autosomal dominant

References
Cantu JM, Sanchez-Corona J, Fragoso R, et al.: A "new" autosomal dominant genodermatosis characterized by hyperpigmented spots and palmoplantar hyperkeratosis. Clin Genet 1978; 14:165–168.
Fulk CS: Primary disorders of hyperpigmentation. J Am Acad Dermatol 1984;10:1–16.

CARCINOID SYNDROME

Manifestations and Major Findings
carcinoid tumors arising from APUD (*A*mine *P*recursor *U*ptake and *D*ecarboxylation) cells which secrete serotonin, kallikrein, histamine
asthma
heart disease (fibrosis of endocardium)
diarrhea
abdominal pain
syncope
shock
5-HIAA (5-hydroxyindole acetic acid) in urine
tumors most common in appendix, small intestine, rectum, and bronchus

Clinical features evident only if tumor involves the liver, bronchus, or ovary.

Cutaneous Manifestations
flushing (face and upper trunk) in paroxysms
periorbital edema
pellagra-like rash (from acquired tryptophan deficiency)
scleroderma-like changes on the lower extremities
hyperpigmentation
facial cyanosis (after years)
telangiectasias

> **References**
> **Altman AR, Tschen JA, Rice L:** Treatment of malignant carcinoid syndrome with a long-acting somatostatin analogue. Arch Dermatol 1989; 125:394–396.
> **Castiello RJ, Lynch PJ:** Pellagra and the carcinoid syndrome. Arch Dermatol 1972; 105:574–577.
> **Gregory B, Ho VC:** Cutaneous manifestations of gastrointestinal disorders. J Am Acad Dermatol 1992; 26:153–166.
> **Maton PN:** The carcinoid syndrome. J Am Med Assoc 1988; 260:1602-1605.

CARDIOCUTANEOUS SYNDROME
see LEOPARD SYNDROME

CARDIOFACIOCUTANEOUS SYNDROME, CFC SYNDROME

Manifestations and Major Findings
Noonan syndrome-like features, but genetically distinct
ptosis
short stature
cardiac abnormalities
pulmonary defects
mental retardation

Characteristic Facies
round face
macrocephaly
hypertelorism/prominent eyes
dysplastic teeth
broad nose
posteriorly rotated ears

Cutaneous Manifestations
sparse, curly, short hair
decreased or absent eyelashes and eyebrows
dysplastic nails/koilonychia
hyperkeratotic patches on helix of ears, knees, and scattered over the body
keratosis pilaris
palmoplantar keratoderma
hyperplasia and dystrophy of sweat ducts
café au lait macules
pigmented nevi
syringocystadenoma papilliferum
acanthosis nigricans
hemangiomas
ichthyosis
skin redundancy on hands or feet/lymphedema
seborrheic dermatitis
eczema

autosomal dominant

> **References**
> **Borradori L, Blanchet-Bardon C:** Skin manifestations of cardio-facio-cutaneous syndrome. J Am Acad Dermatol 1993; 28:815–819.
> **Mathews CA, George P, Hood AF:** Cardiofaciocutaneous syndrome. Arch Dermatol 1993; 129:46–47.
> **Piérard GE, Soyeur-Broux M, Estrada JA, Piérard-Franchimont C, et al.:** Cutaneous presentation of the cardio-facio-cutaneous syndrome. J Am Acad Dermatol 1990; 22:920–922.

CARNEY SYNDROME,
NAME SYNDROME, CARNEY COMPLEX, LAMB SYNDROME *see also* NAME SYNDROME

Manifestations and Major Findings
cardiocutaneous syndrome characterized by pigmented skin lesions and atrial myxomas
lentigines (mucocutaneous)
atrial myxomas (may be fatal)
mucocutaneous myxomas
blue nevi
congenital melanocytic nevi
schwannomas

ENDOCRINE ABNORMALITIES
endocrine overactivity
Cushing syndrome
sexual precocity in boys
acromegaly
thyroid hyperplasia or adenomas
pigmented nodular adrenocortical disease
testicular tumors
uterine myxomas and other hamartomas

autosomal dominant or sporadic inheritance

> **References**
> Atherton DJ, Pitcher DW, Wells RS, Macdonald DM: A syndrome of various cutaneous pigmented lesions, myxoid neurofibromata and atrial myxoma: the "NAME" syndrome. Br J Dermatol 1980; 103:421–429.
> Carney JA, Gordon H, Carpenter PC, Shenoy BV, Go VLW: The complex of myxomas, spotty pigmentation, and endocrine overactivity. Medicine 1985; 64:270–283.
> Carney JA, Headington JT, Su WPD: Cutaneous myxomas. Arch Dermatol 1986; 122:790–798.
> Carney JA, Hruska LS, Beauchamp GD, Gordon H: Dominant inheritance of the complex of myxomas, spotty pigmentation, and endocrine overactivity. Mayo Clin Proc 1986; 61:165–172.
> Handley J, Carson D, Sloan J, Walsh M, et al.: Multiple lentigines, myxoid tumours and endocrine overactivity; four cases of Carney's complex. Br J Dermatol 1992; 126:367–371.
> Rhodes AR, Silverman RA, Harrist TJ, Perez-Atayde AR: Mucocutaneous lentigines, cardiomucocutaneous myxomas, and multiple blue nevi: The "LAMB" syndrome. J Am Acad Dermatol 1984; 10:72–82.
> Uhle P, Norvell SS: Generalized lentiginosis. J Am Acad Dermatol 1988; 18:444–447.
> Young WF, Carney JA, Musa BU, Wulffraat NM, Lens JW, Drexhage HA: Familial Cushing's Syndrome due to primary pigmented nodular adrenocortical disease. N Engl J Med 1989; 321:1659-1664.

CARPAL TUNNEL SYNDROME

Manifestations and Major Findings
Pain and paresthesia of the hand in the distribution of the median nerve, caused by compression of the median nerve by flexor retinaculum fibers
reddish discoloration of the fingers, bullae, and necrosis
nail dystrophy

> **References**
> Tosti A, Morelli R, D'Alessandro R, et al.: Carpal tunnel syndrome presenting with ischemic skin lesions, acroosteolysis, and nail changes. J Am Acad Dermatol 1993; 29:287–290.

CARRION DISEASE,
BARTONELLOSIS

Manifestations and Major Findings
infection caused by *Bartonella bacilliformis*
transmitted by *Phlebotomus* (bloodsucking sandfly)
endemic in Peru
epidemics in neighboring Latin American countries
This disease may present as two forms: Oroya fever – sudden onset of fever, anemia, hepatosplenomegaly, petechiae; or verruga peruana – papules, nodules, hemangiomatous lesions.

> **References**
> LeBoit PE, Berter TG, Egbert BM, et al.: Epithelioid hemangioma-like vascular proliferation in AIDS. Manifestation of cat-scratch disease bacillus or infection? Lancet 1988; 1:960-963.

CARTILAGE–HAIR HYPOPLASIA,
McKUSICK SYNDROME, METAPHYSEAL CHONDRODYSPLASIA (McKUSICK TYPE)

Manifestations and Major Findings
fine sparse hair, often fragile
metaphyseal chondrodysplasia (short limbs)
mild bowing of legs
wide irregular metaphyses
defective cell-mediated immunity
neutropenia
hyperextensible digits
small nails
abnormal elastic tissue
more common in Amish and Finnish

autosomal recessive

> **References**
> Brennan TE, Pearson RW: Abnormal elastic tissue in cartilage–hair hypoplasia. Arch Dermatol 1988; 124:1411–1414   ▷ ▷ ▷

> > >
Lux SE, Johnston RB, August CS, Say B, et al.: Chronic neutropenia and abnormal cellular immunity in cartilage–hair hypoplasia. N Engl J Med 1970; 282:231–236.
McKusick VA, Eldridge R, Hostetler JA, Ruangwit U, et al.: Dwarfism in the Amish. Bull Johns Hopkins Hosp 1964; 116:285–326.
Polmar SH, Pierce GF: Cartilage Hair Hypoplasia: immunological aspects and their clinical implications. Clin Immunol Immunopathol 1986; 40:87–93.

CASTLEMAN DISEASE, CASTLEMAN TUMOR

Manifestations and Major Findings
multicentric giant lymph node hyperplasia
usually involves mediastinal lymph nodes
may progress to malignant lymphoma
associated with erosive lichen planus, and pemphigus vulgaris

> **References**
> **Ashinoff R, Cohen R, Lipkin G:** Castleman's tumor and erosive lichen planus: coincidence or association? J Am Acad Dermatol 1989; 21:1076–1080.
> **Hanson CA, Frizzera G, Pattan DF, Peterson BA, et al.:** Clonal rearrangement for immunoglobulin and T-cell receptor genes in systemic Castleman's disease. Am J Pathol 1988; 131:84–91.
> **Sterling GB:** Kaposi's sarcoma and Castleman's disease. J Am Acad Dermatol 1990; 22:144.

CAT-CRY SYNDROME
see CRI-DU-CHAT SYNDROME

CAT-SCRATCH DISEASE

Manifestations and Major Findings
caused by *Rochalimaea henselae* or *Afipia felis*
history of animal (usually cat) contact with presence of scratch or inoculation of skin, eye, or mucous membrane
red, tender papule at site of cat-scratch (incubation 3–30 days) which becomes vesicular, then crusted
regional lymphadenopathy
systemic manifestations – fever, malaise, headache, anorexia
rare enanthems, morbilliform eruptions, petechial exanthem, or granulomatous lesions
encephalopathy (rare)
course usually benign

> **References**
> **Burnett JW:** Cat scratch disease. Cutis 1991; 48:443–444.
> **Calzavara-Pinton PG, Facchetti F, Carlino A, DePanfilis G:** Multiple scattered granulomatous skin lesions in Cat Scratch Disease. Cutis 1992; 49:318–320.
> **English CK, Wear DJ, Margileth AM, Lissner CR, et al.:** Cat-scratch disease. Isolation and culture of the bacterial agent. J Am Med Assoc 1988; 259:1347–1352.
> **Margileth AM:** Dermatologic manifestations and update of cat scratch disease. Pediatr Dermatol 1988; 5:1–9.

CAUDA EQUINA SYNDROME

Manifestations and Major Findings
compression of nerves or vasculature of the cauda equina
presents as leg weakness and incontinence

> **References**
> **Rozich J, Holley HP, Henderson F, Gardner J, et al.:** Cauda equina syndrome secondary to disseminated zygomycosis. J Am Med Assoc 1988; 260:3638–3640.

CERAMIDASE DEFICIENCY
see FARBER SYNDROME

CEREBRAL GIGANTISM SYNDROME see SOTOS SYNDROME

CEREBROHEPATORENAL SYNDROME see ZELLWEGER SYNDROME

CHAGAS DISEASE, AMERICAN TRYPANOSOMIASIS

Manifestations and Major Findings
Trypanosoma cruzi infection (parasitic)

transmitted by triatomid (reduviid bug) – assassin or kissing bugs

ACUTE DISEASE
fever, headache, myalgias
facial or unilateral eyelid edema (Romaña sign)
meningoencephalitis
myocarditis
exanthem

SUBACUTE AND CHRONIC DISEASE
myocarditis
megacolon
megaesophagus

> **References**
> Hagar JM, Rahimtoola SH: Chagas' heart disease in the United States. N Engl J Med 1991; 325:763–768.
> Kirchhoff LV, Neva FA: Chagas' disease in Latin American immigrants. J Am Med Assoc 1985; 254:3058-3060.
> Libow LF, Beltrani VP, Silvers DN, Grossman ME: Post-cardiac transplant reactivation of Chagas' disease diagnosed by skin biopsy. Cutis 1991; 48:37–40.

CHANARIN–DORFMAN SYNDROME
see DORFMAN–CHANARIN SYNDROME

CHAND SYNDROME, CHANDS

Manifestations and Major Findings
*c*urly *h*air
*a*nkyloblepharon
*n*ail *d*ysplasia (hypoplastic)

autosomal recessive

> **References**
> Baughman FA: CHANDS: The curly hair–ankyloblepharon–nail dysplasia syndrome. Birth Defects 1971; VII (8):100–102.
> Toriello HV, Lindstrom JA, Waterman DF, Baughman FA: Re-evaluation of CHANDS. J Med Genet 1979; 16:316–317.

CHARGE SYNDROME

Manifestations and Major Findings
*c*oloboma
*h*eart disease
*a*tresia choanae
*r*etarded growth
*g*enital hypoplasia
*e*ar anomalies/deafness

OTHER FINDINGS
micrognathia
cleft palate
facial palsy
swallowing difficulty
tracheoesophageal fistula

> **References**
> Pagon RA, Graham JM, Zonana J, Yong SL: Coloboma, congenital heart disease, and choanal atresia with multiple anomalies: CHARGE association. J Pediatr 1981; 99:223–227.

CHÉDIAK–HIGASHI SYNDROME
see also ALBINISM

Manifestations and Major Findings
oculocutaneous albinism
• silver hair (Fig. 24)
giant lysosomal granules in leukocytes, melanocytes, platelets, and other cells
photophobia, pale ocular fundi, and decreased lacrimation
recurrent pyogenic sinopulmonary and cutaneous infections, particularly staphylococcal and streptococcal infections

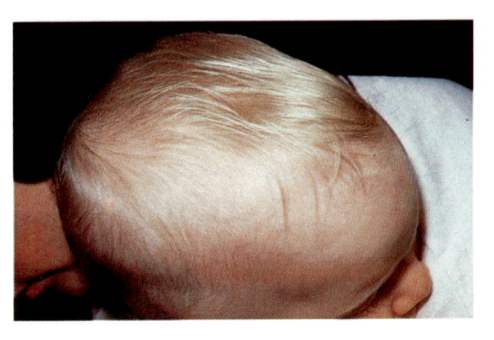

• *Figure 24 Silver hair; a characteristic finding in Chédiak–Higashi syndrome.*

bleeding tendency
neutropenia
neutrophil dysfunction
neurologic symptoms
–clumsiness
–nystagmus
–abnormal gait
–seizures
–paresthesias
early fatality (secondary to hemorrhage or infection)

OTHER FINDINGS
hepatosplenomegaly
lymphadenopathy
gingivitis
oral ulcerations
ultraviolet-induced cell killing abnormality

autosomal recessive

References
Anderson LL, Paller AS, Malpass D, Schmidt ML, et al.: Chediak–Higashi syndrome in a black child. Pediatr Dermatol 1991; 9:31–36.
Bolognia JL, Pawelek JM: Biology of hypopigmentation. J Am Acad Dermatol 1988; 19:217–255.

CHEILITIS GRANULOMATOSA
see MIESCHER GRANULOMATOSIS

CHILD SYNDROME CONGENITAL HEMIDYSPLASIA WITH ICHTHYOSIFORM NEVUS AND LIMB DEFECTS see also DISORDERS OF CORNIFICATION (DOC 16)

Manifestations and Major Findings
congenital hemidysplasia
ichthyosiform (psoriasiform) nevus
limb defects ranging from digital hypoplasia to agenesis of the extremity
sharp midline demarcation of unilateral ichthyosis
patchy cutaneous involvement on contralateral side
face spared
unilateral alopecia
stippled epiphyses
other organ involvement (central nervous system, musculoskeletal, viscera, cardiac)

X-linked dominant disorder, lethal in males

References
Emami S, Rizzo WB, Hanley KP, Taylor JM, et al.: Peroxisomal abnormality in fibroblasts from involved skin of CHILD Syndrome. Arch Dermatol 1992; 128:1213–1222.
Happle R: How many epidermal nevus syndromes exist? J Am Acad Dermatol 1991; 25:550–556.
Happle R: Ptychotropism as a cutaneous feature of the CHILD syndrome. J Am Acad Dermatol 1990; 23:763–766.
Hebert AA, Esterly NB, Holbrook KA, Hall JC: The CHILD syndrome: histologic and ultrastructural studies. Arch Dermatol 1987; 123:503–509.

'CHINESE RESTAURANT' SYNDROME

Manifestations and Major Findings
development of chest pain
flushing
burning sensation over the face
chest pressure
headaches
occurs 10–20 minutes after eating monosodium L-glutamate (dose may vary between individuals)

References
Altman DF (1992). Food poisoning. In Wyngaarden JB, Smith LH and Bennett JC (eds.) Cecil Textbook of Medicine, 19th edition, p.730–733. (Philadelphia: WB Saunders).

CHLORPROMAZINE SYNDROME

Manifestations and Major Findings
pigmentation induced by ingestion of chlorpromazine
slate-gray pigmentation on sun-exposed areas, may become purplish
cataracts
corneal opacities

pigmentation of conjunctivae
melanosome complexes within lysosomes of dermal macrophages and chlorpromazine in macrophages, endothelial cells, and Schwann cells

CHONDRODYSPLASIA PUNCTATA SYNDROMES

Types of Chondrodysplasia Punctata and Features

1 Conradi–Hünermann syndrome
moderate form (Happle type)
ichthyosis with thick, yellow scales (in whorls) which clear in 3–6 months
asymmetric skeletal defects
asymmetric calcific epiphyseal stippling in newborn
flat facies with depressed nasal bridge
joint contractures
kyphoscoliosis
follicular atrophoderma
scarring alopecia (patchy)
dry, lusterless hair
cataracts
normal mentation
X-linked dominant

mild form
calcific stippling of epiphyses – mild and symmetrical, resolves with time
typical facies
shortened columella
depressed nasal bridge
flattened nasal tip
no skin changes
no cataracts
variable mental retardation
short stature
autosomal dominant

2 rhizomelic chondrodysplasia punctata
coronal clefts in lateral X-rays of vertebral bodies
severe symmetrical shortening of proximal extremities and contractures
microcephaly
cataracts (bilateral)
ichthyosiform lesions on skin (mild)
alopecia
spasticity/contractures of multiple joints
characteristic facies
flat nasal root/bridge
upward-slanting palpebral fissures
lymphedema of the face in newborn period
severe psychomotor retardation
congenital heart disease
early fatality
deficiency of peroxisomal enzyme acyl-CoA dihydroxyacetone-phosphate acyltransferase
autosomal recessive

References
Borochowitz Z: Generalized chondrodysplasia punctata with shortness of humeri and brachymetacarpy: humero-metacarpal (HM) type: variation or heterogeneity? Am J Med Genet 1991; 41:417–422.
Kalter DC, Atherton DJ, Clayton PT: X-linked dominant Conradi–Hünermann Syndrome presenting as congenital erythroderma. J Am Acad Dermatol 1989; 21:248–256.
O'Brien TJ: Chondrodysplasia punctata (Conradi Disease). Int J Dermatol 1990; 29:472–476.
Silengo MC, Luzzatti L, Silverman FN: Clinical and genetic aspects of Conradi–Hünermann disease. J Pediatr 1980; 97:911–917.

CHONDROECTODERMAL DYSPLASIA SYNDROME
see ELLIS–VAN CREVELD SYNDROME

CHRIST–SIEMENS–TOURAINE SYNDROME
see ECTODERMAL DYSPLASIA; HYPOHIDROTIC

CHRONIC FATIGUE SYNDROME

Manifestations and Major Findings
chronic or recurrent and disabling illness
abnormal antibody reactivity to Epstein–Barr virus
erythema multiforme

References
Drago F, Romagnoli M, Loi A, Rebora A: Epstein–Barr virus-related persistent erythema multiforme in chronic fatigue syndrome. Arch Dermatol 1992; 128:217–222.

CHRONIC GRANULOMATOUS DISEASE

Manifestations and Major Findings
leukocytes ingest bacteria but do not kill them (defect in production of superoxide anion)
severe recurrent granulomatous reactions to catalase-positive organisms requiring H_2O_2 production (i.e. *Staphylococcus aureus* and other bacteria)
nitroblue tetrazolium (dye-reduction) test negative
neonatal pustulosis
periorificial eczema
skin abscesses and nodules (ulcerated)
oral ulcers with stomatitis
draining lymphadenopathy
hepatosplenomegaly
recurrent pneumonia with lung abscesses
diarrhea with malabsorption and fistulae
osteomyelitis, particularly with *Aspergillus*
peripheral leukocytosis
elevated immunoglobulins
short stature
female carriers may have lupus-like skin lesions
phagocyte cytochrome b missing or abnormal in X-linked disease

X-linked recessive or autosomal recessive

References
Ezekowitz RAB, Dinauer MC, Jaffe HS, Orkin SH, et al.: Partial correction of the phagocyte defect in patients with X-linked chronic granulomatous disease by subcutaneous interferon gamma. N Engl J Med 1988; 319:146–151.
Garioch JJ, Sampson JR, Seywright M, Thomson J: Dermatoses in five related female carriers of X-linked chronic granulomatous disease. Br J Dermatol 1989; 121:391–396.
Mizuno Y, Hara T, Nakamura M, Ueda K, et al.: Classification of chronic granulomatous disease on the basis of monoclonal antibody-defined cytochrome b deficiency. J Pediatr 1988; 113:458–462.
Schapiro BL, Newburger PE, Klempner MS, Dinauer MC: Chronic granulomatous disease presenting in a 69-year-old man. N Engl J Med 1991; 325:1786–1790. ▷ ▷ ▷
The International Chronic Granulomatous Disease Cooperative Study Group: A controlled trial of interferon gamma to prevent infection in chronic granulomatous disease. N Engl J Med 1991; 324:509–516.
Yeaman GR, Froebel K, Galea G, Ormerod A, et al.: Discoid lupus erythematosus in an X-linked cytochrome-positive carrier of chronic granulomatous disease. Br J Dermatol 1992; 126:60–65.

CHURG–STRAUSS SYNDROME,
ALLERGIC GRANULOMATOSIS, ALLERGIC ANGIITIS, CHURG–STRAUSS GRANULOMA

Manifestations and Major Findings
triad of findings
– history of severe asthma or allergic rhinitis
– pulmonary infiltrates
– peripheral blood eosinophilia (may exceed 80%)

OTHER FINDINGS
- erythematous, papulonodular, vasculitic skin lesions on extensor surfaces of extremities (Fig. 25) and scalp resembling urticaria, purpura, ulcerations, erythema multiforme
livedo reticularis
disseminated necrotizing vasculitis (small arteries, veins, capillaries) with granulomatous infiltrates
gastrointestinal symptoms – bloody diarrhea
myocardial granulomas (may be fatal)
neuropathy (mononeuritis multiplex)
seizures
arthralgias
anticytoplasmic antibodies (p-ANCA) usually present
onset usually 20–40 years of age
sudden death may occur

References
Crotty CP, DeRemee RA, Winkelmann RK: Cutaneous clinicopathologic correlation of allergic granulomatosis. J Am Acad Dermatol 1981; 5:571–581.
Finan MC, Winkelmann RK: The cutaneous extravascular necrotizing granuloma (Churg–Strauss granuloma) and systemic disease: a review of 27 cases. Medicine 1983; 62:142–158. ▷ ▷ ▷

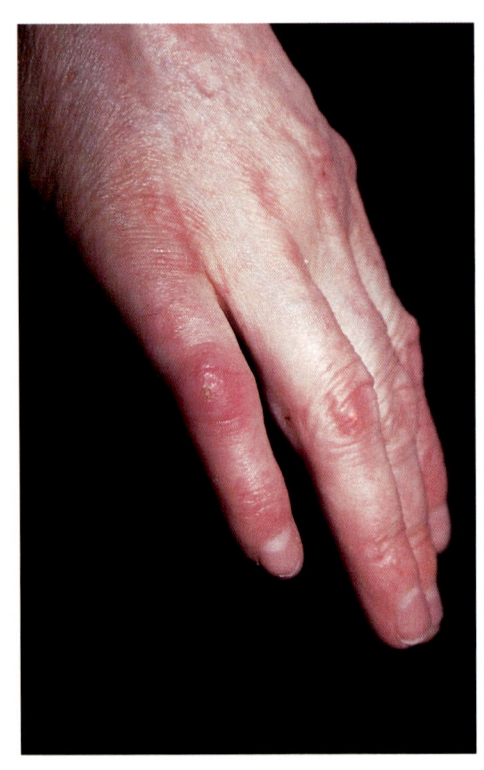

• *Figure 25* Erythematous, papulonodular, vasculitic skin lesions of the extensor surface of the hand in Churg–Strauss syndrome.

▷ ▷ ▷
Lanham JG, Elkon KB, Pusey CD, Hughes GR: Systemic vasculitis with asthma and eosinophilia: a clinical approach to the Churg–Strauss syndrome. Medicine 1984; 63:65–81.
Schwartz RA, Churg J: Churg–Strauss syndrome (a review). Br J Dermatol 1992; 127:199–204.
Yevich I: Necrotizing vasculitis with granulomatosis. Int J Dermatol 1988; 27:540–546.

CICATRICIAL PEMPHIGOID
see BRUNSTING–PERRY SYNDROME

CLEIDOCRANIAL DYSOSTOSIS

Manifestations and Major Findings
aplasia of the clavicles (partial or complete)
small thorax with oblique ribs
late ossification of cranial sutures
delayed eruption of teeth with dental anomalies
supernumerary teeth
prognathism
short stature (mild)
brachycephaly with bossing
deafness (conductive)
hand anomalies with asymmetric finger length
skeletal abnormalities with delayed ossification of bones, scoliosis, and cercival ribs

autosomal dominant with wide variability

CLOUSTON SYNDROME
see ECTODERMAL DYSPLASIA; HIDROTIC

COATS DISEASE

Manifestations and Major Findings
telangiectasias of face, conjunctivae, nail beds, and breasts
retinal telangiectasias with massive exudation and retinal detachment

References
Allen HB, Parlette HL: Coats Disease. A condition that may mimic the Sturge–Weber Syndrome. Arch Dermatol 1973; 108:413–415.

COBB SYNDROME,
CUTANEOMENINGOSPINAL ANGIOMATOSIS

Manifestations and Major Findings
vascular malformations of the spinal cord
port-wine stain (capillary malformation) or angiokeratoma of corresponding dermatome
neurologic signs of cord compression or anoxia

OTHER FINDINGS
angioma of the vertebrae
renal angiomas
kyphoscoliosis

sporadic inheritence

References
Jessen RT, Thompson S, Smith EB: Cobb syndrome. Arch Dermatol 1977; 113:1587–1590.

COCARDE NEVUS

Manifestations and Major Findings
acquired nevocellular nevus with target-like (rosette) appearance
central nevus, nonpigmented zone, peripheral pigmented halo

> **References**
> Guzzo C, Johnson B, Honig P: Cocarde nevus: a case report and review of the literature. Pediatr Dermatol 1988; 5:250–253.

COCKAYNE SYNDROME

Manifestations and Major Findings
premature aging
microcephaly
photosensitivity – scaly erythema, begins at 1 year of age
short stature
mental retardation (progressive)
disproportionately large hands, feet, and ears
atrophy of the subcutaneous fat of the face with sunken eyes
extensive demyelination of peripheral nerves and central nervous system

OTHER FINDINGS
bullae
ocular defects
 –cataracts
 –retinal degeneration
 –optic atrophy
progressive deafness
early canities
flexion contractures
short life expectancy
kyphosis
fibroblasts sensitive to ultraviolet irradiation and certain chemicals
increased sister chromatid exchanges
not prone to cancer

autosomal recessive

> **References**
> Beauregard S, Gilchrest BA: Syndromes of premature aging. Dermatol Clin 1987; 5:109–121.
> Schmickel RD, Chu EHY, Trosko JE, Chang CC: Cockayne syndrome: a cellular sensitivity to ultraviolet light. Pediatrics 1977; 60:135–139.
> Sugarman GI, Landing BH, Reed WB: Cockayne syndrome: clinical study of two patients and neuropathologic findings in one. Clin Pediatr 1977; 16:225–232.

COCKAYNE–TOURAINE SYNDROME see EPIDERMOLYSIS BULLOSA; DYSTROPHIC

COFFIN–SIRIS SYNDROME, FIFTH DIGIT SYNDROME

Manifestations and Major Findings
hypoplastic or absent nails on the fifth fingers and toes (constant finding)
small or hypoplastic nails (affecting all nails)
distal phalanx of the fifth finger and toe either absent or hypoplastic
sparse scalp hair
microdontia
developmental delay
CNS malformations
delayed bone growth
hypoplasia of the patella
hypertrichosis of the body
lax joints
hypotonia
cleft palate
recurrent respiratory infections
congenital heart disease
gastrointestinal ulcers with perforation

Characteristic Facies
widening of nose and/or mouth
microcephaly
prominent lips
low nasal bridge
bushy eyebrows and eyelashes

> **References**
> Kucirka SJ, Scher RK: Heritable nail disorders. Dermatol Clin 1987; 5:179–191.

CONFLUENT AND RETICULATED PAPILLOMATOSIS

see GOUGEROT–CARTEAUD SYNDROME

CONGENITAL ADRENAL HYPERPLASIA, ADRENAL VIRILISM SYNDROME

Congenital adrenal hyperplasia causes increased androgen production due to 21-hydroxylase, 11-β-hydroxylase, or 3-β-hydroxysteroid dehydrogenase deficiency.

Manifestations and Major Findings
ambiguous genitalia in females
hyperpigmentation of the genitalia
virilization
failure to thrive
vomiting
salt-losing crises
shock
in late onset (in females)
–acne
–hirsutism
–menstrual disorders
–most common defect associated with late onset is 21-hydroxylase deficiency

autosomal recessive

> **References**
> **Feingold KR, Elias PM:** Endocrine-skin interactions. J Am Acad Dermatol 1988; 19:1–20.
> **Pang S, Pollack MS, Marshall RN, Immken L:** Prenatal treatment of congenital adrenal hyperplasia due to 21-hydroxylase deficiency. N Engl J Med 1990; 322:111–115.
> **Pang S, Wallace MA, Hofman L, Thuline HC, Dorche C, et al.:** Worldwide experience in newborn screening for classical congenital adrenal hyperplasia due to 21-hydroxylase deficiency. Pediatrics 1988; 81:866–874.
> **Savage MO:** Congenital adrenal hyperplasia. Clin Endocrinol 1985; 14:893–909.
> **Sperling LC, Heimer WL:** Androgen biology as a basis for the diagnosis and treatment of androgenic disorders in women. I. J Am Acad Dermatol 1993; 28:669–683.

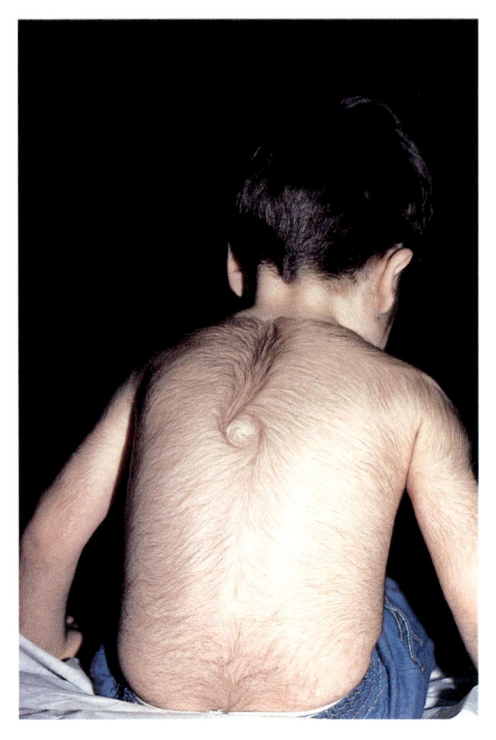

• *Figure 26 Congenital hypertrichosis lanuginosa; extreme hypertrichosis of the body.*

CONGENITAL HYPERTRICHOSIS LANUGINOSA, WOLFMAN SYNDROME

Manifestations and Major Findings
• extreme hypertrichosis (hairiness) (Fig. 26) beginning in childhood or birth
hair over entire body lengthens with age, except palms and soles
dental abnormalities – hypodontia and anodontia
external ear abnormalities

autosomal dominant

> **References**
> **Barth JH, Wilkinson JD, Dawber RPR:** Prepubertal hypertrichosis. Arch Dis Child 1987; 63:666–667.
> **Beighton P:** Congenital hypertrichosis lanuginosa. Arch Dermatol 1970; 101:669–672.
> **Partridge JW:** Congenital hypertrichosis lanuginosa: neonatal shaving. Arch Dis Child 1987; 62:623–625.

CONRADI–HÜNERMANN SYNDROME see CHONDRODYSPLASIA PUNCTATA SYNDROMES *and* DISORDERS OF CORNIFICATION

CORNELIA DE LANGE SYNDROME

see DE LANGE SYNDROME

COUMARIN NECROSIS

Manifestations and Major Findings
- necrosis, mainly affecting the skin and subcutaneous tissue in areas of abundant fat (breasts, buttocks, thighs) (Fig. 27)

usually appears 3–5 days after coumarin therapy starts

associated with heterozygous protein C deficiency (*see* protein C deficiency)

> **References**
> Bauer KA: Coumarin-induced skin necrosis. Arch Dermatol 1993; 129:766–768.
> Gladson CL, Groncy P, Griffin JH: Coumarin necrosis, neonatal purpura fulminans, and protein C deficiency. Arch Dermatol 1987; 123:1701a–1706a.
> Gold JA, Watters AK, O'Brien E: Coumarin versus heparin necrosis. J Am Acad Dermatol 1987; 16:148–149.
> Schramm W, Spannagl M, Bauer KA, Rosenberg RD, et al.: Treatment of coumarin-induced skin necrosis with a monoclonal antibody purified protein C concentrate. Arch Dermatol 1993; 129:753–756.

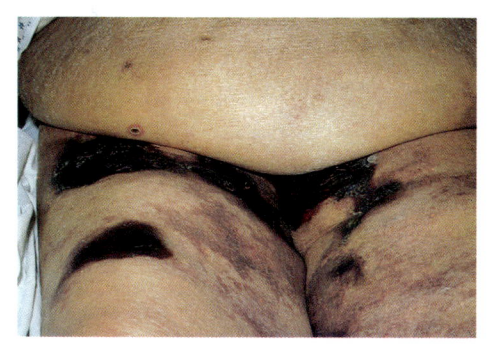

- *Figure 27 Coumarin necrosis of the skin and subcutaneous tissue of the thighs and abdomen.*

COWDEN DISEASE, MULTIPLE HAMARTOMA SYNDROME

Manifestations and Major Findings
multiple hamartomatous lesions of ectodermal, endodermal, and mesodermal origin
trichilemmomas (especially facial)
facial papules, often grouped around the mouth, nose, or ears
oral papillomatosis (cobblestoning)
keratoses – acral, palmoplantar

OTHER FINDINGS
strong association with malignancy of breast and thyroid
lipomas
angiomas
neuromas
epidermal cysts
craniomegaly
adenoid facies
high-arched palate
hamartomatous polyps in gastrointestinal tract
ovarian cysts
adenocarcinoma of the uterus
angioid streaks
thyroid adenoma or goiter
fibrocystic breast disease
kyphosis
bone cysts
pectus excavatum

autosomal dominant

> **References**
> Allen BS, Fitch MH, Smith JG: Multiple hamartoma syndrome. J Am Acad Dermatol 1980; 2:303–308.
> Barax CN, Lebwohl M, Phelps RG: Multiple hamartoma syndrome. J Am Acad Dermatol 1987; 17:342–346.
> Gregory B, Ho VC: Cutaneous manifestations of gastrointestinal disorders. J Am Acad Dermatol 1992; 26:153–166.
> Salem OS, Steck WD: Cowden's disease (multiple hamartoma and neoplasia syndrome). J Am Acad Dermatol 1983; 8:686–696.
> Starink TM: Cowden's disease: analysis of fourteen new cases. J Am Acad Dermatol 1984; 11:1127–1141.

CRANDALL SYNDROME
see also PILI TORTI SYNDROMES

Manifestations and Major Findings
pili torti (twisted hair shafts)
progressive sensorineural deafness
hypogonadism after puberty
deficiencies of lutenizing and growth hormones

X-linked recessive

> **References**
> Crandall BF, Samec L, Sparkes RS, Wright SW: A familial syndrome of deafness, alopecia and hypogonadism. J Pediatr 1973; 82:461–465.

CRANIOFACIAL DYSOSTOSIS
see CROUZON SYNDROME

CREST SYNDROME, CRST SYNDROME

Manifestations and Major Findings
*c*alcinosis cutis
*R*aynaud phenomenon
*e*sophageal involvement
• *s*clerodactyly (Fig. 28)
*t*elangiectasias (mat-like)
anticentromere antibody-positive
a milder form of scleroderma than progressive systemic sclerosis

> **References**
> Kurzhals G, Meurer M, Krieg T, Reimer G: Clinical association of autoantibodies to fibrillarin with diffuse scleroderma and disseminated telangiectasia. J Am Acad Dermatol 1990; 23:832–836.
> Uitto J, Jiminez S: Fibrotic skin diseases. Arch Dermatol 1990; 126:661–664.

CRI-DU-CHAT SYNDROME, CAT-CRY SYNDROME, 5P SYNDROME

Manifestations and Major Findings
characteristic high-pitched, cat-like, whining cry
microcephaly
cleft palate

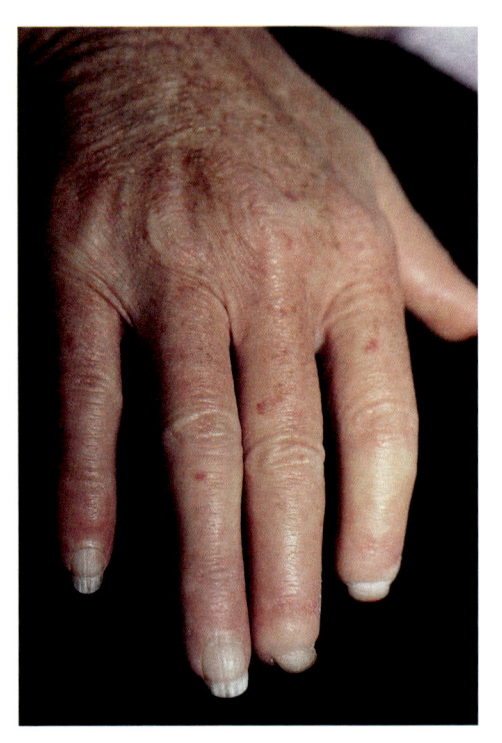

• *Figure 28 Sclerodactyly in CREST syndrome. Note the loss of fingertips and telangiectasias.*

severe mental retardation
growth retardation
congenital heart disease
simian crease
premature canities (graying of hair)

Characteristic Facies
down-slanting palpebral fissures
epicanthal folds
hypertelorism
malformed ears with preauricular skin tags
micrognathia
narrow forehead

partial deletion of short arm of chromosome 5

CROCODILE TEARS SYNDROME, BOGORAD SYNDROME, GUSTATORY LACRIMATION

Manifestations and Major Findings
paroxysmal lacrimation during eating as a sequel of facial palsy

caused by VII cranial nerve lesion (central to the geniculate ganglion) with misdirected regeneration of autonomic fibers
ectropion

CROHN DISEASE, REGIONAL ILEITIS

Manifestations and Major Findings
chronic granulomatous disorder of the small intestines
cobblestone nodularities of oral mucosa
oral ulcerations

Cutaneous Manifestations
perianal abscesses and fistulae as an extension of intestinal disease
erythema nodosum
erythema multiforme
• pyoderma gangrenosum (Fig. 29)
cutaneous vasculitis
erythema elevatum diutinum
epidermolysis bullosa acquisita
acne fulminans
zinc deficiency from malabsorption
numerous eroded cutaneous granulomas (metastatic Crohn disease)

References
Ahrenstedt O, Knutson L, Nilsson B, Nilsson-Ekdahl K, et al.: Enhanced local production of complement components in the small intestines of patients with Crohn's disease. N Engl J Med 1990; 322:1345–1349.

Borradori L, Saada V, Rybojad M, Flageul B, et al.: Oral intraepidermal IgA pustulosis and Crohn's disease. Br J Dermatol 1992; 126:383–386.
Gregory B, Ho VC: Cutaneous manifestations of gastrointestinal disorders. Part II. J Am Acad Dermatol 1992; 26:371–383.
Lifshitz AY, Stern F, Kaplan B, Sofer E, et al.: Pellagra complicating Crohn's disease. J Am Acad Dermatol 1992; 27:620.
Shum DT, Guenther L: Metastatic Crohn's disease. Arch Dermatol 1990; 126:645–648.
Walker KD, Badame AJ: Erythema elevatum diutinum in a patient with Crohn's disease. J Am Acad Dermatol 1990; 22:948–952.

CRONKHITE–CANADA SYNDROME

Manifestations and Major Findings
gastrointestinal polyposis (hamartomas)
generalized alopecia (thin and sparse hair), with total hair loss later
diffuse and spotty hyperpigmentation – especially on the hands, palms, and volar aspects of the fingers
sparing of mucous membranes
nail dystrophy with triangular nail plate and shedding
malabsorption
diarrhea
weight loss
abdominal pain
adult onset
neurological symptoms

References
Cronkhite LW, Canada WJ: Generalized gastrointestinal polyposis. An unusual syndrome of polyposis, pigmentation, alopecia and onychotrophia. N Engl J Med 1955; 252:1011–1015.
Daniel ES, Ludwig SL, Lewin KJ, et al.: The Cronkhite–Canada syndrome: an analysis of clinical and pathological features and therapy in 55 patients. Medicine 1982; 61:293–308.
Gregory B, Ho VC: Cutaneous manifestations of gastrointestinal disorders. Part I. J Am Acad Dermatol 1992; 26:153–166.
Herzberg AJ, Kaplan DL: Cronkhite–Canada syndrome. Int J Dermatol 1990; 29:121–125.
Rappaport LB, Sperling HV, Stravrides A: Colon cancer in the Cronkhite–Canada syndrome. J Clin Gastroenterol 1986; 8:199–202.

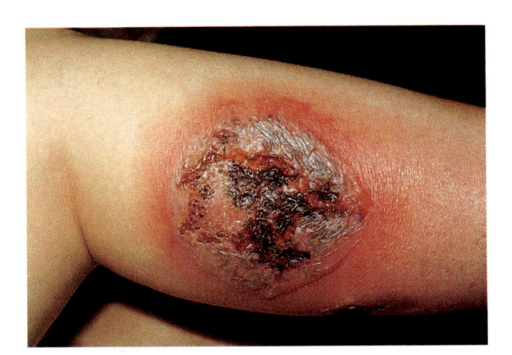

• *Figure 29* Pyoderma gangrenosum; a cutaneous manifestation of Crohn disease.

CROSS SYNDROME,
CROSS–McKUSICK–BREEN SYNDROME, OCULOCEREBRAL SYNDROME WITH HYPOPIGMENTATION *see also* ALBINISM

Manifestations and Major Findings
tyrosinase-positive albinism
white to pink skin color
hair with yellow, metallic sheen
spasticity
athetosis
severe mental retardation
high-pitched cry
gingival fibromatosis
high-arched palate

OCULAR ABNORMALITIES
blue-gray irides
microphthalmia
small opaque corneas
nystagmus
cataracts

autosomal recessive

> **References**
> Bolognia JL, Parwelek JM: Biology of hypopigmentation. J Am Acad Dermatol 1988; 19:217–255.

CROUZON SYNDROME,
CRANIOFACIAL DYSOSTOSIS

Manifestations and Major Findings
shallow orbits with exophthalmos
premature craniosynostosis
frontal bossing
maxillary hypoplasia

autosomal dominant

> **References**
> Orlow SJ: Cutaneous findings in craniofacial malformation syndromes. Arch Dermatol 1992; 128:1379–1386.

CROW–FUKASE SYNDROME
see POEMS SYNDROME

CRST SYNDROME
see CREST SYNDROME

CURTH–MAKLIN SYNDROME
see DISORDERS OF CORNIFICATION; DOC 8

CUSHING SYNDROME

Manifestations and Major Findings
glucocorticoid excess – endogenous or exogenous
truncal obesity
slender limbs
hirsutism
hyperpigmentation
telangiectasias
thin, fragile, atrophic skin
acneiform eruptions
striae
'moon facies' with plethora
'buffalo hump'
diabetes
hypertension
osteoporosis
compression fractures

> **References**
> Feingold KR, Elias PM: Endocrine–skin interactions. J Am Acad Dermatol 1988; 19:1–20.
> Findling JW: The Cushing syndromes, an enlarging clinical spectrum. N Engl J Med 1989; 321:1677–1678.

CUTIS HYPERELASTICA
see EHLERS–DANLOS SYNDROME

CUTIS LAXA

Manifestations and Major Findings
elastic fibers are sparse, short, fragmented, clumped with deficiency of elastin
skin recoils very slowly after stretching

Types of Cutis Laxa and Features

1 generalized cutaneous involvement
intrauterine growth retardation
skin hangs in loose folds from birth and becomes inelastic
generalized elastic tissue abnormality predisposing to:
– inguinal hernias
– lax joints
– bronchiectasis with pulmonary emphysema
– mitral valve prolapse
– aortic aneurysm
– gastrointestinal diverticula
– prolapse of the rectum or uterus
– bladder or urinary tract diverticula
scant body hair
dental caries
osteoporosis
genital abnormalities
autosomal dominant (milder) or autosomal recessive (severe)

2 X-linked cutis laxa, occipital horn syndrome
affects males
characteristic facies:
– hooked nose
– long philtrum
mild skin laxity
joint hypermobility
skeletal abnormalities:
– thoracic malformations
– carpal synostoses
bladder neck obstruction
chronic diarrhea
personality disorders
low serum copper levels
decreased lysyl oxidase activity
X-linked recessive

3 acquired cutis laxa
Type I Primary Generalized Elastolysis
onset at any age
may begin with an urticarial or papulovesicular eruption
progressive development of loose skin (initially on the face and neck)
systemic complications:
– inguinal and hiatal hernias
– emphysema
– aortic dilation
– diverticula of colon
Type I acquired cutis laxa may be associated with penicillamine, penicillin, complement deficiency, systemic lupus erythematosus, or amyloidosis.
Type II
acute inflammatory skin lesions followed by localized cutis laxa

References
Byers PH, Siegel RC, Holbrook KA, Narayanan AS, et al.: X-linked cutis laxa. N Engl J Med 1980; 303:61–65.
Fisher BK, Page E, Hanna W: Acral localized acquired cutis laxa. J Am Acad Dermatol 1989; 21:33–40.
Kitano Y, Nishida K, Okada N, Mimaki T, et al.: Cutis laxa with ultrastructural abnormalities of elastic fiber. J Am Acad Dermatol 1989; 21:378–380.
Pope FM 1993. Cutis Laxa. In McKusick's Heritable Disorders of Connective Tissue, 5th edition, p.253–279. (St Louis: Mosby-Year Book).

D

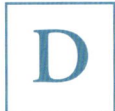

DANDY–WALKER COMPLEX

Manifestations and Major Findings
aplasia or hypoplasia of cerebellar vermis
cystic dilatation of the fourth ventricle with enlargement of the posterior fossa
hydrocephalus
associated with facial hemangiomas

References
Hirsch J-F, Pierre-Kahn A, Renier D, et al.: The Dandy–Walker malformation: a review of 40 cases. J Neurosurg 1984; 61:515–522.
Kadonaga JN, Barkovich AJ, Edwards MSB, Frieden IJ: Neurocutaneous melanosis in association with the Dandy–Walker complex. Pediatr Dermatol 1991; 9:37–43.
Reese V, Frieden IJ, Paller AS, Esterly NB, et al.: Association of facial hemangiomas with Dandy–Walker and other posterior fossa malformations. J Pediatr 1993; 122:379–384.

DARIER DISEASE, KERATOSIS FOLLICULARIS, DARIER–WHITE DISEASE

Manifestations and Major Findings
- firm, greasy, yellow-brown, crusted, malodorous papules (Fig. 30) in seborrheic and flexural areas

white cobblestoning of mucous membranes
- nail changes (Fig. 31)

  –white or red longitudinal bands
  –V-shaped nicks at distal margin
  –subungual hyperkeratoses

keratoses or minute pits on palms and soles
immunologic impairment of T cells in some patients
mental disturbances
aggravated by sunlight or heat

autosomal dominant

References
Burge SM, Wilkinson JD: Darier–White disease: a review of the clinical features in 163 patients. J Am Acad Dermatol 1992; 27:40–50.
Munro CS: The phenotype of Darier's disease: penetrance and expressivity in adults and children. Br J Dermatol 1992; 127:126–130.
Oxholm A, Oxholm P, Bang Fd, Horrobin DF: Abnormal essential fatty acid metabolism in Darier's disease. Arch Dermatol 1990; 126:1308–1311.

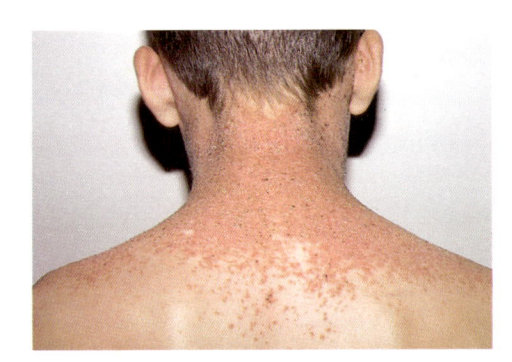

- *Figure 30 Darier disease; characteristic greasy papules on a patient's neck and shoulders.*

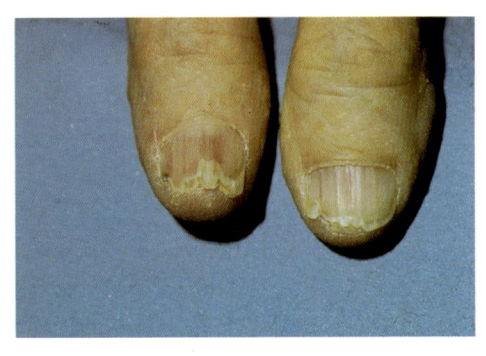

- *Figure 31 Darier disease; nail changes showing longitudinal bands and marginal nicks.*

DEGOS DISEASE, MALIGNANT ATROPHIC PAPULOSIS

Manifestations and Major Findings
endovasculitis affecting the skin, gastrointestinal tract, central nervous system, eye, and other organs
crops of asymptomatic dome-shaped papules which develop into • depressed atrophic scars with porcelain-white centers and telangiectatic rims (Fig. 32)
gastrointestinal lesions may lead to acute abdominal symptoms and fatal peritonitis
histology shows wedge-shaped infarction with lymphocytic vasculitis

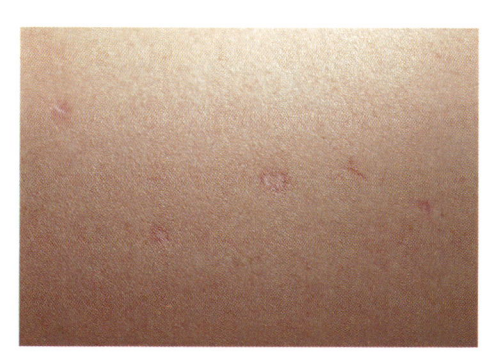

• *Figure 32 Depressed atrophic scars in Degos disease develop from asymptomatic dome-shaped papules.*

References
Degos R: Malignant atrophic papulosis. Br J Dermatol 1979; 100:21–35.
Demitsu T, Nakajima K, Okuyama R, Tadaki T: Malignant atrophic papulosis (Degos' syndrome). Int J Dermatol 1992; 31:99–102.
Plantin P, Labouche F, Sassolas B, Delaire P, Guillet G: Degos' disease: a 10 year follow-up of a patient without visceral involvement. J Am Acad Dermatol 1989; 21:136–137.
Su WPD, Schroeter AL, Lee DA, et al.: Clinical and histologic findings in Degos' syndrome (malignant atrophic papulosis). Cutis 1985; 35:131–138.

DE LANGE SYNDROME, CORNELIA DE LANGE SYNDROME, BRACHMAN–DE LANGE SYNDROME

Manifestations and Major Findings
characteristic low-pitched, weak, growling cry
growth retardation (prenatal onset)
mental retardation (may be severe)
hypoplastic nipples
hypoplastic genitalia

Characteristic Facies
small nose
mid-facial 'cyanosis'
anteverted nostrils
low hairline
micrognathia
characteristic lips and mouth – thin lips with small midline 'beak' of upper lip and corresponding notch in lower lip
bushy and confluent eyebrows (synophrys)
long and curly eyelashes
dilated veins on the temples or forehead

Cutaneous Manifestations
hypertrichosis, especially on the lower back and face
cutis marmorata
hemangiomas
deficient epidermal ridge patterns

SKELETAL ABNORMALITIES
small hands and feet
short, broad first metacarpal
low-set thumbs
syndactyly
hypoplasia of hand and limbs

References
Pashayan H, Whelan D, Guttman S, et al.: Variability of the de Lange syndrome: report of 3 cases and genetic analysis of 54 families. J Pediatr 1969; 75:853–858.
Salazar FN: Dermatological manifestations of the Cornelia de Lange syndrome. Arch Dermatol 1966; 94:38–43.
Schuster DS, Johnson SAM: Cutaneous manifestations of the Cornelia de Lange syndrome. Arch Dermatol 1966; 93:702–707.
Schwartz ID, Schwartz KJ, Kousseff BG, Bercu BB, Root AW: Endocrinopathies in Cornelia de Lange syndrome. J Pediatr 1990; 117:920–923.

DELLEMAN–OORTHUYS SYNDROME,
OCULOCEREBROCUTANEOUS SYNDROME

Manifestations and Major Findings
orbital cysts
microphthalmia
porencephaly or cerebral malformations
 (e.g. agenesis of the corpus callosum)
skull defects
eyelid colobomas
skin tags in the periorbital region
aplasia cutis congenita (scalp, neck,
 lumbosacral areas)

> **References**
> Delleman JW, Oorthuys JWE: Orbital cyst in addition to congenital cerebral and focal dermal malformations: a new entity? Clin Genet 1981; 19:191–198.
> Delleman JW, Oorthuys JWE, Bleeker-Wagemakers EM, ter Haar BGA, et al.: Orbital cyst in addition to congenital cerebral and focal dermal malformations: a new entity. Clin Genet 1984; 25:470-472.
> Happle R: Lethal genes surviving by mosaicism: a possible explanation for sporadic birth defects involving the skin. J Am Acad Dermatol 1987; 16:899–906.

DERCUM DISEASE, ADIPOSIS DOLOROSA, LIPOMATOSIS DOLOROSA

Manifestations and Major Findings
• multiple, painful, symmetrical lipomas (Fig. 33)

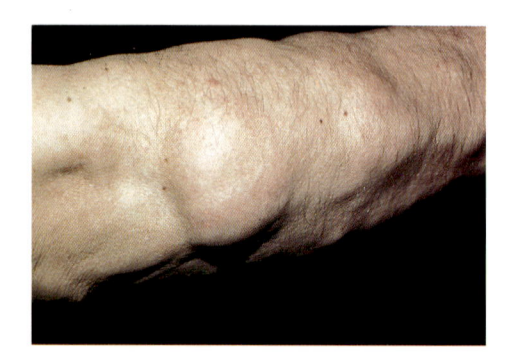

• *Figure 33 Multiple, painful, symmetrical lipomas in Dercum disease.*

obesity
ecchymoses
psychoneurotic symptoms
more common in women
amenorrhea

autosomal dominant in some families

> **References**
> Held JL, Andrew JA, Kohn SR: Surgical amelioration of Dercum's disease: a report and review. J Dermatol Surg Oncol 1989; 15:1294–1296.

DERMATITIS HERPETIFORMIS,
DUHRING–BROCQ DISEASE

Manifestations and Major Findings
• vesiculobullous, intensely pruritic eruption on the extensor surfaces (Fig. 34)
granular IgA deposits in dermal papillae (+C3)

OTHER FINDINGS
oral blisters
gluten-sensitive enteropathy (asymptomatic)
HLA-B8, -DR3, and -DQW2 antigens

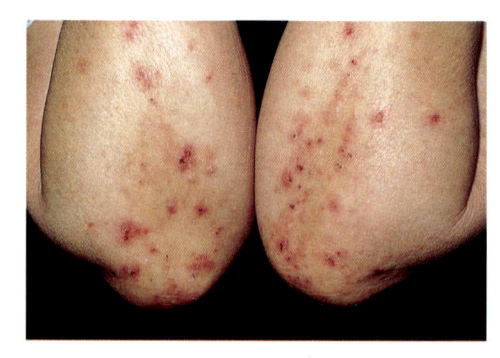

• *Figure 34 Dermatitis herpetiformis; vesiculobullous, intensely pruritic eruption on the extensor surfaces.*

DERMATOFIBROSIS LENTICULARIS DISSEMINATA
see BUSCHKE–OLLENDORFF SYNDROME

DERMOCHONDROCORNEAL DYSTROPHY see FRANÇOIS SYNDROME

DE SANCTIS–CACCHOINE SYNDROME, XERODERMIC IDIOCY SYNDROME
see also XERODERMA PIGMENTOSUM

Manifestations and Major Findings
xeroderma pigmentosum
- most severely affected in Group A, milder in Group D
- defect in DNA excision–repair system

severe progressive neurologic degeneration (begins in childhood)
- choreoathetosis
- ataxia
- mental deficiency (severe)

microcephaly
short stature
immature sexual development
neural deafness
increased incidence of skin cancer and leukemia

autosomal recessive

> **References**
> Kraemer KH, Lee MM, Scotto J: Xeroderma pigmentosum (review). Arch Dermatol 1987; 123:241–250.

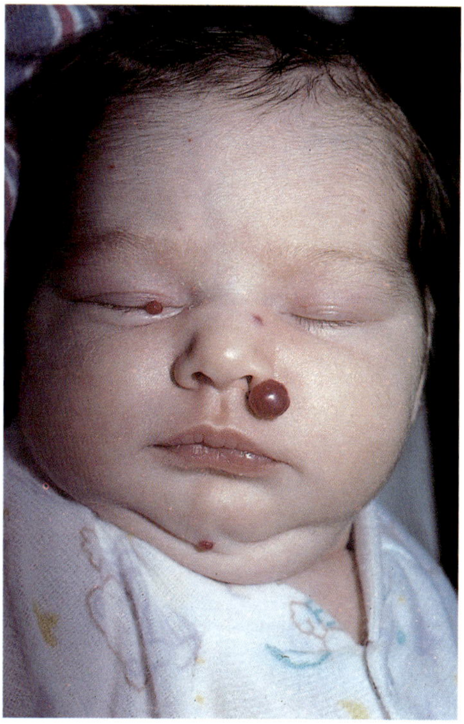

DIFFUSE NEONATAL HEMANGIOMATOSIS

Manifestations and Major Findings
triad of findings
- hepatomegaly
- congestive heart failure
- • cutaneous hemangiomas (usually numerous and small) (Fig. 35)

OTHER FINDINGS
neonatal onset
other organs may be involved (brain, intestines, lungs, tongue)
hemorrhage into organs
interference of functions of vital organs (brain, lungs)

> **References**
> Golitz LE, Rudikoff J, O'Meara OP: Diffuse neonatal hemangiomatosis. Pediatr Dermatol 1986; 3:145–152. ▷ ▷ ▷

• *Figure 35 Diffuse neonatal hemangiomatosis; lesions are usually numerous and small.*

> ▷ ▷ ▷
> Special Symposia. The management of disseminated eruptive hemangiomata in infants. Pediatr Dermatol 1984; 1:312–317.

DIGEORGE SYNDROME, THIRD AND FOURTH PHARYNGEAL POUCH SYNDROME

Manifestations and Major Findings
absence of T cells
thymic hypoplasia or aplasia
increased susceptibility to infections (oral candidiasis)
absence of parathyroid glands causing tetany from neonatal hypocalcemia
bifid uvula
cleft palate
cardiac anomalies
- interrupted aortic arch
- right aortic arch

Cutaneous Manifestations
seborrheic dermatitis
atopic dermatitis (eczema)
cutaneous abscesses

Characteristic Facies
laterally displaced inner canthi
short down-slanting palpebral fissures
small ears with notched pinnae
micrognathia

autosomal dominant inheritance in some cases

References
Archer E, Chuang T-Y, Hong R: Severe eczema in a patient with DiGeorge's syndrome. Cutis 1990; 45:455–459.
Cohen MM: Origins of recognizable syndromes: etiologic and pathogenetic mechanisms and the process of syndrome delineation. J Pediatr 1989; 115:161–163.
Keppen LD, Fasules JW, Burks AW, Gollin SM, et al.: Confirmation of autosomal dominant transmission of the DiGeorge malformation complex. J Pediatr 1988; 113:506–508.
Stevens CA, Carey JC, Shigeoka AO: DiGeorge anomaly and velocardiofacial syndrome. Pediatrics 1990; 85:526–530.

DILANTIN HYPERSENSITIVITY SYNDROME *see* HYDANTOIN SYNDROME

DILANTIN SYNDROME
see FETAL HYDANTOIN SYNDROME

DILATED PORE OF WINER
see WINER PORE

DISORDERS OF CORNIFICATION (DOC), ICHTHYOSIS

Disorders of Cornification; Types and Features

1 **DOC 1 (vulgaris type), ichthyosis vulgaris**
common disorder
onset usually 3–12 months of age

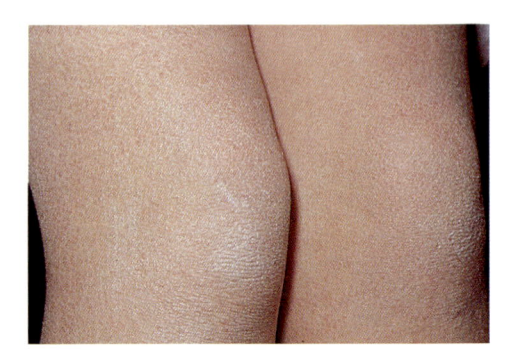

• *Figure 36* Ichthyosis vulgaris (DOC 1) showing fine and light scaling.

• scales, fine and light in color (Fig. 36)
scaling most prominent on the extremities and extensor surfaces
flexures spared
keratosis pilaris
histology shows absent granular layer and retention hyperkeratoses
associated with atopy
increased palmar/plantar markings
improves in summer and with age
autosomal dominant

2 **DOC 2 (steroid sulfatase deficiency), recessive X-linked ichthyosis**
onset 0–3 months of age
mild to moderate severity
• scales, brown and adherent (dirty appearance) (Fig. 37)
generalized involvement, milder on face
may involve the flexures and neck
slightly thickened, scaly palms and soles
asymptomatic corneal opacities
histology shows hyperkeratosis with acanthosis and increased or normal granular layer

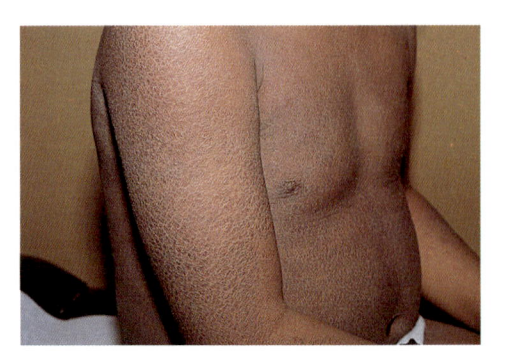

• *Figure 37* Steroid sulfatase deficiency (DOC 2) showing brown, adherent scaling.

Dermatologic Syndromes 55

deficiency of steroid sulfatase (arylsulfatase C) in the placenta, skin, and blood
cholesterol sulfate build-up in scales
diagnostic lipoprotein electrophoresis – rapid mobility of low-density lipoproteins
cryptorchidism
testicular carcinoma associated with Xg[a] blood group

X-linked recessive (males only)

3 DOC 3 (bullous type), epidermolytic hyperkeratosis, bullous congenital ichthyosiform erythroderma (see also epidermolytic hyperkeratosis)
blisters or erosions at birth
generalized scaling develops in later infancy
scales are warty, ridged, and columnar
spontaneous erosions throughout life where scales have been removed
secondary infection resulting in malodor
histology shows intracellular vacuolar degeneration of upper spinous/granular cell layers, and large clumped keratohyalin granules
keratins 1 and 10 affected – chromosomes 12q and 17q

autosomal dominant or sporadic

4 DOC 4 (lamellar-recessive type), lamellar ichthyosis
collodion baby at birth

- large, dark, plate-like scales (generalized) (Fig. 38)
mild erythroderma
ectropion
eclabium
dystrophic nails
alopecia
no abnormality of mucosa or teeth
decreased sweating
fissuring between scales
histology shows massive orthohyperkeratosis and mild/moderate acanthosis
decreased transit time of epidermal cells with increased mitotic activity
alteration of scale lipids

autosomal recessive

5 DOC 5 (congenital erythrodermic type), nonbullous congenital ichthyosiform erythroderma, lamellar ichthyosis
- usually born with collodion membrane (Fig. 39)
generalized scaling and erythroderma
scales on face, trunk, and scalp (fine and white)
scales on legs (large, plate-like, and dark)
ectropion
corneal dystrophy
sparse hair
nail dystrophy
small stature (occasional)
mental retardation (occasional)
biopsy is nondiagnostic
marked decrease in transit time of epidermal cells with increased mitotic activity

autosomal recessive or dominant

6 DOC 6 (lamellar-dominant type), autosomal dominant lamellar ichthyosis
erythroderma absent or very mild
palmoplantar keratoderma prominent
resembles DOC 4 or DOC 5

autosomal dominant

▷ ▷ ▷

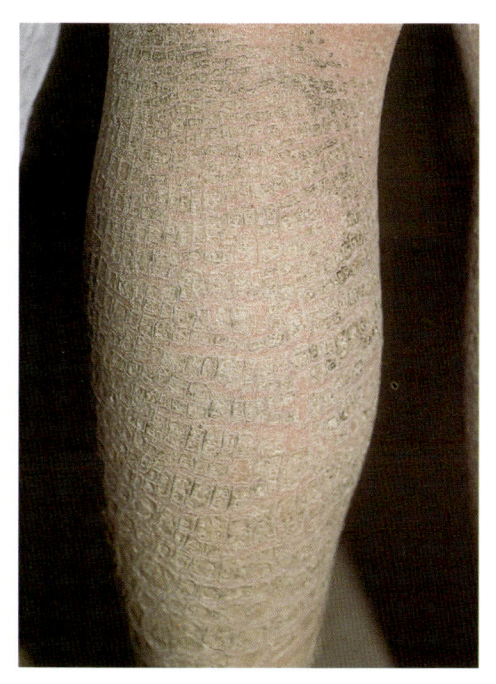

- *Figure 38* Scales found in lamellar ichthyosis (DOC 4) are large, dark, and plate-like.

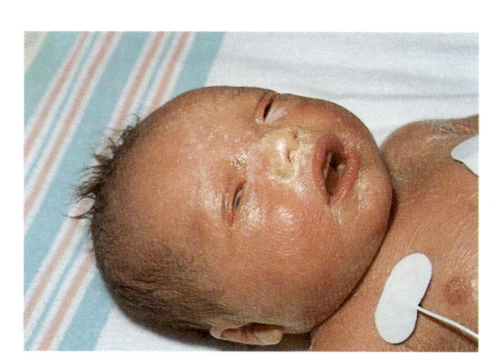

- *Figure 39* Collodion baby with nonbullous congenital ichthyosiform erythroderma; note the thick membrane on the skin and ectropion.

▷ ▷ ▷

7 DOC 7 (harlequin type), harlequin fetus
born with massive hyperkeratotic plates resembling the diamond pattern on a harlequin's costume
distorted facial features with ectropion, eclabium, rudimentary ears and nose
absence of lamellar bodies on electron microscopy
autosomal recessive

8 DOC 8 (Curth-Macklin type), ichthyosis hystrix
resembles DOC 3 (bullous type) except blistering does not occur
- scales are warty, quill-like projections (swirling) (Fig. 40)
severe palmoplantar keratoderma
'porcupine men'
autosomal dominant

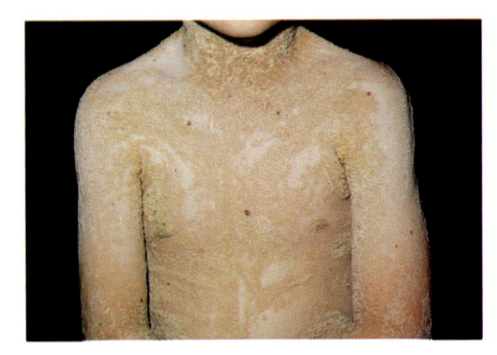

- *Figure 40 Swirling patterns of warty, quill-like projections in Curth–Macklin type ichthyosis hystrix.*

> **References**
> Curth HO, Macklin MT: The genetic basis of various types of ichthyosis in a family group. Am J Hum Genet 1954; 6:371–381.
> Kanerva L, Karvonen J, Oikarinen A, et al.: Ichthyosis hystrix (Curth–Macklin). Light and electron microscopic studies performed before and after etretinate treatment. Arch Dermatol 1984; 120:1218–1223.

9 DOC 9 (Netherton type), ichthyosis linearis circumflexa (*see also* **Netherton syndrome**)
trichorrhexis invaginata (bamboo hair) – defect in keratinization of the internal root sheath
ichthyosis linearis circumflexa (serpiginous double-edged scale)
atopy
pruritus
aminoaciduria
other hair defects – pili torti, trichorrhexis nodosa
autosomal recessive

10 DOC 10 (Sjögren–Larsson type) (*see also* **Sjögren–Larsson syndrome**)
begins in first months of life or as a collodion baby
triad of findings – spastic diplegia or tetraplegia, mental retardation, and ichthyosis
scaling as in DOC 4 or 5, accentuated in flexures and on abdomen
fatty alcohol: NAD oxidoreductase (FAO) deficiency
autosomal recessive

11 DOC 11 (phytanic acid storage type), Refsum disease, heredopathia atactica polyneuritiformis (*see also* **Refsum disease**)
atypical retinitis pigmentosa
deficiency of phytanic acid α-hydroxylase
cerebellar ataxia
peripheral neuropathy
acquired scaling as in ichthyosis vulgaris (DOC 1)
develops insidiously after 20 years of age
autosomal recessive

12 DOC 12 (neutral lipid storage type), neutral lipid storage disease, Dorfman–Chanarin syndrome (*see also* **Dorfman–Chanarin syndrome**)
generalized ichthyosis resembling congenital erythrodermic type (DOC 5)
accumulation of neutral triglyceride vacuoles in many tissues – muscle, liver, CNS, and leukocytes
myopathy
leukocytes with numerous lipid vacuoles on peripheral blood smear
most common in the Middle Eastern or Mediterranean peoples
deafness
cataracts
fatty liver
mild mental retardation
mild growth retardation
histology shows lipid vacuoles in basal cell layer, muscle, liver, leukocytes and CNS
autosomal recessive

13 DOC 13 (multiple sulfatase deficiency) (*see also* **multiple sulfatase deficiency syndrome**)
impaired activity of all lysosomal sulfatases, including steroid sulfatase
scaling as in recessive X-linked ichthyosis (DOC 2)
neurodegenerative disease
hepatosplenomegaly
skeletal changes
mental retardation
presence of neutrophil storage granules
autosomal recessive

14 DOC 14 (trichothiodystrophy type), Tay syndrome, IBIDS syndrome (*see also* trichothiodystrophy)
*i*chthyosiform erythroderma
*b*rittle hair
*i*ntellectual impairment
*d*ecreased fertility
*s*hort stature
palmoplantar keratoderma
sulfur-deficient hair
photosensitivity with DNA excision–repair defect in some patients
characteristic light and dark banding of hair under polarizing microscope

15 DOC 15 (keratitis–deafness type), KID syndrome, aypical ichthyosiform erythroderma with deafness (*see also* KID syndrome)
*k*eratitis (progressive)
*i*chthyosiform erythroderma with rugose plaques on the cheeks, periocular areas, and limbs
*d*eafness (neurosensory)
sparse eyebrows and eyelashes
thickened palms with stippled appearance
squamous cell carcinoma (late development)
autosomal dominant

16 DOC 16 (unilateral hemidysplasia type), CHILD syndrome (*see also* CHILD syndrome)
*c*ongenital *h*emidysplasia with *i*chthyosiform (psoriasiform) nevus and *l*imb *d*efects
X-linked dominant

17 DOC 17 (chondrodysplasia punctata syndromes), Conradi–Hünermann syndrome (*see also* chondrodysplasia punctata syndromes)
scaling in whorl-like pattern (early) followed by follicular atrophoderma
stippled epiphyses
unusual facies
shortening of humerus and femur
skeletal deformities
lens opacities

18 DOC 18 (erythrokeratodermia variabilis type) (*see also* erythrokeratodermia variabilis)
patchy erythema of variable intensity which migrates
fixed plaques of erythema with hyperkeratosis on extensor surfaces

19 DOC 19 (erythrokeratolysis hiemalis type), Oudsthoorn disease (*see also* Oudsthoorn disease)
cyclic attacks of symmetric erythematous plaques with peeling
onset in infancy or adolescence
improves with age
worsens in winter, or during fever or surgery

20 DOC 20 (erythrokeratodermia progressiva symmetrica type), Gottron syndrome (*see also* Gottron syndrome)
fixed erythematous hyperkeratotic symmetric plaques
spares the trunk
onset in infancy, then stabilizes
palmoplantar involvement

21 DOC 21 (peeling skin type), familial continuous skin peeling (*see also* peeling skin syndrome)
periodic shedding of stratum corneum in sheets
erythroderma
autosomal recessive

22 DOC 22 (Darier type), keratosis follicularis (*see also* Darier disease)
papular hyperkeratotic crusted lesions in seborrheic distribution
nails show white or red longitudinal streaks and notching at the distal edge
cobblestoning of the oral mucosa
autosomal dominant

23 DOC 23 (Giroux–Barbeau type) (*see also* Giroux–Barbeau syndrome)
focal erythematosus, hyperkeratotic plaques, resembling erythrokeratodermia variabilis (DOC 18)
onset in infancy
progressive neurologic disorder after 40 years of age
occurs in French Canadians

24 DOC 24 (keratosis follicularis spinulosa decalvans type)
pronounced follicular hyperkeratosis leading to progressive scarring alopecia
atopy
photophobia
keratitis

References
Abdel-Hafez K, Safer AM, Selim MM, Rehak A: Familial continual skin peeling. Dermatologica 1983; 166:23–31.
Levy SB, Goldsmith LA: The peeling skin syndrome. J Am Acad Dermatol 1982; 7:606–613.
Rand RE, Baden HP: The ichthyoses – a review. J Am Acad Dermatol 1983; 8:285–305.
Smacks DP, Korge BP, James WD: Keratin and keratinization. J Am Acad Dermatol 1994; 30:85–102.
Williams ML, Elias PM: From basket weave to barrier. Arch Dermatol 1993; 129:626–629.

DOHI, ACROPIGMENTATION SYMMETRICA OF
see ACROPIGMENTATION SYMMETRICA OF DOHI

DONAHUE SYNDROME,
LEPRECHAUNISM

Manifestations and Major Findings
low birthweight
severely retarded somatic and mental development
lipodystrophy (congenital) or absence of fat
- hypertrichosis, especially facial (Fig. 41)
large genitalia
absence of detectable high-affinity, low-capacity insulin receptors with insulin resistance and hyperinsulinemia
- acanthosis nigricans (Fig.41)
loosely folded skin
malnutrition
often early death

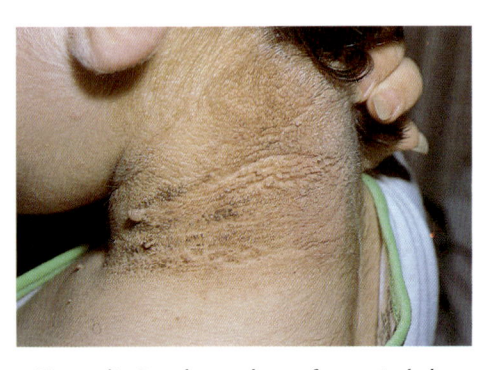

- *Figure 41 Donahue syndrome; features include facial hypertrichosis and acanthosis nigricans.*

Characteristic Facies
broad nose
low set and large ears
widely spaced eyes

> **References**
> **Donahue WL, Uchida I:** Leprechaunism; a euphemism for a rare familial disorder. J Pediatr 1954; 45:505–519.

DONOVANOSIS, GRANULOMA INGUINALE, GRANULOMA VENEREUM, ULCERATING GRANULOMA OF THE PUDENDA

Manifestations and Major Findings
chronic, mildly contagious, progressively destructive granulomatous disease of the genitalia and surrounding skin
caused by *Calymmatobacterium granulomatis* (previously *Donovania granulomatis*)
usually acquired by sexual contact (low infectivity)
widespread in tropics and subtropics
tissue scrapings show Donovan bodies within characteristic large mononuclear cells
earliest lesion is a firm papule or nodule which breaks down to form a nonpainful ulcer

> **References**
> **Niemel PLA, Engelkens HJH, Van der Meijden WI, Stolz E:** Donovanosis (granuloma inguinale) still exits. Int J Dermatol 1992; 31:244–246.

DORFMAN–CHANARIN SYNDROME, CHANARIN–DORFMAN SYNDROME, NEUTRAL LIPID STORAGE DISEASE
see also DISORDERS OF CORNIFICATION; DOC 12

Manifestations and Major Findings
lipid metabolism disorder with accumulation of neutral triglyceride vacuoles
foamy, vacuolated lipid droplets in basal cell and granular layers of the epidermis, leukocytes, bone marrow, muscle, liver, and central nervous system
generalized ichthyosis resembling congenital erythrodermic type
mild to moderate erythema – scaling resembles nonbullous congenital ichthyosiform erythroderma (DOC 5)
hepatosplenomegaly
myopathy
deafness (neurosensory)
cataracts
ectropion
nystagmus
mild to moderate mental retardation

microcephaly
growth retardation
most common in Middle Eastern, Jewish, or Mediterranean people

autosomal recessive

> **References**
> Nanda A, Sharma R, Kanwar AJ, Kaur S, Dash S: Dorfman–Chanarin syndrome. Int J Dermatol 1990; 29:349–351.
> Srebrnik A, Tur E, Perluk C, Elman M, et al.: Dorfman–Chanarin Syndrome. J Am Acad Dermatol 1987; 17:801–808.
> Venencie PY, Armengaud D, Foldès C, Vieillefond A, et al.: Ichthyosis and neutral lipid storage disease (Dorfman–Chanarin Syndrome). Pediatr Dermatol 1988; 5:173–177.

DOWLING–DEGOS DISEASE

Manifestations and Major Findings
reticulate macular or papular pigmentation in the axillary, groin and other flexural areas
onset in childhood or later, and progressive
seborrheic keratoses

OTHER FINDINGS
follicular plugging (comedo-like lesions)
pitted scars near the angles of the mouth
mental retardation
more common in women

autosomal dominant or sporadic

> **References**
> Fulk CS: Primary disorders of hyperpigmentation. J Am Acad Dermatol 1984; 10:1–16.
> Kershenovich J, Langenberg A, Odom RB, LeBoit PE: Dowling–Degos' disease mimicking chloracne. J Am Acad Dermatol 1992; 27:345–348.
> Kikuchi I, Crovato F, Rebora A: Haber's syndrome and Dowling–Degos syndrome. Int J Dermatol 1988; 27:96–97.
> Weber LA, Kantor GR, Bergfeld WF: Reticulate pigmented anomaly of the flexures (Dowling–Degos Disease): a case report associated with hidradenitis suppurativa and squamous cell carcinoma. Cutis 1990; 45:446–450.

DOWLING–MEARA SYNDROME
see EPIDERMOLYSIS BULLOSA SIMPLEX HERPETIFORMIS

DOWN SYNDROME, TRISOMY 21 SYNDROME, MONGOLISM

Manifestations and Major Findings
hypotonia
mental retardation (mild to moderate)
short stature
anomalous auricles
excess skin on the back of the neck
dysplasia of the pelvis – shallow acetabular angle with small iliac wings (shaped like elephant's ears)
single palmar crease (simian crease)
congenital heart defects, especially endocardial cushion defects
Brushfield spots (speckling of the iris with lack of peripheral patterning)
cataracts
acute leukemia
duodenal atresia
epilepsy
hypoplastic teeth
joint laxity
Alzheimer disease after 40 years of age
atlantoaxial dislocation
• dysplasia of the midphalanx of fifth finger (Fig. 42)
clinodactyly

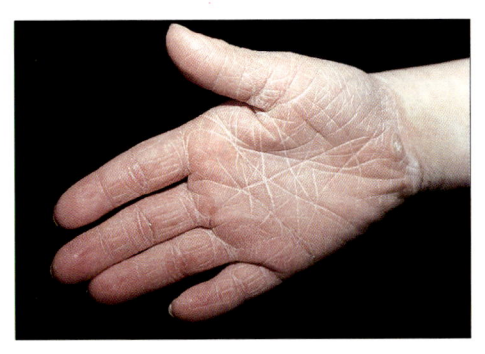

• *Figure 42 Hyperlinearity of the palms with atopic dermatitis in a patient with Down syndrome.*

Characteristic Facies
flat facies
brachycephaly
protrusion of the tongue
epicanthal folds

Cutaneous Manifestations
soft and velvety skin in early childhood
dry skin in late childhood
premature wrinkling of the skin
cutis marmorata
acrocyanosis
atopic dermatitis
elastosis perforans serpiginosa
fungal infections (tinea)
syringomas
alopecia areata
vitiligo
angular cheilitis

trisomy 21 (as an additional autosomal chromosome or translocation)

References
Carey AB, Park HK, Burke WA: Multiple eruptive syringomas associated with Down's syndrome (letter). J Am Acad Dermatol 1988; 19:759–760.
Maroon M, Tyler W, Marks VJ: Calcinosis cutis associated with syringomas: a transepidermal elimination disorder in a patient with Down syndrome. J Am Acad Dermatol 1990; 23:372–375.
Olson JC, Bender JC, Levinson JE, Oestreich A, Lovell DJ: Arthropathy of Down syndrome. Pediatrics 1990; 86:931–936.
Scherbenske JM, Benson PM, Rotchford JP, James WD: Cutaneous and ocular manifestations of Down syndrome. J Am Acad Dermatol 1990; 22:933–938.

DRESBACH SYNDROME
see SICKLE CELL DISEASE

DUBOWITZ SYNDROME

Manifestations and Major Findings
Small stature (prenatal onset)

Characteristic Facies
microcephaly
high, sloping forehead
facial asymmetry
bilateral epicanthal folds
blepharophimosis
micrognathia
ptosis
low-set, dysplastic, or prominent ears
prominent nose

OTHER FINDINGS
eczematous dermatitis
thick skin
sparse hair (especially lateral eyebrows)
clinodactyly
preaxial polydactyly
hypospadias/cryptorchidism
normal intelligence or severe mental retardation
immunodeficiency
leukemia/lymphoma

autosomal recessive

References
Dubowitz V: Familial low birthweight dwarfism with an unusual facies and a skin eruption. J Med Genet 1965; 2:12–17.
Vieluf D, Korting HC, Braun-Falco O, Walther J-U: Dubowitz syndrome: atopic dermatitis, low birth weight dwarfism and facial dysmorphism. Dermatologica 1990; 180:247–249.
Winter RM: Dubowitz syndrome. J Med Genet 1986; 23:11.

DUHRING–BROCQ DISEASE
see DERMATITIS HERPETIFORMIS

DUMPING SYNDROME,
POSTGASTRECTOMY SYNDROME

Manifestations and Major Findings
flushing
sweating
dizziness
weakness
vasomotor collapse

occurs after eating in patients with shunts in the upper gastrointestinal tract

DUPUYTREN CONTRACTURE

Manifestations and Major Findings
bilateral contracting fibrosis of palmar fascia
palmar nodules usually develop over ulnar half of the hand
dimpling or puckering of palmar skin over the head of the fourth metacarpal
tingling, edema, changes in temperature, and sweating of the hand
knuckle pads
more common in middle-aged men
Dupuytren contracture is associated with alcoholic cirrhosis, epilepsy, diabetes mellitus, Peyronie disease, and keloid scarring.

autosomal dominant

DURY–VAN BOGAERT SYNDROME

Manifestations and Major Findings
spastic diplegia
epilepsy
mental retardation
cutis marmorata
acrocyanosis
dystrophy of the nails
hypertrichosis (occasional)

DYSCHROMATOSIS SYMMETRICA HEREDITARIA see ACROPIGMENTATION SYMMETRICA OF DOHI

DYSKERATOSIS CONGENITA,
ZINSSER–COLE–ENGMAN SYNDROME

Manifestations and Major Findings
reticulate hyperpigmentation or poikiloderma (especially flexural areas)
- dystrophy of the nails (after 5 years of age) (Fig. 43)

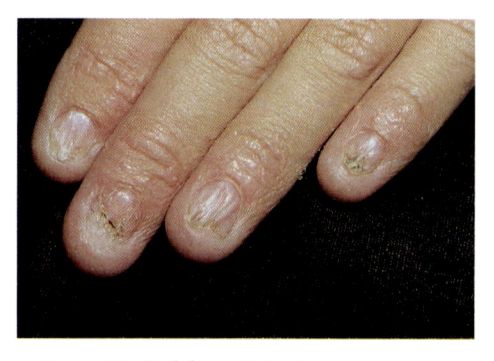

• *Figure 43 Nail dystrophy in dyskeratosis congenita.*

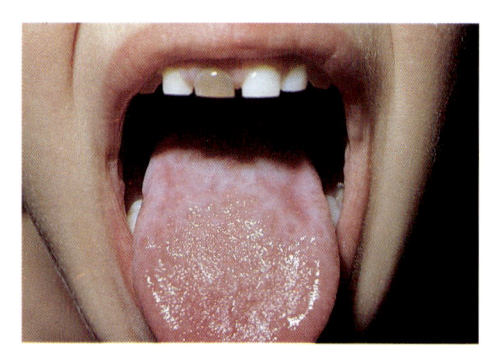

• *Figure 44 Premalignant leukoplakia of the tongue in dyskeratosis congenita.*

- premalignant leukoplakia (Fig. 44) with or without bullae of the oral, anal, esophageal, and/or urethral mucosae

OTHER FINDINGS
bone marrow hypofunction and aplasia with pancytopenia, blood dyscrasia, and anemia
sparse, fine hair with alopecia and canities (premature graying)
blepharitis
ectropion
epiphora
hyperkeratosis and/or hyperhidrosis of the palms and soles
squamous cell carcinoma development in areas of leukoplakia
adenocarcinoma of the mucosal surfaces or other malignancies
sister chromatid exchanges
mean age of diagnosis at 10 years

hypogenitalism
splenomegaly
mental retardation (mild)
mild growth retardation
male predominance

autosomal recessive or X-linked; gene assignment to Xq28

> **References**
> **Connor JM, Gatherer D, Gray FC, Pirrit LA, et al.:** Assignment of the gene for dyskeratosis congenita to Xq28. Hum Genet 1986; 72:348–351.
> **Davidson HR, Connor JM:** Dyskeratosis congenita. J Med Genet 1988; 25:843–846.
> **Esterly NB:** Nail dystrophy in dyskeratosis congenita and chronic graft-vs-host disease (letter) Arch Dermatol 1986; 122:506–507.
> **Phillips RJ, Judge M, Webb D, Harper JI:** Dyskeratosis congenita: delay in diagnosis and successful treatment of pancytopenia by bone marrow transplantation. Br J Dermatol 1992; 127:278–280.

DYSPLASTIC NEVUS SYNDROME,
B–K MOLE SYNDROME, FAMILIAL ATYPICAL MOLE–MALIGNANT MELANOMA SYNDROME (FAMMM SYNDROME), FAMILIAL MELANOMA SYNDROME, ATYPICAL MOLE SYNDROME

Manifestations and Major Findings
abnormal melanocytic nevi
– increased numbers, predominantly on the upper trunk and extremities
– variable size (5–15 mm)
– variable outline and color
abnormal pattern of melanocytic growth
hypermutability of fibroblasts and lymphoblasts
increased incidence of melanoma
conjunctival melanoma or melanosis

autosomal dominant (familial form); sporadic form has similar clinical findings

> **References**
> **Ackerman AB, Mihara I:** Dysplasia, dysplastic melanocytes, dysplastic nevi, the dysplastic nevus syndrome, and the relationship between dysplastic nevi and malignant melanomas. Hum Pathol 1985; 16:87–91.
> **Bataille V, Boyle J, Hungerford JL, Newton JA:** Three cases of primary acquired melanosis of the conjunctiva as a manifestation of the atypical mole syndrome. Br J Dermatol 1993; 128:86–90.
> **Clark WH:** The dysplastic nevus syndrome. Arch Dermatol 1988; 124:1207–1210.
> **Clark WH, Reimer RR, Greene M, Ainsworth AM, et al.:** Origin of familial malignant melanomas from heritable melanocytic lesions. Arch Dermatol 1978; 114:732–738.
> **Kopf AW, Friedman RJ, Rigel DS:** Atypical mole syndrome. J Am Acad Dermatol 1990; 22:117–118.
> **Sagebiel RW:** The dysplastic melanocytic nevus. J Am Acad Dermatol 1989; 20:496–501.

E

ECTODERMAL DYSPLASIA

see also ECTRODACTYLY–ECTODERMAL DYSPLASIA–CLEFTING (EEC) SYNDROME, OROFACIODIGITAL SYNDROME TYPE I, FREIRE–MAIA SYNDROME, RAPP–HODGKIN SYNDROME, ANKYLOBLEPHARON–ECTODERMAL DYSPLASIA–CLEFTING (AEC) SYNDROME, HALLERMANN–STREIFF SYNDROME, JOHANSON–BLIZZARD SYNDROME, FRANCESCHETTI–JADASSOHN SYNDROME, ELLIS-VAN CREVELD SYNDROME, BASAN TYPE ECTODERMAL DYSPLASIA

References
Berg D, Weingold DH, Abson KG, Olsen EA: Sweating in ectodermal dysplasia syndromes. Arch Dermatol 1990; 126:1075–1079.
Rajagopalan K, Tay CH: Hidrotic ectodermal dysplasia. Arch Dermatol 1977;113:481–485.
Solomon LM, Cook B, Klipfel W: The ectodermal dysplasias. Dermatol Clin 1987; 5:231–237.
Wilkinson RD, Schopflocher P, Rozenfeld M: Hidrotic ectodermal dysplasia with diffuse eccrine poromatosis. Arch Dermatol 1977; 113:472–476.

ECTODERMAL DYSPLASIA (HIDROTIC), CLOUSTON SYNDROME

Manifestations and Major Findings
generalized hypotrichosis (sparse, fine, blond, brittle hair)
nail dystrophy
– thickened nails
– striations
– discoloration
– slow growth
hyperkeratosis of the palms and soles with pebbling (especially fingertips)

OTHER FINDINGS
paronychial infections
normal teeth
mental retardation (mild)
normal sweating
more common in French Canadian families

autosomal dominant

ECTODERMAL DYSPLASIA (HYPOHIDROTIC), ANHIDROTIC ECTODERMAL DYSPLASIA, CHRIST–SIEMENS–TOURAINE SYNDROME

Manifestations and Major Findings
sweat glands – partial or complete absence with heat intolerance
• hypodontia, anodontia, and conical incisors (Fig. 45)
fine, sparse, light, and twisted terminal hairs and eyebrows
brittle, thin, ridged nails

Characteristic Facies
thick everted lips
frontal bossing
large pointed ears
saddle nose
sunken cheeks
maxillary hypoplasia

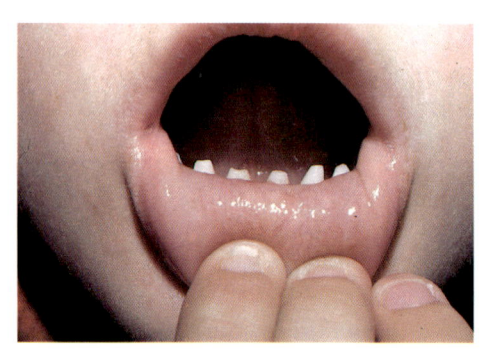

Figure 45 Conical incisors are common dental features of hypohidrotic ectodermal dysplasia, as are thin, brittle nails.

OTHER FINDINGS

frequent bronchitis and pneumonia
recurrent otitis media
depressed cell-mediated immunity
elevated IgE
rhinitis is common
no sense of smell or taste
unexplained fever in infancy and childhood
poorly developed mucous glands in respiratory and gastrointestinal tract
atopic dermatitis
soft, dry, finely-wrinkled skin (especially around the eyes)
sweating on back in pattern of Blaschko lines
dry mouth
salivary gland inflammation and/or ectasia of the ducts
decreased lacrimation
breathy voice caused by an abnormality of the mucosa of the laryngeal folds

RARE FINDINGS

mental retardation (mild)
short stature
hearing loss
hypoplasia or aplasia of the breasts
photophobia
corneal and lenticular opacities
neonatal scaling

X-linked recessive or autosomal recessive

Carrier females may show dental defects, hair abnormalities, reduced sweating, and dermatoglyphic abnormalities.

References
Berg D, Weingold DH, Abson KG, Olsen EA: Sweating in ectodermal dysplasia syndromes. Arch Dermatol 1990; 126:1075–1079.
Clarke A: Hypohidrotic ectodermal dysplasia. J Med Genet 1987; 24:659–663.
Norval EJG, van Wyk CW, Basson NJ, Coldrey J: Hypohidrotic ectodermal dysplasia: A genealogic, stereomicroscope, and scanning electron microscope study. Pediatr Dermatol 1988; 5:159–166.
Solomon LM, Cook B, Klipfel W: The ectodermal dysplasias. Dermatol Clin 1987; 5:231–237.
Sybert VP: Hypohidrotic ectodermal dysplasia: argument against an autosomal recessive form clinically indistinguishable from X-linked hypohidrotic ectodermal dysplasia (Christ–Siemens–Touraine Syndrome). Pediatr Dermatol 1989; 6:76–81.

ECTRODACTYLY–ECTODERMAL DYSPLASIA–CLEFTING SYNDROME, EEC SYNDROME

Manifestations and Major Findings
- lobster-claw deformity (ectrodactyly, syndactyly) (Fig. 46)
ectodermal dysplasia
 –sparse, wiry, hypopigmented hair
 –peg-shaped teeth with defective enamel
 –dystrophic, misshapen nails
 –sweat glands may or may not be abnormal
cleft lip and/or palate
midface hypoplasia

OTHER FINDINGS

breathy voice caused by abnormal mucosa of the laryngeal folds
hypoplastic nipples
fair, thin, xerotic skin
brown macules over trunk and limbs
telangiectasias
small, low-set ears
ocular abnormalities
 –corneal scarring leading to blindness
 –blue irides
 –photophobia

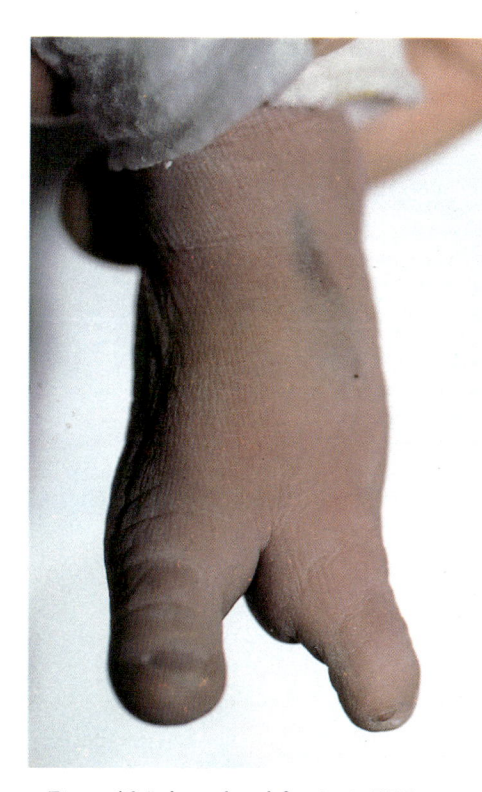

Figure 46 Lobster-claw deformity in EEC syndrome.

–blepharitis
–abnormalities of the lacrimal ducts (stenosis)
mental retardation

autosomal dominant

> **References**
> **Fried K:** Ectrodactyly–ectodermal dysplasia–clefting (EEC) syndrome. Clin Genet 1972; 3:396–400.
> **Solomon LM, Cook B, Klipfel W:** The ectodermal dysplasias. Dermatol Clin 1987; 5:231–237.
> **Solomon LM, Keuer EJ:** The ectodermal dysplasias. Problems of classification and some newer syndromes. Arch Dermatol 1980; 116:1295–1299.

ECZEMA HERPETICUM
see KAPOSI VARICELLIFORM ERUPTION

EEC SYNDROME see ECTRODACTYLY–ECTODERMAL DYSPLASIA–CLEFTING SYNDROME

EHLERS–DANLOS SYNDROME (EDS), CUTIS HYPERELASTICA

Manifestations and Major Findings
hyperextensibility of the joints – subluxation, genu recurvatum, kyphoscoliosis
• hyperelasticity and friability of skin (Fig. 47)
fragility of blood vessels and bowel wall
• atrophic scarring (Fig. 48)
molluscoid pseudotumors (blue/gray spongy tumors)

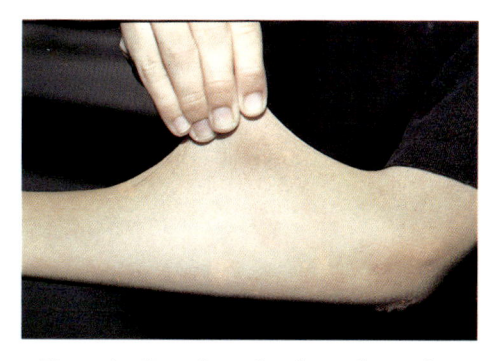

Figure 47 Hyperelastic skin due to abnormal collagen in Ehlers–Danlos syndrome.

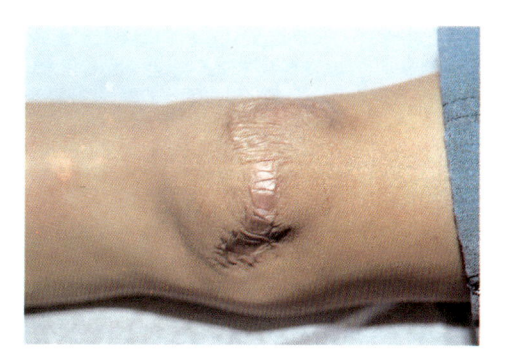

Figure 48 Atrophic scarring is a common finding in Ehlers–Danlos syndrome.

varicose veins in early life
irregular collagen fibers in bone with decreased mineralization
premature birth due to ruptured fetal membranes
Findings vary according to type.

Types of Ehlers–Danlos Syndrome and Features

I gravis type (classic, severe)
skin fragility and hyperextensibility
soft, velvety skin
joint hypermobility
easily bruised skin
atrophic scars
can be seen in premature newborns
varicose veins
Biochemical defect unknown.
autosomal dominant

II mitis type (classic, mild)
similar to Ehlers–Danlos syndrome gravis, but less severe
easily bruised skin
floppy mitral valve
Biochemical defect unknown.
autosomal dominant

III hypermobile type
large and small joint hypermobility (marked) and dislocations
soft skin
Biochemical defect unknown.
autosomal dominant

IV vascular type
arterial, bowel, and uterine rupture
marked skin fragility with thin, translucent skin
easily bruised skin
absence of skin and joint extensibility
tendency to form keloids
characteristic facial appearance with parchment-like skin and very thin nose
reduced life expectancy
Biochemical defect: abnormal type III collagen synthesis, secretion, or structure; deletions and point mutations in the gene.
autosomal dominant or autosomal recessive

V X-linked type
similar to Ehlers–Danlos syndrome mitis
Biochemical defect unknown
X-linked recessive

VI ocular–scoliotic type
marked joint and skin involvement
scleral and corneal fragility
keratoconus
intraocular hemorrhage
scoliosis
hypotonia
Biochemical defect: decreased lysyl hydroxylase activity.
autosomal recessive

VII arthrochalasis multiplex congenita type
extreme joint hypermobility with congenital hip dislocation
short stature
excessive, soft skin particularly on the limbs
normal scarring
micrognathia
Biochemical defect: deletion of exons in type I collagen genes that encode the amino-terminal propeptide cleavage sites in the dominant type.
autosomal dominant
Biochemical defect: amino-terminal protease deficiency in the recessive type.
autosomal recessive

VIII periodontal type
moderate joint and skin involvement
periodontitis
gingival regression
tooth loss
Biochemical defect unknown.
autosomal dominant

IX occipital horn syndrome, X-linked cutis laxa (see also cutis laxa)
inguinal hernias
bladder diverticula and rupture
soft, extensible, lax skin
short arms
broad clavicles
limited pronation and supination of the arms
occipital horns develop in adolescence
low serum copper and ceruloplasmin levels
Biochemical defect: lysyl oxidase deficiency with altered copper metabolism: defective cross-links of collagen.
X-linked recessive

X fibronectin type
similar to Ehlers–Danlos syndrome mitis
striae distensae
prominent bruising
abnormal clotting studies
normal skin texture
Biochemical defect: functionally abnormal plasma fibronectin causing platelet aggregation defects.
autosomal recessive

References
Beighton P 1993. The Ehlers–Danlos Syndrome. McKusick's Heritable Disorders of Connective Tissue, 5th edition, p.189–251. (St Louis: Mosby-Year Book).   ▷ ▷ ▷

▷ ▷ ▷
Dembure PP, Janko AR, Priest JH, Elsas LJ: Ascorbate regulation of collagen biosynthesis in Ehlers–Danlos syndrome, type VI. Metabolism 1987; 36:687–691.

Holzberg M, Hewan-Lowe KO, Olansky AJ: The Ehlers–Danlos syndrome: recognition, characterization, and importance of a milder variant of the classic form. J Am Acad Dermatol 1988; 19:656–666.

Nelson DL, King RA: Ehlers–Danlos syndrome type VIII. J Am Acad Dermatol 1981; 5:297–303.

Pope FM, Nicholls AC, Palan A, Kwee ML, et al.: Clinical features of an affected father and daughter with Ehlers–Danlos syndrome type VIIB. Br J Dermatol 1992; 126:77–82.

Superti-Furga A, Gugler E, Gitzelmann R, Steinmann B: Ehlers–Danlos syndrome type IV: A multi-exon deletion in one of the two COL 3A1 alleles affecting structure, stability, and processing of type III procollagen. J Biol Chem 1988; 263:6226–6232.

Uitto J, Shamban A: Heritable skin diseases with molecular defects in collagen or elastin. Dermatol Clin 1987; 5:63–84.

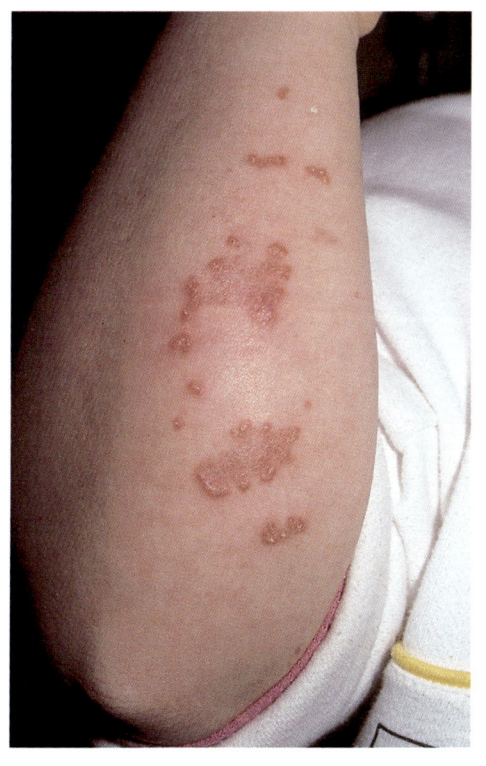

• *Figure 49 Elastosis perforans serpiginosa; erythematous, scaly, keratotic papules in serpiginous formations are seen in this patient with Down syndrome.*

ELASTOSIS PERFORANS SERPIGINOSA

Manifestations and Major Findings
- erythematous, scaly, keratotic papules arranged in serpiginous lines (Fig. 49)
  perforation of dermal elastic fibers through the epidermis
  lesions enlarge by developing peripheral papules which involute in the atrophic center

Elastosis perforans serpiginosa can be seen in normal patients or may be associated with Down syndrome, Ehlers–Danlos syndrome, osteogenesis imperfecta, pseudoxanthoma elasticum, Rothmund–Thomson syndrome, Marfan syndrome, or penicillamine therapy.

References
Mehregan AH: Perforating dermatoses: A clinicopathologic review. Int J Dermatol 1977; 16:19–27.

ELEJALDE SYNDROME,
NEUROECTODERMAL MELANOLYSOSOMAL DISEASE

Manifestations and Major Findings
silvery hair
severe dysfunction of central nervous system
 – mental retardation
 – developmental retardation
 – severe hypotonia
abnormal intracytoplasmic inclusions in all tissues
abnormal melanosomes clumped in hair shafts
tanning of skin where exposed to the sun

OTHER FINDINGS
plagiocephaly
micrognathia
crowded teeth
high-arched palate
pectus excavatum
cryptorchidism
severe myopia

autosomal recessive

References
Elejalde BR, Holguin J, Valencia A, Gilbert EF: Mutations affecting pigmentation in man: 1. Neuroectodermal melanolysosomal disease. Am J Med Genet 1979; 3:65–80.

ELLIS–VAN CREVELD SYNDROME,
CHONDROECTODERMAL DYSPLASIA SYNDROME

Manifestations and Major Findings
ectodermal dysplasia of nails, teeth, and hair
– small, thin, short, ridged nails
– small, defective, peg-shaped teeth or natal
– sparse, brittle hair
normal sweating
short upper lip
chondrodysplasia of the long bones (causing short arms and legs)
short stature
polydactyly
hypertelorism
congenital cardiac disease (atrial septal defect)
mental retardation
occasional abnormalities of the liver, kidneys, urinary tract, and central nervous system

autosomal recessive (most common in Amish families)

References
DaSilva EO, Janovitz D, de Albuquerque SC: Ellis–Van Creveld syndrome: report of 15 cases in an inbred kindred. J Med Genet 1980; 17:349–356.
Mahoney MJ, Hobbins JC: Prenatal diagnosis of chondroectodermal dysplasia (Ellis–van Creveld syndrome) with fetoscopy and ultrasound. N Engl J Med 1977; 297:258–260.

EOSINOPHILIA–MYALGIA SYNDROME

Manifestations and Major Findings
associated with consumption of L-tryptophan
myalgias (intense)
muscle weakness
fatigue
eosinophilia (eosinophil count > 2000/mm^3)
respiratory symptoms – dyspnea, cough
hepatomegaly
edema
heart failure
arrhythmias
polyneuropathy

Cutaneous Manifestations
peripheral edema
alopecia
maculopapular or vesicular eruptions
scleroderma-like thickening (later)
eosinophilic fasciitis

References
Blavrelt A, Falanga V: Idiopathic and L-tryptophan-associated eosinophilia fasciitis before and after L-tryptophan contamination. Arch Dermatol 1991; 127:1159–1166.
Hertzman PA, Blevins WL, Mayer J, Greenfield B, Ting M, et al.: Association of the eosinophilia-myalgia syndrome with the ingestion of tryptophan. N Engl J Med 1990; 322:869–873.
Kaufman LD, Seidman RJ, Phillips ME, Gruber BL: Cutaneous manifestations of the L-tryptophan-associated eosinophilia-myalgia syndrome: a spectrum of sclerodermatous skin disease. J Am Acad Dermatol 1990; 23:1063–1069.
Medsger TA: Tryptophan-induced eosinophilia-myalgia syndrome. N Engl J Med 1990; 322:926–928.
Oursler JR, Farmer ER, Roubenoff R, Mogavero HS, et al.: Cutaneous manifestations of the eosinophilia-myalgia syndrome. Br J Dermatol 1992; 127:138–146.
Swygert LA, Maes EF, Sewell LE, Miller L, et al.: Eosinophilia-myalgia syndrome. Results of national surveillance. J Am Med Assoc 1990; 264:1698–1703.
Uitto J, Varga J, Peltonen J, Jiminez SA: Eosinophilia-myalgia syndrome. Int J Dermatol 1992; 31:223–228.

EOSINOPHILIC CELLULITIS
see WELLS SYNDROME

EOSINOPHILIC FASCIITIS,
SHULMAN SYNDROME

Manifestations and Major Findings
rapid onset of tenderness, pain, and swelling of extremities, face, or abdomen (occasionally involved)

spares the hands – no Raynaud phenomenon nor sclerodactyly
recent history of exertion
early skin edema followed by sclerodermoid changes in previously edematous areas
absent visceral involvement
myalgias
arthralgias
joint contractures
peripheral blood eosinophilia common (eosinophil count > 1000 /mm^3)
hypergammaglobulinemia
dramatic response to systemic prednisone therapy

References
Coyle HE, Chapman RS: Eosinophilic fasciitis (Shulman syndrome) in association with morphoea and systemic sclerosis. Acta Derm Venereol (Stockh) 1980; 60:181–182.
Falanga V, Medsger TA: Frequency, levels, and significance of blood eosinophilia in systemic sclerosis, localized scleroderma, and eosinophilic fasciitis. J Am Acad Dermatol 1987; 17:648–656.
Fu TS, Soltani K, Sorensen LB, Levinson D, et al.: Eosinophilic fasciitis. J Am Med Assoc 1978; 240: 451–453.

EOSINOPHILIC PUSTULAR FOLLICULITIS see OFUJI SYNDROME

EPIDERMAL NEVUS SYNDROME,
FEUERSTEIN–MIMS SYNDROME, SCHIMMELPENNING SYNDROME

Manifestations and Major Findings
epidermal nevi (may or may not be extensive)
endocrine abnormalities
kidney anomalies
cardiac abnormalities
oral involvement
– malformations of the teeth
– hypodontia
systemic malignancies (rare)

SKELETAL ABNORMALITIES
kyphosis/scoliosis
vitamin D-resistant rickets
syndactyly
bone cysts
short limbs
hemihypertrophy

CENTRAL NERVOUS SYSTEM ABNORMALITIES
developmental delay
mental retardation
seizures
deafness
cortical atrophy
hydrocephalus
porencephaly
hamartomas
spastic hemiparesis or tetraparesis
cerebrovascular malformations

OCULAR ABNORMALITIES
eyelid involvement of the epidermal nevus
colobomas of the eyelid, iris, or retina
conjunctival dermoid cysts
microphthalmia
corneal opacities
cataracts

Cutaneous Abnormalities
vascular malformations
hypochromic nevi
café au lait macules
nevus sebaceus

References
Baker RS, Ross PA, Baumann RJ: Neurologic complications of the epidermal nevus syndrome. Arch Neurol 1987; 44:227–232.
Eichler C, Flowers FP, Ross J: Epidermal nevus syndrome: case report and review of clinical manifestations. Pediatr Dermatol 1989; 6:316–320.
Goldberg LH, Collins SAB, Siegel DM: The epidermal nevus syndrome: case report and review. Pediatr Dermatol 1987; 4:27–33.
Happle R: How many epidermal nevus syndromes exist? J Am Acad Dermatol 1991; 25:550–556.
Mostafa WZ, Satti MB: Epidermal nevus syndrome: a clinicopathologic study with six-year follow-up. Pediatr Dermatol 1991; 8:228–230.
Rogers M, McCrossin I, Commers C: Epidermal nevi and the epidermal nevus syndrome. J Am Acad Dermatol 1989; 20:476–488.

EPIDERMODYSPLASIA VERRUCIFORMIS, LEWANDOWSKY–LUTZ SYNDROME

Manifestations and Major Findings
macules and papules simulate flat warts or tinea versicolor and may become confluent
associated with human papilloma virus (HPV) types 3, 5, 8, 9, 12, 14, 15, 17, 19–25, 28, 29, etc.)
sun-exposed areas most commonly affected
flat, verrucous lesions on the dorsa of arms, elbows, and knees
malignant transformation into squamous cell carcinoma
early death
impairment of cell-mediated immunity

autosomal recessive, autosomal dominant, or X-linked dominant

References
Kaspar TA, Wagner RF, Jablonska S, Niimura M, et al.: Prognosis and treatment of advanced squamous cell carcinoma secondary to epidermodysplasia verruciformis: a worldwide analysis of 11 patients. J Dermatol Surg Oncol 1991; 17:237–240.
Majewski S, Malejczyk J, Jablonska S, Misiewicz J, et al.: Natural cell-mediated cytotoxicity against various target cells in patients with epidermodysplasia verruciformis. J Am Acad Dermatol 1990; 22:423–427.

EPIDERMOLYSIS BULLOSA

Types of Epidermolysis Bullosa (EB) and Features

EPIDERMOLYSIS BULLOSA SIMPLEX
1 **EB simplex (localized), Weber–Cockayne syndrome**
    acrally located temperature-sensitive blistering
    associated with hyperhidrosis of palms/soles
    early onset (or rarely late)
    occasional oral involvement during childhood
    no extracutaneous involvement
    autosomal dominant; chromosome 17

2 **EB simplex with anodontia/hypodontia, Kallin syndrome**
    onset in infancy (3 months to 1 year)
    blistering affects hands and/or feet
    alopecia with brittle hair
    oral erosions
    thickened nails
    anodontia/hypodontia
    autosomal recessive

3 **dominant EB simplex (generalized), Köbner syndrome**
    temperature-sensitive blistering
    nail dystrophy (rare)
    plantar calluses common
    oral involvement
    occasional growth retardation
    no extracutaneous involvement
    autosomal dominant

4 **EB simplex herpetiformis, Dowling–Meara syndrome**
    onset in first 3 months of life
    • herpetiform (grouped) blistering (Fig. 50)
    severe involvement at birth with progressive improvement
    skin improves during episodes of fever
    clumping of tonofilaments on electron microscopy
    caused by defect in basilar (K5, K14) keratin filaments
    autosomal dominant; chromosomes 12 and 17

5 **EB simplex with mottled pigmentation**
    truncal mosaic pigmentation present at birth – fading with time
    generalized blisters in infancy – improves with age
    punctate hyperkeratosis of the palms and soles
    variable nail dystrophy

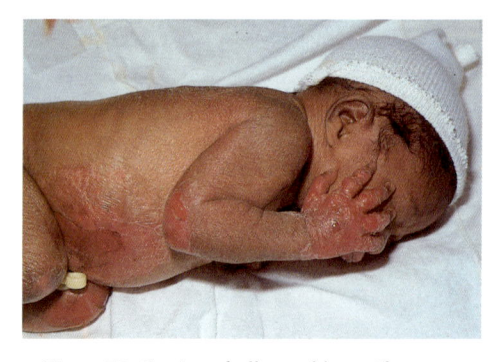

• *Figure 50 Erosions, bullae and herpetiform blistering of a neonate with epidermolysis bullosa simplex herpetiformis (Dowling–Meara syndrome).*

oral erosions (perinatal)
excessive caries
autosomal dominant

6 EB simplex superficialis
onset from birth to 2 years of age
milia, scarring, and atrophy common
nail involvement common
oral erosions
conjunctival vesiculation infrequent
autosomal dominant

7 dominant EB simplex, Ogna type
tendency for generalized bruising
onychogryphosis of the great toes
linked to erythrocyte glutamic-pyruvic transaminase (GPT) gene locus
hemorrhagic blisters/erosions
no oral involvement
autosomal dominant; chromosome 8q

8 EB simplex with/without neuromuscular disease
onset at birth or early infancy
milia infrequent
atrophic scarring common
alopecia (scarring)
nail dystrophy
oral involvement very common
neuromuscular disease
—muscular dystrophy
—congenital myasthenia gravis
keratitis (rare)
autosomal recessive

9 EB simplex Mendes DaCosta variant
tense bullae – mainly on the trunk and limbs – formed by trauma (not spontaneous)
reticulate pigmentation with atrophy, involving the face and limbs (poikiloderma)
alopecia
microcephaly
growth retardation
mental retardation
short conical fingers
acrocyanosis
nail dystrophy
X-linked recessive

JUNCTIONAL EPIDERMOLYSIS BULLOSA

1 localized junctional EB inversa
neonatal blistering with pyoderma-like lesions
age 3 months to 5 years, clear of lesions
school-age blistering, spares hands, feet, elbows, and knees
dystrophic or absent nails
oral and laryngeal involvement
corneal involvement
albostriate lesions reported
involvement of intertriginous areas
dysplastic teeth
gastrointestinal tract involvement infrequent
autosomal recessive

2 localized junctional EB minimus
onset at birth
distribution over the hands, feet, and pretibial areas with blisters
absent nails frequent
oral lesions common
enamel hypoplasia
nasal mucosa involved
autosomal recessive

3 localized junctional EB progressiva (neurotropica), Gedde–Dahl syndrome
delayed onset (5–8 years)
progresses with age, mainly on the hands, feet, elbows, and knees
occasional deafness
dystrophic or absent nails
oral erosions
enamel hypoplasia
mild finger contractures
hypoacusis frequent
loss of lingual papillae
amorphous deposits in lamina lucida
autosomal recessive

4 localized junctional EB (other)
onset at birth
involvement of hands, feet, and pretibial areas
oral lesions common
dystrophic or absent nails
plantar blisters are painful and heal poorly
enamel hypoplasia
nasal mucosal erosions
autosomal recessive

5 generalized junctional EB gravis, letalis, Herlitz syndrome
severe generalized involvement
characteristic hypertrophic perioral and perinasal granulation tissue
death common within the first few years of life
severe growth retardation
severe anemia
oral, esophageal, gastrointestinal, laryngeal, and genitourinary involvement
scarring and atrophy common
dystrophic or absent nails
defective dental enamel with pits
ocular involvement infrequent
pyloric stenosis
autosomal recessive ▷ ▷ ▷

72 Dermatologic Syndromes

▷ ▷ ▷
6 generalized junctional EB mitis, non-Herlitz variant
- large blisters (Fig. 51) (often hemorrhagic at birth)
teeth with enamel defects
improvement with age
atrophic alopecia of the scalp (infrequent)
absence of axillary and pubic hair
dystrophic or absent nails
oral involvement with erosions, microstomia, and ankyloglossia
laryngeal involvement
gastrointestinal involvement infrequent
autosomal recessive

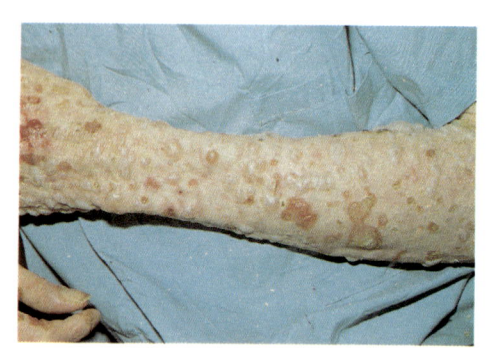

• *Figure 51 Large blisters in generalized junctional epidermolysis bullosa mitis.*

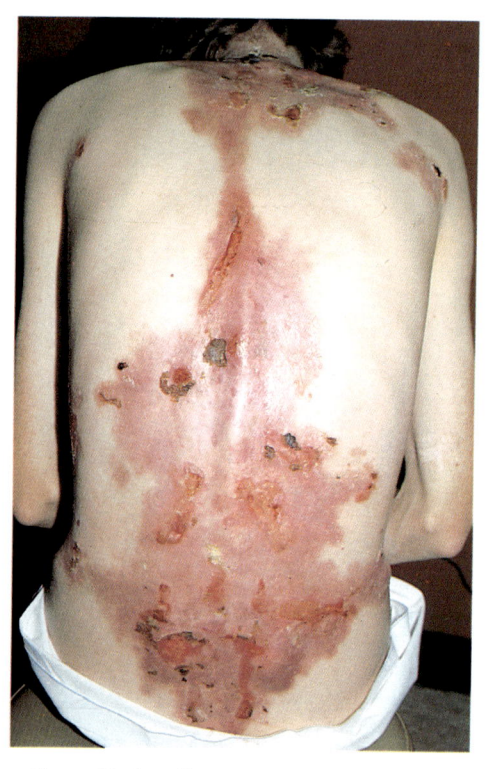

• *Figure 52 Atrophic scarring in recessive dystrophic epidermolysis bullosa inversa.*

7 generalized cicatricial junctional EB
onset at birth
generalized distribution (especially acral)
atrophy and scarring common
scarring alopecia
oral erosions
enamel hypoplasia
pseudosyndactyly (mitten deformities)
esophageal, laryngeal, and ocular involvement
kidney involvement infrequent
autosomal recessive

DYSTROPHIC EPIDERMOLYSIS BULLOSA
1 localized recessive dystrophic EB inversa
onset at birth
worst affected areas are intertriginous sites (neck, groin, axillae)
- milia, scarring, and atrophy (Fig. 52)
nail dystrophy variable
oral involvement severe
excessive caries
acral musculoskeletal deformities variable
esophageal involvement
keratitis
autosomal recessive

2 localized acral dominant dystrophic EB (minimus)
onset in early childhood
acral distribution
mild erosions and blisters – absent after early childhood
milia and scarring absent
nail dystrophy (especially toes)
no oral involvement
no growth retardation
no extracutaneous involvement
autosomal dominant

3 localized pretibial dominant dystrophic EB, Kuske–Portugal syndrome
late onset (11–24 years of age)
exclusively affects pretibial areas and dorsa of feet
occasional association with albopapuloid lesions
milia absent
scarring and atrophy
no oral involvement
autosomal dominant

4 localized centripetal recessive dystrophic EB
onset at birth
acral distribution with characteristic progressive centripetal spread

milia, scarring, and atrophy
dystrophic or absent nails
no extracutaneous involvement
autosomal recessive

5 localized dominant dystrophic EB (other)
acral involvement
onset in early childhood

6 generalized dominant dystrophic albopapuloid EB , Pasini variant
onset at birth
extensive blistering
- albopapuloid lesions (Fig. 53)
- dystrophic or absent nails (Fig. 53)
oral involvement (mild)
fibroblast glycosaminoglycan accumulation in one family
milia and scarring common
growth retardation occasional
esophageal involvement occasional
squamous cell carcinoma in unhealed erosions
anchoring fibrils are rudimentary and reduced in number over all skin
autosomal dominant

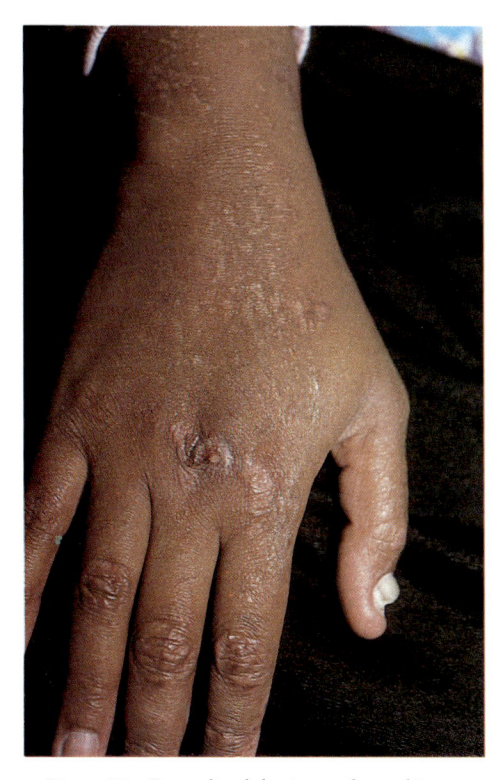

- *Figure 53* Generalized dominant dystrophic albopapuloid epidermolysis bullosa; dystrophic nails are a feature as are the albopapuloid lesions.

7 generalized dominant dystrophic EB, Cockayne–Touraine syndrome
onset at birth
blistering on extensor surfaces and generalized scarring, possibly hypertrophic
oral lesions uncommon and mild
rarely involves trunk
anchoring fibrils are rudimentary in involved skin only
milia and scarring common
dystrophic or absent nails
esophageal involvement
keratitis (infrequent)
squamous cell carcinoma in unhealed erosions
autosomal dominant

8 generalized dominant dystrophic EB, Bart syndrome (see also Bart syndrome)
blisters at birth which later resolve
congenital aplasia cutis
oral lesions
nail involvement
autosomal dominant

9 transient bullous dermolysis of the newborn
onset at birth
generalized distribution
milia, scarring, and atrophy minimal
mild/variable mechanical fragility
disappearance of apparent clinical disease within first year of life
autosomal dominant or possible autosomal recessive

10 generalized recessive dystrophic EB gravis, Hallopeau–Siemens variant, generalized gravis, sublethal variant, mutilans
onset at birth
severe, generalized blistering
mitten deformity (digital fusion) and contractions
mucosal involvement severe
decreased life expectancy
growth retardation severe
anchoring fibrils absent or defective
squamous cell carcinoma in old unhealed ulcers
marked fragility of the skin
severe anemia
keratitis
esophageal, small intestinal, anal, urethral, kidney, bladder, and vaginal involvement
autosomal recessive

11 generalized recessive dystrophic EB mitis
less severe involvement than in Hallopeau–Siemens variant
no mitten hands
generalized distribution
milia, scarring, and atrophy

▷ ▷ ▷

▷ ▷ ▷
dystrophic or absent nails
mild oral involvement
growth retardation absent
autosomal recessive

References
Bruckner-Tuderman L, Vogel A, Ruegger S, Odermatt B, et al.: Epidermolysis bullosa simplex with mottled pigmentation. J Am Acad Dermatol 1989; 21:425–432.
Fine J-D, Bauer EA, Briggaman RA, Carter DM, et al.: Revised clinical and laboratory criteria for subtypes of inherited epidermolysis bullosa. J Am Acad Dermatol 1991; 24:119–135.
Fine J-D, Johnson L, Wright T: Epidermolysis bullosa simplex superficialis. Arch Dermatol 1989; 125:633–638.
Fine J-D, Johnson L, Wright T, Horiguchi Y: Epidermolysis bullosa simplex: identification of a kindred with autosomal recessive transmission of the Weber–Cockayne variety. Pediatr Dermatol 1989; 6:1–5.
Fine J-D, Stenn J, Johnson L, Wright T: Autosomal recessive epidermolysis bullosa simplex. Arch Dermatol 1989; 125:931–938.
Fulk CS: Primary disorders of hyperpigmentation. J Am Acad Dermatol 1984; 10:1–16.
Haber RM, Hanna W: Epidermolysis bullosa progressiva. J Am Acad Dermatol 1987; 16:195–200.
Haber RM, Hanna W, Ramsay CA, Boxall LBH: Hereditary epidermolysis bullosa. J Am Acad Dermatol 1985; 13:252–278.
Hacham-Zadeh S, Rappersberger K, Livshin R, Konrad K: Epidermolysis bullosa herpetiformis Dowling–Meara in a large family. J Am Acad Dermatol 1988; 18:702–706.
Lichtenwald DJ, Hanna W, Sander DN, Jakubovic HR, et al.: Pretibial epidermolysis bullosa: report of a case. J Am Acad Dermatol 1990; 22:346–350.
Pearson RW: Clinicopathologic types of epidermolysis bullosa and their nondermatological complications. Arch Dermatol 1988; 124:718–725.
Sasai Y, Saito N, Seiji M: Epidermolysis bullosa dystrophica et albo-papuloidea. Arch Dermatol 1973; 108:554–557.

EPIDERMOLYSIS BULLOSA ACQUISITA

Manifestations and Major Findings
acral distribution of blisters – usually trauma induced
adult onset of disease (or childhood)
milia and scar formation
hyperpigmentation
mucosal involvement variable
histology shows
 –separation below the lamina densa
 –IgG and complement deposits below the lamina densa by immunoelectron microscopy
 –possible IgA and IgM deposits
Epidermolysis bullosa acquisita may be associated with Crohn disease, ulcerative colitis, multiple myeloma, amyloidosis, lymphoma, chronic lymphocytic leukemia, carcinomas, systemic lupus erythematosus, and rheumatoid arthritis.

References
McCuaig CC, Chan LS, Woodley DT, Rasmussen JE, et al.: Epidermolysis bullosa acquista in childhood. Arch Dermatol 1989; 125:944–949.
Thiers BH: The mechanobullous diseases. Hereditary epidermolysis bullosa and epidermolysis bullosa acquisita. J Am Acad Dermatol 1981; 5:745–748.
Zhu X-J, Niimi Y, Brystryn J-C: Epidermolysis bullosa acquisita. Arch Dermatol 1990; 126: 171–174.

EPIDERMOLYTIC HYPERKERATOSIS, BULLOUS CONGENITAL ICHTHYOSIFORM ERYTHRODERMA, VÖRNER DISEASE (LOCALIZED TO PALMS AND SOLES)
see also DISORDERS OF CORNIFICATION; DOC 3

Manifestations and Major Findings
widespread blistering or erosions at birth
scaling replaces blistering later
scales are brown, verrucous, and columnar
• flexures have accentuated, rippled hyperkeratosis (Fig. 54)
palmoplantar keratoderma
frequent pyogenic infections inducing blisters and malodor
face shows milder involvement without ectropion
histology demonstrates clumping of keratin filaments
increased transit time of epidermal cells
keratin gene abnormality (K1 and K10)

autosomal dominant; chromosome 12q and 17q

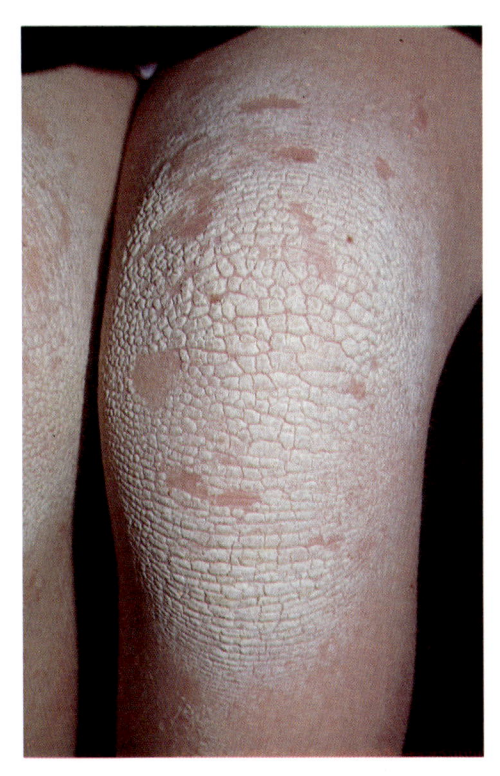

Figure 54 Columnar, rippled hyperkeratosis on the knee of a patient with epidermolytic hyperkeratosis.

References
Nazzaro V, Ermacora E, Santucci B, Caputo R: Epidermolytic hyperkeratosis: generalized form in children from parents with systematized linear form. Br J Dermatol 1990; 122:417–422.
Williams ML, Elias PM: Genetically transmitted, generalized disorders of cornification. Dermatol Clin 1987; 5:155–178.

EPITHELIOMA ADENOIDES CYSTICUM OF BROOKE see BROOKE SYNDROME

ERYTHEMA INDURATUM
see BAZIN DISEASE

ERYTHEMA INFECTIOSUM
see FIFTH DISEASE

ERYTHROKERATODERMIA VARIABILIS, MENDES DACOSTA DISEASE, KERATOSIS RUBRA FIGURATA see also DISORDERS OF CORNIFICATION; DOC 18

Manifestations and Major Findings
fixed, sharply marginated, keratotic plaques – usually on the extensor surfaces
- variable erythemas (Fig. 55) (independent of plaques)

may include palms and soles
normal hair, nails, and mucous membranes
close linkage to Rh locus on short arm of chromosome 1

autosomal dominant or recessive

References
Gewirtzman GB, Winkler NW, Dobson RL: Erythrokeratodermia variabilis. Arch Dermatol 1978; 114:259–261.
Luy JT, Jacobs AH, Nickoloff BJ: A child with erythematous and hyperkeratotic patches. Arch Dermatol 1988; 124:1271–1276.
Macfarlane AW, Chapman SJ, Verbov JL: Is erythrokeratoderma one disorder? A clinical and ultrastructural study of two siblings. Br J Dermatol 1991; 124:487–491.

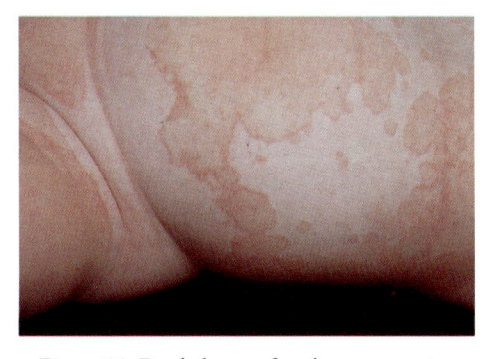

Figure 55 Fixed plaques of erythema present in erythrokeratodermia variabilis.

ERYTHROKERATOLYSIS HIEMALIS
see OUDSTHOORN DISEASE

ERYTHROPLASIA OF QUEYRAT

Manifestations and Major Findings
squamous cell carcinoma *in situ* of the penis
slightly raised, sharply outlined, red, velvety plaque on the mucous membranes – usually the glans penis
plaque may become malignant
histologically identical to Bowen disease

ESCOBAR SYNDROME
see MULTIPLE PTERYGIUM SYNDROME

ESSENTIAL FATTY ACID DEFICIENCY

Manifestations and Major Findings
linoleic acid deficiency
severe scaly dermatosis
extensive percutaneous water loss
hyperproliferation of the epidermis
sebaceous gland hypertrophy
growth retardation
thin, discolored, or absent hair
increased infections
poor wound healing
thrombocytopenia

> **References**
> **Horrobin DF:** Essential fatty acids in clinical dermatology. J Am Acad Dermatol 1989; 20: 1045–1053.
> **Lee EJ, Gibson RA, Simmer K:** Transcutaneous application of oil and prevention of essential fatty acid deficiency in preterm infants. Arch Dis Child 1993; 68:27–28.
> **Ziboh VA, Chapkin RS:** Biologic significance of polyunsaturated fatty acids in the skin. Arch Dermatol 1987; 123:1686a–1690a.

EVANS SYNDROME

Manifestations and Major Findings
idiopathic thrombocytopenic purpura
autoimmune hemolytic anemia
intermittent neutropenia
course is usually chronic and relapsing
antibodies frequently directed at red blood cells, platelets, neutrophils, and lymphocytes

Cutaneous Manifestations
ecchymoses
petechiae
pallor
jaundice

Evans syndrome may be associated with systemic lupus erythematosus, mixed connective tissue disease, thrombotic thrombocytopenic purpura, and sarcoidosis.

> **References**
> **Pui C-H, Williams J, Wang W:** Evans syndrome in childhood. J Pediatr 1980; 97:754–758.

F

FABRY DISEASE, FABRY–ANDERSON SYNDROME, ANDERSON–FABRY DISEASE, ANGIOKERATOMA CORPORIS DIFFUSUM

Manifestations and Major Findings
deficiency of lysosomal hydrolase α-galactosidase A
ceramide trihexoside accumulation in blood vessels
hypertension
coronary artery disease
renal failure
varicose veins
lipid-laden macrophages in urine – 'Maltese cross'
hypogonadism
usually fatal by 40 years of age
Diagnosis of Fabry disease is by finding decreased α-galactosidase A in plasma and cultured fibroblasts.

OCULAR FINDINGS
asymptomatic corneal opacities (cornea verticillata)
blood vessel tortuosity (corneal and retinal)
posterior capsular cataracts
retinal edema

NEUROLOGICAL FINDINGS
severe acral paresthesias (episodic)
cerebrovascular accidents
febrile episodes
weakness
headaches
seizures

Cutaneous Manifestations
angiokeratomas (1–2 mm), mainly on lower trunk and oral mucosa (present by puberty)
clusters of punctate telangiectasias, usually in axillae and on upper chest
scant body hair
polyarteritis nodosa
hypohidrosis
skin histology shows lamellar bodies in the endothelial cells

X-linked recessive

References
Chesser RS, Gentry RH, Fitzpatrick JE: Perioral telangiectases: a new cutaneous finding in Fabry's disease. Arch Dermatol 1990; 126:1655.
Kang WH, Chun SI, Lee S: Generalized anhidrosis associated with Fabry's disease. J Am Acad Dermatol 1987; 17:883–887.
Paller AS: Vascular disorders. Dermatol Clin 1987; 5:239–250.
Utecht LM, Vidmar DA, Cobb MW: Fabry's disease. J Assoc Military Dermatol 1990; 16:6–9.
von Scheidt W, Eng CM, Fitzmaurice TF, Erdmann E, et al.: An atypical variant of Fabry's disease with manifestations confined to the myocardium. N Engl J Med 1991; 324:395–399.

FACIODIGITOGENITAL DYSPLASIA *see* AARSKOG SYNDROME

FAMILIAL DYSAUTONOMIA SYNDROME *see* RILEY–DAY SYNDROME

FAMILIAL MEDITERRANEAN FEVER

Manifestations and Major Findings
intermittent, irregular, self-limiting fever lasting 24–48 h
arthritis
abdominal pain/peritonitis
pleurisy
synovitis
neuropathy
renal amyloidosis
most common in Sephardic Jews, Armenians, and Arabs

Cutaneous Manifestations
erysipelas-like lesions on legs
urticaria
leukocytoclastic vasculitis

autosomal recessive

> **References**
> Breathnach SM: Amyloid and amyloidosis. J Am Acad Dermatol 1988; 18:1–16.

FAMILIAL MELANOMA SYNDROME *see* DYSPLASTIC NEVUS SYNDROME

FANCONI APLASTIC ANEMIA,
FANCONI SYNDROME, EHRLICH–FANCONI SYNDROME, CONGENITAL PANCYTOPENIA

Manifestations and Major Findings
severe progressive refractory hypoplastic anemia and pancytopenia
usually diagnosed at 4–10 years of age
hypoplasia or aplasia of the thumb, carpal bones, or radius
absent radial pulse
short stature
low birth weight
mental retardation
renal anomalies
–aplasia
–duplication
–ectopia
–horseshoe kidney
testicular hypoplasia
splenic hypoplasia
ear anomalies and/or deafness
congenital heart disease
chromosome breaks and rearrangements
defective DNA repair
high incidence of leukemia, hepatocellular carcinoma, squamous cell carcinoma of the anus, vulva, and oral mucosa

Characteristic Facies
microphthalmia
ptosis
strabismus
microcephaly

Cutaneous Manifestations
generalized brown pigmentation of skin (pronounced in intertriginous areas)
hypopigmented or hyperpigmented macules
café au lait macules

autosomal recessive

> **References**
> Fulk CS: Primary disorders of hyperpigmentation. J Am Acad Dermatol 1984; 10:1–16.
> Swift MR, Hirschhorn K: Fanconi's anemia: inherited susceptibility to chromosome breakage in various tissues. Ann Intern Med 1966; 65:496–503.

FARBER SYNDROME, DISSEMINATED LIPOGRANULOMATOSIS, CERAMIDASE DEFICIENCY, FARBER LIPOGRANULOMATOSIS

Manifestations and Major Findings
lipid storage disease – ceramide accumulation in the joints, central nervous system, heart, lungs, and lymph nodes
joint abnormalities
–pain
–swelling
–contractures
aphonia, dysphonia, or hoarseness
mental retardation
motor retardation
cherry-red spots on macula retinae
pulmonary infections

Cutaneous Manifestations

cutaneous nodules (periarticular) leading to painful and progressively deformed joints
skin infiltrated with papules, plaques, and nodules, especially around ears and occipital regions
perianal telangiectatic plaques

autosomal recessive

> **References**
> Chanoki M, Ishii M, Fukai K, et al.: Farber's lipogranulomatosis in siblings: light and electron microscopic studies. Br J Dermatol 1989; 121: 779–785.

FAVRE–RACOUCHOT SYNDROME

Manifestations and Major Findings

senile atrophy of the skin in areas of solar elastosis
numerous periorbital comedones
epidermal cysts

> **References**
> Sharkey MJ, Keller RA, Grabski WJ, McCollough ML: Favre–Racouchot syndrome. Arch Dermatol 1992; 128:615–616.

FELTY SYNDROME

Manifestations and Major Findings

chronic deforming rheumatoid arthritis
neutropenia
splenomegaly

OTHER FINDINGS
lymphadenopathy
hepatomegaly
fever
weight loss
anemia
thrombocytopenia
cutaneous abnormalities
–hyperpigmentation
–multiple, painful leg ulcers
–skin nodules
–pyoderma gangrenosum

FERGUSON–SMITH TYPE KERATOACANTHOMA
see also KERATOACANTHOMA

Manifestations and Major Findings

multiple self-healing keratoacanthomas
lesions begin in the second decade
lesions commonly occur on sun-exposed areas, and may cluster around the nose and ears, or palms and soles
scarring typical after resolution of lesions
lesions may develop singly or in crops of about a dozen at a time
Keratoacanthomas are well-differentiated squamous tumors, resembling squamous cell carcinomas, that spontaneously involute.

autosomal dominant

> **References**
> Higuchi M, Tanikawa E, Nomura H, Hachisuka H, et al.: Multiple keratoacanthomas with peculiar manifestations and course. J Am Acad Dermatol 1990; 23:389–392.

FETAL ALCOHOL SYNDROME

Manifestations and Major Findings

caused by maternal ingestion of alcohol during pregnancy
prenatal and postnatal growth deficiency
mental retardation
speech and language disorders
hearing loss
cardiac malformations
central nervous system malformations
skeletal abnormalities
renal abnormalities

Cutaneous Manifestations

hemangiomas
hypertrichosis
nail dysplasia with thinning

Characteristic Facies

microcephaly
maxillary hypoplasia
elongated philtrum

cleft palate
abnormal pinnae with prominent crus of the helix
narrow palpebral fissures
micrognathia

> **References**
> **Church MW, Gerkin KP:** Hearing disorders in children with fetal alcohol syndrome: findings from case reports. Pediatrics 1988; 82:147–154.
> **Clarren SK:** Recognition of fetal alcohol syndrome. J Am Med Assoc 1981; 245:2436–2439.
> **Crain LS, Fitzmaurice NE, Mondry C:** Nail dysplasia and fetal alcohol syndrome. Am J Dis Child 1983; 137:1069–1072.

FETAL HYDANTOIN SYNDROME,
FETAL DILANTIN SYNDROME

Manifestations and Major Findings
growth retardation
mental retardation

DIGITAL ABNORMALITIES
hypoplasia of the distal phalanges
absent or hypoplastic nails
pigmented or streaked nails
finger-like thumb
abnormal palmar creases

OTHER FINDINGS
umbilical or inguinal hernias
hypospadias
bifid scrotum
webbed neck
cardiac defects
renal abnormalities
skeletal malformations

Characteristic Facies
ocular abnormalities
 –hypertelorism
 –epicanthal folds
microcephaly
cleft lip and/or palate
prominent low-set ears
hypertrichosis

> **References**
> **Buehler BA, Delimont D, van Waes M, Finnell RH:** Prenatal prediction of risk of the fetal hydantoin syndrome. N Engl J Med 1990; 322:1567–1572.
> **Johnson RB, Goldsmith LA:** Dilantin digital defects. J Am Acad Dermatol 1981; 5:191–196.
> **Nanda A, Kaur S, Bhakoo ON, Kapoor MM, et al.:** Fetal hydantoin syndrome: a case report. Pediatr Dermatol 1989; 6:130–133.
> **Van Dyke DC, Hodge SE, Heide F, Hill LR:** Family studies in fetal phenytoin exposure. J Pediatr 1988; 113:301–306.

FETAL VARICELLA SYNDROME,
CONGENITAL VARICELLA SYNDROME

Manifestations and Major Findings
maternal varicella or zoster infection during pregnancy (first two trimesters)
small for gestational age
prematurity
skin lesions – cicatrical areas in a dermatomal distribution
gastrointestinal abnormalities
genitourinary abnormalities
females more commonly affected

NEUROLOGIC ABNORMALITIES
limb paresis
hydrocephalus
cortical atrophy
seizures
Horner syndrome
bulbar dysphagia
mental retardation

OCULAR ABNORMALITIES
chorioretinitis
anisocoria
nystagmus
microphthalmia
cataracts

SKELETAL ABNORMALITIES
hypoplasia of limbs or fingers/toes
equinovarus/calcaneovalgus
hypoplasia of ribs
scoliosis

> **References**
> Alkalay AL, Pomerance JL, Rimoin DL: Fetal varicella syndrome. J Pediatr 1987; 111:320–323.

FIFTH DIGIT SYNDROME
see COFFIN–SIRIS SYNDROME

FIFTH DISEASE, ERYTHEMA INFECTIOSUM, HUMAN PARVOVIRUS B19 INFECTION

Manifestations and Major Findings
arthropathy of large joints (more common in adults)
usually benign course
malaise
mild fever
peripheral blood eosinophilia
transient erythrocyte aplastic crisis with anemia in patients with sickle cell disease
fetal death or wastage in infection during pregnancy

Cutaneous Manifestations
'slapped cheek' appearance
- reticulated (lace-like) erythematous rash (Fig. 56) on trunk and extremities lasting 6–10 days
purpura
dark-red macules on mucous membranes

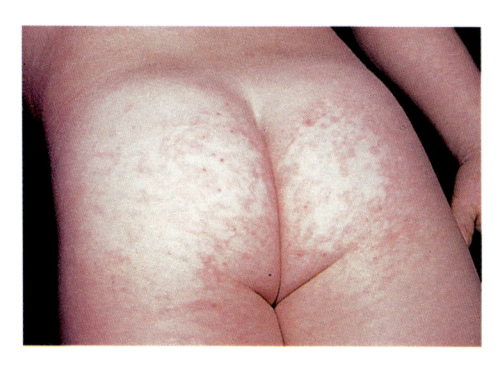

- *Figure 56* Reticulated, lace-like, erythematous rash in fifth disease.

> **References**
> Morbidity and Mortality Weekly Report (CDC). Risks associated with human parvovirus B19 infection. Arch Dermatol 1989; 125:475–480.
> Plotkin SA, Halsey NA, Lepow ML, Marcuse EK, et al.: Parvovirus, erythema infectiosum, and pregnancy. Pediatrics 1990; 85:131–133.
> Ware R: Human parvovirus infection. Pediatr 1989; 114:343–348.

FISCH SYNDROME

Manifestations and Major Findings
deafness
preature canities (graying of hair)
partial heterochromia irides

> **References**
> Ortonne JP: Piebaldism, Waardenburg's syndrome, and related disorders. Dermatol Clin 1988; 6:205–216.

FISH ODOR SYNDROME, TRIMETHYLAMINURIA

Manifestations and Major Findings
odor of fish in sweat, urine, and breath
dietary management helpful

> **References**
> Rothschild JG, Hansen RC: Fish odor syndrome: trimethylaminuria with milk as chief dietary factor. Pediatr Dermatol 1985; 3:38–39.

FLEGEL DISEASE, HYPERKERATOSIS LENTICULARIS PERSTANS

Cutaneous Manifestations
chronic, persistent, asymptomatic, reddish-brown, hyperkeratotic 1–5 mm papules
lesions usually on legs, dorsal aspect of hands, arms, and occasionally trunk
removal of scale causes slight bleeding
onset in adulthood

autosomal dominant

References
Fathy S, Azadeh B: Hyperkeratosis lenticularis perstans. Int J Dermatol 1988; 27:120–121.
Langer K, Zonzits E, Konrad K: Hyperkeratosis lenticularis perstans (Flegel's disease). J Am Acad Dermatol 1992; 27:812–816.
Pearson LH, Smith JG, Chalker DK: Hyperkeratosis lenticularis perstans (Flegel's disease). J Am Acad Dermatol 1987; 16:190–195.

FOCAL DERMAL HYPOPLASIA,
GOLTZ SYNDROME

Manifestations and Major Findings
laryngeal papillomas
mental retardation
defects of the teeth, heart, central nervous system, and genitourinary system

SKELETAL ABNORMALITIES
syndactyly
clinodactyly
polydactyly
absence or hypoplasia of the digits
osteopathia striata
clefting
scoliosis
spinal defects
asymmetry of the body

OCULAR ABNORMALITIES
colobomas
microphthalmia
strabismus
lens subluxation
photophobia

Cutaneous Manifestations
linear streaks of skin atrophy with herniation of adipose tissue
localized aplasia cutis
alopecia or sparse, brittle hair
- fibrovascular papillomas, often periorificial (Fig. 57)
- reticular hypopigmentation and/or hyperpigmentation (Fig. 58)
dystrophy of the nails

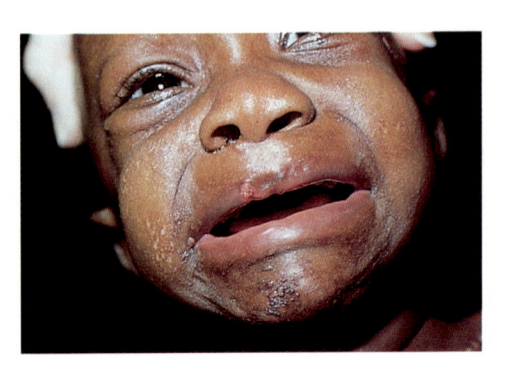

• *Figure 57* Periorificial fibrovascular papillomas, and asymmetric nasal alae are seen in this infant with focal dermal hypoplasia.

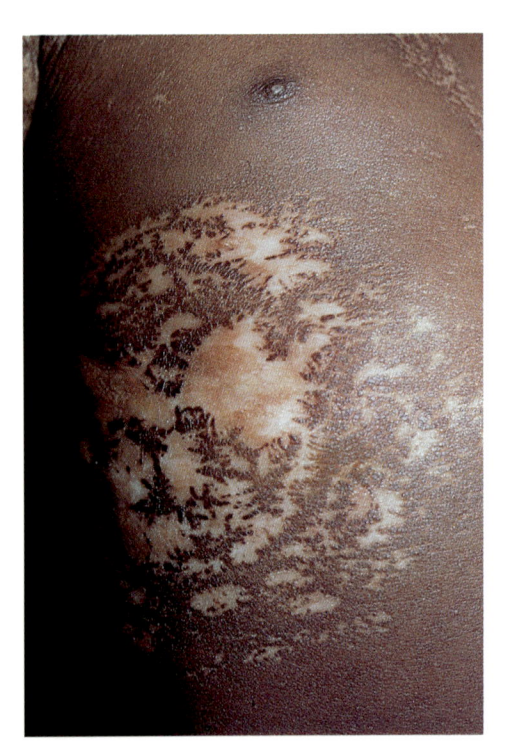

• *Figure 58* Reticular, depressed hypopigmented areas are a finding in focal dermal hypoplasia where the dermis is thin.

Characteristic Facies
triangular facies
rounded skull
pointed chin
- notching and asymmetry of nasal alae (Fig. 57)
radial folds around nose

X-linked dominant

> **References**
> Büchner SA, Itin P: Focal dermal hypoplasia syndrome in a male patient. Arch Dermatol 1992; 128:1078–1082.
> Goltz RW: Focal dermal hypoplasia syndrome. An update. Arch Dermatol 1992; 128:1108–1111.
> Kilmer SL, Grix AW, Isseroff RR: Focal dermal hypoplasia: four cases with widely varying presentations. J Am Acad Dermatol 1993; 28:839–843.
> Pujol RM, Casanova JM, Pérez M, Matias-Guiu X, et al.: Focal dermal hypoplasia (Goltz syndrome): report of two cases with minor cutaneous and extracutaneous manifestations. Pediatr Dermatol 1992; 9:112–116.

FOCAL EPITHELIAL HYPERPLASIA
see HECK DISEASE

FOGO SELVAGEM, BRAZILIAN PEMPHIGUS FOLIACEUS, WILDFIRE

Manifestations and Major Findings
endemic pemphigus foliaceus in central and southern South America
primarily affects adolescents and young adults in rural communities
flaccid bullae in generalized distribution
mucous membranes spared
hyperpigmentation
hyperkeratosis
histology shows
 –subcorneal acantholysis
 –complement and Ig (usually IgG) in epidermal intercellular spaces
circulating IgG autoantibodies

> **References**
> de Messias IT, von Kuster LC, Santamaria J, Kajdacsy-Balla A: Complement and antibody deposition in Brazilian pemphigus foliaceus and correlation of disease activity with circulating antibodies. Arch Dermatol 1988; 124:1664–1668.
> Diaz LA, Sampaio SA, Rivitti EA, Martins CR: Endemic pemphigus foliaceus (fogo selvagem). I. Clinical features and immunopathology. J Am Acad Dermatol 1989; 20:657–669.
> Stanley JR: The enigma of fogo selvagem (editorial). J Am Acad Dermatol 1989; 20:675–676.

FOLLICULAR ATROPHODERMA AND BASAL CELL CARCINOMA SYNDROME *see* BAZEX SYNDROME

FOLLICULAR DEGENERATION SYNDROME, HOT COMB ALOPECIA

Manifestations and Major Findings
mainly affects middle-aged black women
scarring alopecia on the crown of the scalp leaves shiny, smooth, supple scalp skin
use of hot comb, chemical relaxers, or perm solution common
premature desquamation of inner root sheath

> **References**
> Sperling LC, Sau P: The follicular degeneration syndrome in black patients. Arch Dermatol 1992; 128:68–74.

FOLLING DISEASE
see PHENYLKETONURIA

FOURNIER GANGRENE, STREPTOCOCCAL SCROTAL GANGRENE

Manifestations and Major Findings
necrotizing fasciitis of the male genitalia
explosive onset with rapid progression
painful swelling crepitus of scrotum
caused by group A streptococci, multiple organisms, Schwartzman phenomenon, or idiopathic

> **References**
> Bahlmann JCM, Fourie IJH, Arndt TCH: Fournier's gangrene; necrotizing fasciitis of the male genitalia. Br J Urol 1983; 55:85–88.
> Van der Meer JB, van der Wal, Bos WH, Mulder W, et al.: Fournier's gangrene: The human counterpart of the local Schwartzman phenomenon? Arch Dermatol 1990; 126:1376–1377.

FOX–FORDYCE DISEASE

Manifestations and Major Findings
follicular papules and vesicles around the axillae, anogenital region, and breasts
apocrine gland occlusion with itching (apocrine miliaria)
almost exclusively affects women soon after puberty
some remission during pregnancy or while taking oral contraceptives

> **References**
> Giacobetti R, Caro WA, Roenigk HH: Fox–Fordyce disease. Control with tretinoin cream. Arch Dermatol 1979; 115:1365–1366.
> Kronthal HL, Pomeranz JR, Sitomer G: Fox–Fordyce disease. Arch Dermatol 1965; 91:243–245.

FRAGILE X SYNDROME, MARTIN–BELL SYNDROME, MARKER X SYNDROME

Manifestations and Major Findings
fragile site on X chromosome at terminal end of the long arm
normal growth
developmental delay
hyperactivity
autistic behavior (hand-flapping, hand-biting)
shyness
mental retardation
large testes
musculoskeletal findings
– hypotonia
– scoliosis
– flat feet (pes planus)
– hyperextensible joints

Characteristic Facies
large, long, or prominent ears
long face
high, prominent forehead
pale-blue irides
epicanthal folds
high-arched palate
prominent jaw

Cutaneous Manifestations
hyperextensible, loose, velvety/soft skin
abnormal palmar creases
cutis verticis gyrata

X-linked (expression seen more in males)

> **References**
> Chudley AE, Hagerman RJ: Fragile X Syndrome. J Pediatr 1987; 110:821–831.
> Hagerman RJ, Jackson C, Amiri K, Silverman AC, et al.: Girls with Fragile X Syndrome: physical and neurocognitive status and outcome. Pediatrics 1992; 89:395–400.
> Opitz JM, Westphal JM, Daniel A: Discovery of a connective tissue dysplasia in the Martin–Bell Syndrome. Am J Med Genet 1984; 17:101–109.
> Schepis C, Palazzo R, Ragusa RM, et al.: Association of cutis verticis gyrata with fragile X syndrome and fragility of chromosome 12. Lancet 1989; 2:279.
> Shapiro LR: The fragile X syndrome. N Engl J Med 1991; 325:1736–1738.
> Simko A, Hornstein L, Soukup S, Bagamery N: Fragile X syndrome: recognition in young children. Pediatrics 1989; 83:547–552.

FRANCESCHETTI–JADASSOHN SYNDROME, NAEGELI–FRANCESCHETTI–JADASSOHN SYNDROME, MELANOPHORIC NEVUS SYNDROME, NAEGELI SYNDROME

Manifestations and Major Findings
reticulate hyperpigmentation – usually begins at about 2 years of age in previously normal skin
pigmentation accentuated on neck and axillae
pigmentation fades with time
punctate or diffuse keratoderma of the palms and soles
hypohidrosis with heat intolerance
keratosis pilaris
nail dystrophy/malalignment of great toenails
absence of fingerprints
dental enamel defects

autosomal dominant

> **References**
> Fulk CS: Primary disorders of hyperpigmentation. J Am Acad Dermatol 1984; 10:1–16. ▷ ▷ ▷

> > > Griffiths WAD: Reticulate pigmentary disorders – a review. Clin Exp Dermatol 1984; 9:439-450.
> Itin PH, Lautenschlager S, Meyer R, Mevorah B, et al.: Natural history of the Naegeli–Franceschetti–Jadassohn syndrome and further delineation of its clinical manifestations. J Am Acad Dermatol 1993; 28:942–950.

FRANCESCHETTI–ZWAHLEN–KLEIN SYNDROME

see TREACHER COLLINS SYNDROME

FRANÇOIS SYNDROME,
DERMOCHONDROCORNEAL DYSTROPHY

Manifestations and Major Findings
symmetrical xanthoma-like nodules on face and hands (actually fibromas)
osteochondrodystrophy of distal extremity bones causing limitation of movement
corneal dystrophy with white or brownish opacities
fibromatosis of the gingiva
childhood onset

> **References**
> Caputo R, Sambvani N, Monti M, Cavicchini S, et al.: Dermochondrocorneal dystrophy (François syndrome). Arch Dermatol 1988; 124:424–428.

FREIRE-MAIA SYNDROME,
ODONTOTRICHOMELIC SYNDROME

Manifestations and Major Findings
severe hypotrichosis
hypoplastic nails
large nose
large abnormal ears
hypodontia
growth retardation
abnormal electroencephalogram
tyrosinemia

autosomal recessive

> **References**
> Solomon LM, Cook B, Klipfel W: The ectodermal dysplasias. Dermatol Clin 1987; 5:231–237.

FREY SYNDROME

see AURICULOTEMPORAL SYNDROME

FRONTONASAL DYSPLASIA SEQUENCE, MEDIAN CLEFT FACE SYNDROME

Manifestations and Major Findings
defect in midfacial development
incomplete anterior appositional alignment of the eyes
ocular hypertelorism
lateral displacement of the inner canthi
forehead widow's peak
deficit in midline frontal bone
nasal defects vary from notched, broad nasal tip to bifid nostrils
midline dermoid lipomas

FUCOSIDOSIS

Manifestations and Major Findings
absence or diminished activity of α-L-fucosidase
coarse facies (Hurler-like)
growth retardation
hepatosplenomegaly
thoracolumbar kyphosis

NEUROLOGICAL ABNORMALITIES
progressive mental retardation
progressive muscular weakness/hypotonia
spasticity
seizures

Cutaneous Manifestations
hypertrichosis
diffuse angiokeratomas at around 3 years of age
thick skin
decreased or increased sweating
Fucosidosis has infantile, juvenile, and adult clinical forms, and clinical findings are variable.

autosomal recessive

> **References**
> Spranger J: Mini review: inborn errors of complex carbohydrate metabolism. Am J Med Genet 1987; 28:489–499.
> Willems PJ, Garcia CA, DeSmedt MCH, Martin-Jimenez R, et al.: Intrafamilial variability in fucosidosis. Clin Genet 1988; 34:7–14.

FUTCHER LINES

Manifestations and Major Findings

sharp demarcation between dark and light portions of upper arms in darkly pigmented persons

demarcation along anterolateral junction (transition between extensor and flexor surfaces)

> **References**
> Henderson AL: Skin variations in blacks. Cutis 1983; 32:376–377.
> McLaurin CI: Cutaneous reaction patterns in blacks. Dermatol Clin 1988; 6:353–362.

G

G_{M1} GANGLIOSIDOSIS (INFANTILE FORM)

Manifestations and Major Findings
lysosomal β-galactosidase deficiency
failure to thrive
gingival hypertrophy
flexion contractures of the fingers, elbows, and knees
prominent wrists and ankles
hepatosplenomegaly (after 6 months)
macroglossia
cherry-red macula retinae
bony abnormalities
hypotonia
neurologic deterioration
usually fatal by 2 years of age

Cutaneous Manifestations
hyperpigmented macules (mongolian spots)
forehead hypertrichosis
thick skin texture
facial and peripheral edema in early infancy

Characteristic Facies
coarse facies
transverse skin fold below eyes
midface hypoplasia

autosomal recessive

References
Esterly NB, Weissbluth M, Caro WA: Mongolian spots and GM1 gangliosidosis (letter). J Am Acad Dermatol 1990; 22:320. ▷ ▷ ▷

▷ ▷ ▷
Selsor LC, Lesher JL: Hyperpigmented macules and patches in a patient with GM, type 1 gangliosidosis. J Am Acad Dermatol 1989; 20:878–882.
Vélez A, Fuente C, Belinchón I, Martín N, et al.: Congenital segmental dermal melanocytosis in an adult. Arch Dermatol 1992; 128:521–525.

GARDNER–DIAMOND SYNDROME
see AUTOERYTHROCYTE SENSITIZATION SYNDROME

GARDNER SYNDROME

Manifestations and Major Findings
multiple gastrointestinal polyposis (mainly colon) with increased risk for adenocarcinoma
osteomas – especially of mandible, maxilla, and facial bones
• epidermal cysts (Fig. 59)
desmoid tumors
fibromas (skin, subcutaneous tissues, mesentery)
congenital hypertrophy of retinal pigment epithelium

OTHER FINDINGS
increased tetraploidy in skin fibroblasts
dental abnormalities
–supernumerary teeth
–odontomas
–unerupted teeth
lipomas
neurofibromas
ovarian cysts

autosomal dominant; chromosome 5q linked

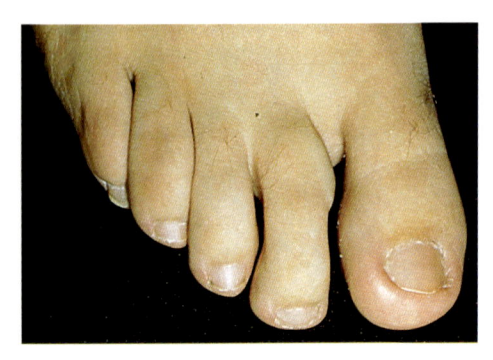

• *Figure 59* Epidermal cyst on the second toe of a patient with Gardner syndrome.

References
Finan MC, Ray MK: Gastrointestinal polyposis syndromes. Dermatol Clin 1989; 7:419–434.
Gregory B, Ho VC: Cutaneous manifestations of gastrointestinal disorders. Part I. J Am Acad Dermatol 1992; 26:153–166.
Kobayashi T, Narahara K, Yokoyama Y, Ueyama S, et al.: Gardner syndrome in a boy with interstitial deletion of the long arm of chromosome 5. Am J Med Genet 1991; 41:460–463.
Kratzer GL, Kasumi A, Krush AJ: Gardner syndrome: study and follow-up of a family. Am J Med Genet 1991; 41:393–397.
Traboulsi EI, Krush AJ, Gardner EJ, Booker SV, et al.: Prevalence and importance of pigmented ocular fundus lesions in Gardner's syndrome. N Engl J Med 1987; 316:661–667.

GARIN–BUJADOUX–BANNWARTH SYNDROME see BANNWARTH SYNDROME

GAUCHER DISEASE

Manifestations and Major Findings
β-glucosidase deficiency
histology shows histiocytes (Gaucher cells) filled with complex lipid in liver, spleen, bones and reticuloendothelial system
hepatosplenomegly
weakness
cuneiform thickenings of ocular conjunctiva
Erlenmeyer flask deformity of femurs
bone pain
pancytopenia
greatly elevated serum acid phosphatase level

Cutaneous Manifestations
patchy pigmentation of the skin resembling chloasma on the face, neck, and hands
symmetrical pigmentation of the lower legs with sharp lower margins and irregular upper margins
mucocutaneous hemorrhage and petechiae
telangiectasia – especially on the upper trunk and face

autosomal recessive

References
Goldblatt J, Beighton P: Cutaneous manifestations of Gaucher disease. Br J Dermatol 1984; 111:331–334.
Peters SP, Lee RE, Glew RH: Gaucher's disease: a review. Medicine 1977; 56:425–442.

GEDDE–DAHL TYPE EPIDERMOLYSIS BULLOSA
see EPIDERMOLYSIS BULLOSA; JUNCTIONAL PROGRESSIVA

GIANOTTI–CROSTI SYNDROME,
PAPULAR ACRODERMATITIS OF CHILDHOOD
see also PAPULOVESICULAR ACROLOCATED SYNDROME

Manifestations and Major Findings
• profuse eruption with sudden onset (Fig. 60)
distinct symmetrical lichenoid papules on the face and extremities
eruption usually spares trunk
eruption nonpruritic or may be pruritic

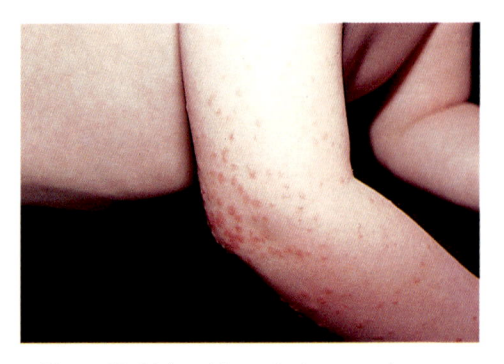

• *Figure 60* Lichenoid papules in an acral distribution in Gianotti–Crosti syndrome.

generalized lymphadenopathy
self-limited course (2–8 weeks)
age of onset usually < 12 years
Gianotti–Crosti syndrome is associated with hepatitis B virus (anicteric subtype ayw), Epstein–Barr virus, Coxsackievirus, parainfluenza virus, echovirus, polio virus, cytomegalovirus, and respiratory syncytial virus.

> **References**
> Caputo R, Gelmetti C, Ermacora E, Gianni E, et al.: Gianotti–Crosti syndrome: a retrospective analysis of 308 cases. J Am Acad Dermatol 1992; 26:207–210.
> Gupta AK, Rasmussen JE: What's new in pediatric dermatology. J Am Acad Dermatol 1988; 18: 239–259.
> Lowe L, Hebert AA, Duvic M: Gianotti–Crosti syndrome associated with Epstein–Barr virus infection. J Am Acad Dermatol 1989; 20:336–338.
> Magyarlaki M, Drobnitsch I, Schneider I: Papular acrodermatitis of childhood (Gianotti–Crosti disease). Pediatr Dermatol 1991; 8:224–227.
> Sagi EF, Linder N, Shouval D: Papular acrodermatitis of childhood associated with hepatitis A virus infection. Pediatr Dermatol 1985; 3:31–33.
> Spear KL, Winkelmann RK: Gianotti–Crosti syndrome. Arch Dermatol 1984;120:891–896.

GILLES DE LA TOURETTE SYNDROME see TOURETTE SYNDROME

GIROUX–BARBEAU SYNDROME,
ERYTHROKERATODERMIA WITH ATAXIA
see also DISORDERS OF CORNIFICATION; DOC 23

Manifestations and Major Findings
ichthyosis resembling erythrokeratodermia variabilis
onset in infancy (with improvements and regressions) often disappearing between ages 25–40 years
slowly progressive neurologic symptoms
– decreased tendon reflexes
– nystagmus
– dysarthria
– gait ataxia after 40 years of age
seen in French Canadians

autosomal dominant

> **References**
> Giroux JM, Barbeau A: Erythrokeratodermia with ataxia. Arch Dermatol 1972; 106:183–188.

GLUCAGONOMA SYNDROME,
NECROLYTIC MIGRATORY ERYTHEMA

Manifestations and Major Findings
glucagonoma of pancreatic α cells
hyperglucagonemia
glossitis
weight loss
diabetes (glucose intolerance)
anemia
hypoaminoacidemia
hypocholesterolemia
conjunctivitis

Cutaneous Manifestations
- necrolytic migratory erythema (Fig. 61) – prolonged, fluctuating, erythematous dermatitis with scaling and erosions – especially on the lower abdomen, groin, and buttocks

candidal infections
brittle nails
alopecia
rash characteristically resolves when tumor is removed

> **References**
> Gregory B, Ho VC: Cutaneous manifestations of gastrointestinal disorders. Part I. J Am Acad Dermatol 1992; 26:153–166. ▷ ▷ ▷

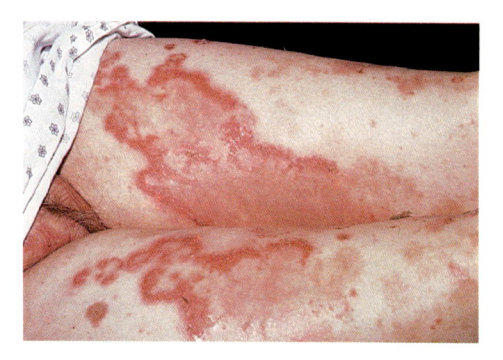

- *Figure 61 Necrolytic migratory erythema of the thighs in glucagonoma syndrome.*

▷ ▷ ▷
Hashizume T, Kiryu H, Noda K, Kano T, et al.: Glucagonoma syndrome. J Am Acad Dermatol 1988; 19:377–383.
Miller SJ: Nutritional deficiency and the skin. J Am Acad Dermatol 1989; 21:1–30.
Vandersteen PR, Scheithauer BW: Glucagonoma syndrome. J Am Acad Dermatol 1985; 12: 1032–1039.

GOLDENHAR SYNDROME, OCULOAURICULOVERTEBRAL DYSPLASIA, FACIOAURICULOVERTEBRAL SYNDROME

Manifestations and Major Findings

abnormal development of both first and second branchial arches
facial asymmetry
malformed ears with accessory auricles and pits
deafness
low hairline on forehead and temples
cleft lip/palate
maxillary hypoplasia
micrognathia
congenital heart disease
normal intelligence

OCULAR ABNORMALITIES
downward slanting fissures
upper eyelid coloboma
microphthalmia
epibulbar dermoid and lipodermoid cysts

VERTEBRAL ABNORMALITIES
usually affects the cervical spine
vertebral hypoplasia
hemivertebrae
scoliosis
spina bifida
rib abnormalities

References
Mellor DH, Richardson JE, Douglas DM: Goldenhar's syndrome: Oculoauriculovertebral dysplasia. Arch Dis Child 1973; 48:537–541.
Rollnick BR, Kaye CI, Nagotoshi K, et al.: Oculoauriculovertebral dysplasia and variants: phenotypic characteristics of 294 patients. Am J Med Genet 1987; 26:361–375.

GOLTZ SYNDROME see FOCAL DERMAL HYPOPLASIA SYNDROME

GONOCOCCAL DERMATITIS SYNDROME

Manifestations and Major Findings

disseminated gonococcal infection caused by *Neisseria gonorrhoeae*
intermittent fever
arthralgia with pain and swelling around one or more joints
• hemorrhagic vesiculopustular vasculitic lesions (Fig. 62) scattered in crops with red halos
mucosal infection (often asymptomatic)
erythema multiforme
erythema nodosum
urticaria

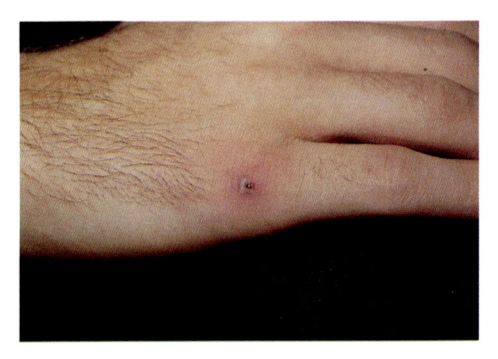

• *Figure 62 Hemorrhagic vesiculopustular vasculitic lesion in gonococcal dermatitis syndrome showing characteristic red halo.*

GORHAM SYNDROME, VANISHING BONE SYNDROME, HEMANGIOMAS WITH OSTEOLYSIS

Manifestations and Major Findings

vascular malformation of the skin and bones causing massive osteolysis
replacement of bone by extensive fibrosis
skeletal lesions usually unilateral
history of prior trauma common
may be fatal in aggressive variants

> **References**
> Carrington PR, Rowley MJ, Fowler M, Megison RP, et al.: Kasabach–Merritt Syndrome with bone involvement: the pseudomalignant sign of Gorham. J Am Acad Dermatol 1993; 29:117–119.
> Choma ND, Biscotti CV, Bauer TW, Mehta AC, Licata AA: Gorham's syndrome: a case report and review of the literature. Am J Med 1987; 83: 1151–1156.
> Gellis SS, Feingold M: Hemangiomas with osteolysis (Gorham's disease: vanishing bone disease). Am J Dis Child 1978; 132:715–716.

GORLIN SYNDROME see BASAL CELL NEVUS SYNDROME

GOTTRON SYNDROME, ACROGERIA

Manifestations and Major Findings
onset in infancy
normal life expectancy
premature aging of extremities
micrognathia
short stature
normal hair
small hands and feet
associated with vascular type Ehlers–Danlos syndrome

Cutaneous Manifestations
atrophic or thickened nails
symmetrical progressive acral erythema and scaling with atrophy and loss of subcutaneous fat
lipoatrophy
prominent vessels on trunk
easy bruising and scar formation
elastosis perforans serpiginosa

autosomal recessive

> **References**
> Beauregard S, Gilchrest BA: Syndromes of premature aging. Dermatol Clin 1987; 5:109–121.
> DeGroot WP, Tafelkruyer J, Woerdemann MJ, et al.: Familial acrogeria (Gottron). Br J Dermatol 1980; 103:213–223.

GOTTRON SYNDROME, SYMMETRICAL PROGRESSIVE ERYTHROKERATODERMIA, PROGRESSIVE SYMMETRICAL ERYTHROKERATODERMIA
see also DISORDERS OF CORNIFICATION; DOC 20

Manifestations and Major Findings
sharply marginated, orange, erythematous plaques – most common on the shoulder girdle, cheeks, buttocks, ankles, and wrists
palmoplantar keratoderma
childhood onset with progression over 1–2 years
pruritus

autosomal dominant

> **References**
> Ruiz-Maldonado R, Tamayo L, del Castillo V, et al.: Erythrokeratoderma progressiva symmetrica: report of 10 cases. Dermatologica 1982; 164:133–141.
> Macfarlane AW, Chapman SJ, Verbov JL: Is erythrokeratodermia one disorder? A clinical and ultrastructural study of two siblings. Br J Dermatol 1991; 124:487–491.

GOTTRON–ARNDT SYNDROME
see SCLEROMYXEDEMA

GOUGEROT–BLUM DISEASE
see PURPURA PIGMENTOSA CHRONICA

GOUGEROT–CARTEAUD SYNDROME, CONFLUENT AND RETICULATED PAPILLOMATOSIS OF GOUGEROT–CARTEAUD

Manifestations and Major Findings
verrucous, flat-topped papules or hyperkeratosis
- lesions become confluent in an irregular network on the trunk, beginning at the midline (Fig. 63)
more common in black females
endocrine abnormalities
–diabetes mellitus
–thyroid disease

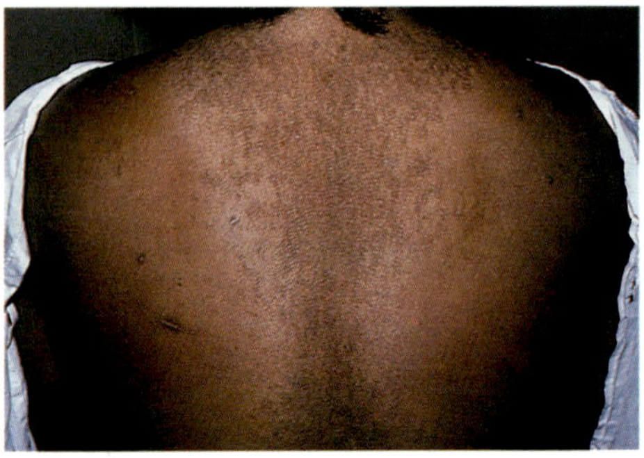

Figure 63 Typical net-like distribution of confluent papillomatosis, beginning at the midline trunk, in Gougerot–Carteaud syndrome.

References
Fulk CS: Primary disorders of hyperpigmentation. J Am Acad Dermatol 1984; 10:1–16.
Hamilton D, Tavofoghi V, Shafer J, Hambrick GW: Confluent and reticulated papillomatosis of Gougerot and Carteaud. J Am Acad Dermatol 1980; 2:401–410.
Hodge JA, Ray MC: Confluent and reticulated papillomatosis: response to isotretinoin. J Am Acad Dermatol 1991; 24:654.
Jimbow M, Talpash O, Jimbow K: Confluent and reticulated papillomatosis: clinical, light and electron microscopic studies. Int J Dermatol 1992; 31:480–483.
Sassolas B, Plantin P, Guillet G: Confluent and reticulated papillomatosis: treatment with minocycline. J Am Acad Dermatol 1992; 26:501–502.

GRAHAM LITTLE SYNDROME,
GRAHAM LITTLE–PICCARDI–LASSUEUR SYNDROME, FELDMAN SYNDROME, LASSUEUR–GRAHAM LITTLE SYNDROME

Manifestations and Major Findings
lichen planus with follicular involvement
acuminate follicular papules with plugging
progressive cicatricial alopecia involving the scalp, axillae, and pubic hair
keratosis pilaris
typically affects women aged 30–70 years

References
Horn RT, Goette DK, Odom RB, et al.: Immunofluorescent findings and clinical changes in two cases of follicular lichen planus. J Am Acad Dermatol 1982; 7:203–207.
Kubba R, Rook A: The Graham Little syndrome. Br J Dermatol 1975; 93 (Suppl. 11):53–55.

GRANULOMA INGUINALE
see DONOVANOSIS

GRANULOMATOUS CHEILITIS
see MELKERSSON–ROSENTHAL SYNDROME

GRAVES DISEASE

Manifestations and Major Findings
hyperthyroidism caused by autoantibodies to receptors for thyroid-stimulating hormone (TSH) on thyroid cells
elevated serum T3 and T4 levels
elevated thyroid radioiodine uptake
depressed serum TSH level
diffuse thyroid enlargement
hyperactivity
nervousness
tremor
hyperreflexia
irritability
weight loss
heat intolerance
ophthalmopathy (exophthalmos)
high-output heart failure
menstrual irregularities
more common in females
Graves disease is associated with other autoimmune endocrine diseases such as myasthenia gravis and pernicious anemia.

Cutaneous Manifestations
pretibial myxedema – localized, edematous, erythematous, waxy plaques mainly located in pretibial areas but may be elsewhere
prominent hair follicles in plaques (*peau d'orange* appearance)

localized hypertrichosis over the plaques
onycholysis

References
Hashizume K, Ichikawa K, Sakurai A, Suzuki S: Administration of thyroxine in treated Graves' disease. N Engl J Med 1991; 324:947–953.
Heymann WR: Cutaneous manifestations of thyroid disease. J Am Acad Dermatol 1992; 26:885–902.

GRAY BABY SYNDROME

Manifestations and Major Findings
gray discoloration of skin caused by markedly increased levels of chloramphenicol in an infant
circulatory collapse
neonates susceptible because of immature hepatic enzymes

References
Prober CG 1991. Antimicrobial therapy. In Rudolph AM (ed.) Rudolph's Pediatrics, 19th edition, p.523–540. (Connecticut: Appleton and Lange).

GREITHER SYNDROME, PROGRESSIVE PALMOPLANTAR KERATODERMA

Manifestations and Major Findings
palmoplantar keratoderma (transgrediens form)
 – involvement of extensor surfaces of hands and feet
onset from 3–8 years of age
spontaneous amputations and deformities
hyperhidrosis or hypohidrosis
total alopecia
loss of teeth
centrofacial lentigines
corneal and lenticular opacities
keratoderma tends to improve in fifth decade

autosomal dominant

References
Fulk CS: Primary disorders of hyperpigmentation. J Am Acad Dermatol 1984; 10:1–16. ▷ ▷ ▷

▷ ▷ ▷
Kansky A, Arzensek J: Is palmoplantar keratoderma of Greither's type a separate nosologic entity? Dermatologica 1979; 158:244–248.
Sybert VP, Dale BA, Holbrook KA: Palmar-plantar keratoderma. J Am Acad Dermatol 1988; 18:75–86.

GRINSPAN SYNDROME

Manifestations and Major Findings
oral lichen planus (bullous form)
cutaneous lichen planus
diabetes mellitus
hypertension

References
Halevy S, Feuerman EJ: Abnormal glucose tolerance associated with lichen planus. Acta Derm Venereol 1979; 59:167–170.

GRISCELLI SYNDROME

Manifestations and Major Findings
acute episodes of fever, neutropenia, and thrombocytopenia
immunodeficiency
–defective T-helper lymphocytes
–reduced humoral immunity with hypogammaglobulinemia
hepatosplenomegaly
no nystagmus or photophobia

Cutaneous Manifestations
pigmentary dilution of skin (mild) and hair (silvery hair)
histology shows
–absence of cutaneous Langerhans cells
–large, irregular clumps of pigment in hair shafts
–1anergy
pyogenic infections

autosomal recessive

References
Griscelli C, Durandy A, Guy-Grand D, Daguillard F, et al.: A syndrome associating partial albinism and immunodeficiency. Am J Med 1978; 65:691–702.

GRÖNBLAD–STRANDBERG SYNDROME see PSEUDOXANTHOMA ELASTICUM

GROVER DISEASE, TRANSIENT ACANTHOLYTIC DERMATOSIS, TRANSIENT AND PERSISTENT ACANTHOLYTIC DERMATOSIS, BENIGN PAPULAR ACANTHOLYTIC DERMATOSIS

Manifestations and Major Findings
acute, discrete, pruritic papules or vesicles mainly on the trunk
typically affects fair skinned, middle-aged to elderly men
exposure to sun, heat, sweating, and ionizing radiation may be precipitating factors
histology shows acantholysis in epidermis
self-limited or intermittent course

References
Chalet M, Grover R, Ackerman AB: Transient acantholytic dermatosis. Arch Dermatol 1977; 113:431–435.
Grover RW: Transient acantholytic dermatosis. Arch Dermatol 1971; 104:26–37.
Heaphy MR, Tucker SB, Winkelmann RK: Benign papular acantholytic dermatosis. Arch Dermatol 1976; 112:814–821.

GRZYBOWSKI TYPE KERATOACANTHOMA
see also KERATOACANTHOMA

Manifestations And Major Findings
numerous, small, eruptive keratoacanthomas (benign squamous tumors)
hundreds of follicular papules measuring 2–3 mm
lesions appear in adult life
oral mucosa and larynx may be involved
pruritus

References
Higuchi M, Tanikawa E, Nomura H, Hachisuka H, et al.: Multiple keratoacanthomas with peculiar manifestations and course. J Am Acad Dermatol 1990; 23:389–392.
Jaber PW, Cooper PH, Greer KE. Generalized eruptive keratoacanthoma of Grzybowski. J Am Acad Dermatol 1993; 29:299–304.
Lloyd KM, Madsen DK, Lin PY: Grzybowski's eruptive keratoacanthoma. J Am Acad Dermatol 1989; 21:1023–1024.
Schwartz RA: The keratoacanthoma: a review. J Surg Oncol 1979; 12:305–317.

GÜNTHER SYNDROME
see PORPHYRIA

H

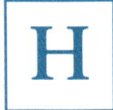

HABER SYNDROME

Manifestations and Major Findings
persistent rosacea-like eruption beginning in childhood
multiple intraepidermal epitheliomas
pitted scars on the face and trunk
pigmented keratotic plaques on trunk and limbs (resembling seborrheic keratoses)

autosomal dominant

> **References**
> Kikuchi I, Crovato F, Rebora A: Haber's syndrome and Dowling–Degos disease. Int J Dermatol 1988; 27:96–97.
> Kikuchi I, Saita B, Inoue S: Haber's syndrome. Arch Dermatol 1981; 117:321–324.
> Seiji M, Otaki N: Haber's syndrome. Familial rosacea-like dermatosis with keratotic plaques and pitted scars. Arch Dermatol 1971; 103:452–455.

HAILEY–HAILEY DISEASE,
CHRONIC BENIGN FAMILIAL PEMPHIGUS

Manifestations and Major Findings
recurrent vesicles, crusts, erosions, and moist vegetations in flexural areas – especially neck, axillae, and groin
usually spares the mucous membranes
usually begins in adolescence
precipitated by skin infections, heat, and sweating
histology shows
– partial acantholysis of the epidermis ('dilapidated brick wall' appearance)
– negative direct immunofluorescence

autosomal dominant

> **References**
> Kartamaa M, Reitamo S: Familial benign chronic pemphigus (Hailey–Hailey Disease). Arch Dermatol 1992; 128:646–648.
> Langenberg A, Berger TG, Cardelli M, Rodman OG, et al.: Genital benign chronic pemphigus (Hailey–Hailey disease) presenting as condylomas. J Am Acad Dermatol 1992; 26:951–955.

HAIR SHAFT ANOMALIES

Types of Hair Shaft Anomalies and Features

1 nonhereditary congenital defects
pili bifurcati
intermittent bifurcation at irregular intervals along the hair shaft
pili multigemini
formation of many hair shafts (2–8) in the same follicular canal
seen mainly on the face and beard area
pseudomonilethrix
artifactual nodes on the hair shaft produced by microscopic slide pressure

2 acquired defects
Pohl–Pinkus marks
isolated narrowings of hair shaft secondary to systemic disease (infection, malnutrition, etc.)
analogous to Beau lines in fingernails
spiral hair (rolled hair)
spiral form of hair
occurs frequently in keratosis pilaris and ichthyosis
trichostasis spinulosa
retention of multiple hairs beneath a follicular plug
5–50 normal, clubbed vellus hairs embedded in a large comedo
trichomalacia
plaques of alopecia with deformed hairs
caused by trauma or trichotillomania

▷ ▷ ▷

▷ ▷ ▷
trichonodosis
knots in hair shafts
occurs in curly-haired persons

3 hair fractures
trichoptilosis
longitudinal fractures of the hair shaft or fraying of the distal end ('split ends')
caused by cosmetic trauma
trichoschisis
clean transverse fractures
occurs in sulfur-deficient hair
fracture associated with localized absence of cuticular cells
trichoclasis
oblique or transverse fractures with irregular borders
usually secondary to cosmetic trauma
'greenstick' fractures of the hair shafts

4 specific dysplasias
monilethrix (beaded hair) see also *monilethrix syndrome*
periodic nonmedullated narrowings of the hair shafts
shafts resemble a beaded necklace
autosomal dominant
trichorrhexis nodosa
transverse fracture of hair shaft
shafts resemble two brushes pushed together
caused by weathering – and rarely by arginosuccinic aciduria (with mental retardation)
see also arginosuccinic aciduria
proximal type – more common in blacks
distal type – more common in whites and orientals
trichorrhexis invaginata (bamboo hair) see also *Netherton syndrome*
nodular alteration resembling a 'ball-and-socket'
seen in Netherton syndrome
hair shafts twist on axis at irregular intervals
pili torti see also *pili torti syndromes*
classical type (Ronchese)
postpubertal type (Beare)
seen in normal individuals as well as in Menkes kinky hair syndrome, Bazex syndrome, Björnstad syndrome, Crandall syndrome, and Salamon syndrome
trichothiodystrophy see also *trichothiodystrophy*
caused by sulfur-deficient hair
polarizing microscopy shows alternating light and dark bands
autosomal recessive

5 defects without fragility of shaft
pili annulati (ringed hair)
alternating dark and light bands along hair shafts
dark bands produced by air bubbles in cuticle and cortex
autosomal dominant

pseudopili annulati
fair hair with flat, twisted areas reflecting light
no underlying cortical defect in hair
wooly hair
fine, sparse, extremely curly hair of oval section
wooly-hair nevus
patch of wooly hair on scalp
pili trianguli et canaliculi see also *uncombable hair syndrome*
uncombable, silvery-blond, wiry hair (spun-glass hair)
difficult to groom
may improve with age
caused by premature keratinization of inner root sheath and canalicular depressions along hair shaft
can occur in other syndromes (progeria, Wilson disease)
autosomal dominant

6 other defects
scalp whorls
scalp hair patterns develop after 10–12 weeks of fetal development, may be multiple

> **References**
> **Birnbaum PS, Baden HP:** Heritable disorders of hair. Dermatol Clin 1987; 5:137–153.
> **Camacho-Martinez F, Ferrando J:** Hair shaft dysplasias. Int J Dermatol 1988; 27:71–80.
> **Price VH:** Disorders of the hair in children. Pediatr Clin N Am 1978; 25:305–320.
> **Reda AM, Rogers RS, Peters MS:** Woolly hair nevus. J Am Acad Dermatol 1990; 22:377–380.
> **Samlaska CP, James WD, Sperling LC:** Scalp whorls. J Am Acad Dermatol 1989; 21:553–556.
> **Stroud JD:** Hair shaft anomalies. Dermatol Clin 1987; 5:581–594.
> **Whiting DA:** Structural abnormalities of the hair shaft. J Am Acad Dermatol 1987; 16:1–25.
> **Zitelli JA:** Pseudomonilethrix. Arch Dermatol 1986; 122:688–690.

HALLERMANN–STREIFF SYNDROME, OCULOMANDIBULOFACIAL SYNDROME, OCULOMANDIBULODYSCEPHALY WITH HYPOTRICHOSIS SYNDROME, FRANÇOIS SYNDROME

Manifestations and Major Findings
short stature
scalp hair becomes sparse and brittle
alopecia along sides and back of head, and along cranial sutures
hypotrichosis of whole body

vitiligo
normal mentation or retardation

OCULAR ABNORMALITIES
microphthalmia
congenital bilateral cataracts

DENTAL ABNORMALITIES
natal teeth
malformed teeth
anodontia
dental hypoplasia

Characteristic Facies
dyscephaly
– brachycephaly
– microcephaly
– frontal bossing
– disproportionately small face with narrow nose
micrognathia
microstomia
centrofacial skin atrophy with telangiectasia
scanty eyebrows and eyelashes

> **References**
> Cohen MM: Hallermann–Streiff Syndrome: a review. Am J Med Genet 1991; 41:488–499.

HALLOPEAU, ACRODERMATITIS CONTINUA OF *see* ACRODERMATITIS CONTINUA OF HALLOPEAU

HALLOPEAU–SIEMENS TYPE EPIDERMOLYSIS BULLOSA
see EPIDERMOLYSIS BULLOSA; DYSTROPHIC

HALLOPEAU TYPE PEMPHIGUS VEGETANS, PYODERMA VEGETANS

Manifestations and Major Findings
variant of pemphigus vulgaris
primary lesions are pustular
- chronic pustular and vegetative lesions (Fig. 64) in axillae and groin
oral lesions common

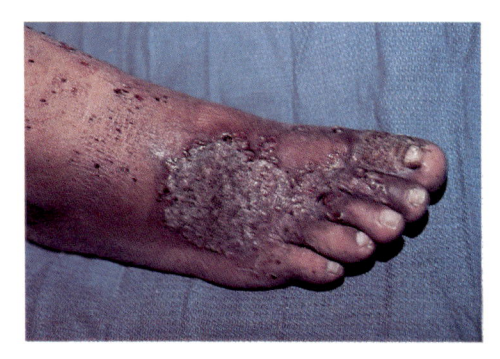

• *Figure 64* Hallopeau type pemphigus vegetans presenting as chronic, pustular, vegetative lesions on the foot.

> **References**
> Nelson CG, Apisarnthanarax P, Bean SF, et al.: Pemphigus vegetans of Hallopeau. Arch Dermatol 1977; 113:942–945.

HALO NEVUS
see SUTTON NEVUS

HAND-FOOT-AND-MOUTH DISEASE

Manifestations and Major Findings
epidemic infection by enteroviruses
– coxsackievirus (usually A16, A2, A4, A5, A7, A10, and other types)
– enterovirus E17
- 1–2 mm vesicular lesions with red halos (usually oval in shape) on palms (Fig. 65), soles, and oral mucosa

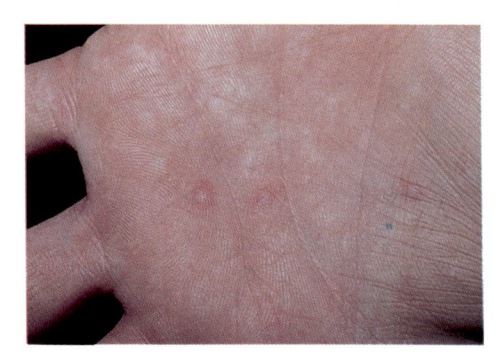

• *Figure 65* Vesicular palmar lesions with red halos are findings in hand-foot-and-mouth disease.

oral scattered vesicles may be painful
lesions often few (< 100)
3–6 day incubation period
mild constitutional symptoms
— malaise
— anorexia
— fever
— diarrhea
self-limited course lasting 3–7 days
encephalitis (rare)

> **References**
> Ishimaru Y, Nakano S, Yamaoka K, et al.: Outbreak of hand, foot and mouth disease caused by Enterovirus 71. Arch Dis Child 1980; 55:583–588.

HAND–SCHÜLLER–CHRISTIAN DISEASE see HISTIOCYTOSIS

HANSEN DISEASE, LEPROSY, HANSENIASIS

Manifestations and Major Findings
chronic infection of skin, peripheral nerves, and other tissues caused by *Mycobacterium leprae*
variable prodrome
most common in tropical/subtropical regions

Types of Leprosy and Features

1 indeterminate leprosy
usually the first signs of infection
macular hypoesthetic lesions
lesions most commonly found on face, extensor surfaces of limbs, buttocks, and trunk
sparing of flexural areas and scalp
paresthesias or numbness common

2 tuberculoid leprosy (TT)
immunologically stable
• well-defined, hypopigmented or erythematous, anesthetic macules (Fig. 66) numbering 1–10
ringed papules with indistinct border
asymmetrical distribution (anywhere)
hair growth impaired
nerve damage with weakness
new lesions characterized by hyperesthesia
marked anesthesia (first loss of temperature, later loss of pain)
early loss of autonomic function in skin and nerve lesions
sweating impaired

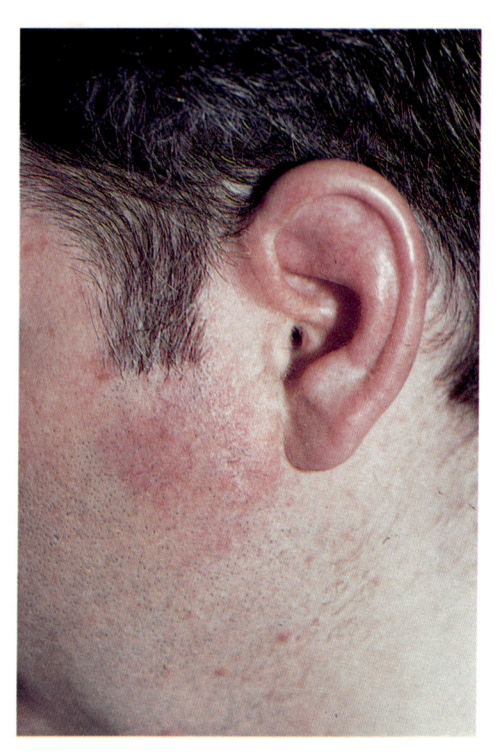

• *Figure 66 A well-defined, erythematous, anesthetic macule on the face in Hansen disease (tuberculoid leprosy stage).*

marked peripheral nerve enlargement
no mucosal or systemic involvement
positive Mitsuda reaction
no *M. leprae* organisms detectable in lesion

3 lepromatous leprosy (LL)
immunologically stable but progressive disease
unrestrained multiplication of *M. leprae*
widespread mucocutaneous membrane lesions
hypopigmented or erythematous macules with ill-defined margins and shiny surface
nodules on face and ears causing leonine facies if untreated
generalized skin thickening (diffuse involvement)
symmetrical distribution with spared areas
slight or ill-defined, late anesthesia – may be extensive over cool areas of the body
late and extensive loss of autonomic function
nerve enlargement slight but widespread
mucosal and systemic involvement common – may be severe during type 2 reactions
numerous *M. leprae* organisms detectable in all affected tissues
early symptoms of lepromatous leprosy
– nasal stuffiness, discharge, and epistaxis
– edema of the legs

4 borderline (dimorphous) leprosy (BB)
intermediate between tuberculoid and lepromatous leprosy
most common type
immunologically unstable – depends on host immune status or treatment and tends to up- and down-grade with time and treatment
nerves widely affected causing
– atrophy of the muscles
– hypoesthesia
– decreased sweating
slit-skin smear shows acid-fast bacilli
Borderline leprosy has three subtypes: borderline tuberculoid (BT), borderline (BB), and borderline lepromatous (BL).

Lepromin Testing

1 lepromin test
intradermal inoculation of standardized extract of lepromatous tissue
not diagnostic
strongly positive in TT leprosy
weakly positive in BT leprosy
negative in BB, BL, and LL leprosy
unpredictable in indeterminate leprosy

2 Fernandez reaction
early lepromin test
read at 48 hours
indicates delayed hypersensitivity to antigens of *M. leprae* or a cross-reacting *Mycobacterium*

3 Mitsuda reaction
late lepromin test (delayed hypersensitivity)
read at 3–4 weeks
papule greater than 4mm indicates a person is capable of mounting an efficient cell-mediated response to *M. leprae*

Reaction States in Leprosy

1 lepra reaction
change in immunologic state – upgrading (reversal) or downgrading (worsening) reaction
acute or insidious pain in affected nerves with loss of function
existing skin lesions enlarge, becoming painful (rarely ulcerating)
edema
reactions occur spontaneously or during treatment

2 erythema nodosum leprosum
systemic involvement with fever and characteristic skin lesions
painful red nodules in skin which may suppurate or ulcerate or form
brawny indurations
more common in lepromatous leprosy
neuritis
uveitis
arthritis
myositis

3 Lucio phenomenon (erythema necroticans)
seen in diffuse lepromatous leprosy with necrotic lesions
irregular erythematous patches form bullae, necrose, and form ulcers
may be fatal
analogous to Arthus reaction

> **References**
> **Binford CH, Meyers WM, Walsh GP:** Leprosy. J Am Med Assoc 1982; 247:2283–2292.
> **Jacobson R:** The face of leprosy in the United States today. Arch Dermatol 1990; 126:1627–1630.
> **Lumpkin LR, Cox GF, Wolf JE:** Leprosy in five armadillo handlers. J Am Acad Dermatol 1983; 9:899–903.
> **Sehgal VN:** Reactions in leprosy, clinical aspects. Int J Dermatol 1987; 26:278–285.
> **Sehgal VN, Srivastava G:** Leprosy in children. Int J Dermatol 1987; 26:557–566.

HAPPY PUPPET SYNDROME
see ANGELMAN SYNDROME

HARADA SYNDROME
see VOGT–KOYANAGI–HARADA SYNDROME

HARLEQUIN FETUS
see also DISORDERS OF CORNIFICATION; DOC 7

Manifestations and Major Findings
massive hyperkeratotic plates on newborn skin resembling the diamond pattern of a harlequin's costume
grotesquely distorted facial features with ectropion, eclabium, and small or absent ears
stillborn/early death
low birth weight/premature
hypoplastic or absent nails
long-term survivors show severe erythroderma

histology shows absence of lamellar bodies by electron microscopy

autosomal recessive

> **References**
> **Dale BA, Holbrook KA, Fleckman P, Kimball JR, et al.:** Heterogeneity in harlequin ichthyosis, an inborn error of epidermal keratinization: variable morphology and structural protein expression and a defect in lamellar granules. J Invest Dermatol 1990; 94:6–18.
> **Fleck RM, Barnadas M, Schulz WW, Roberts LJ, et al.:** Harlequin ichthyosis: an ultrastructural study. J Am Acad Dermatol 1989; 21:999–1006.
> **Rogers M, Scarf C:** Harlequin baby treated with etretinate. Pediatr Dermatol 1989; 6:216–221.

HARTNUP DISEASE

Manifestations and Major Findings
tryptophan malabsorption in the gastrointestinal tract
malabsorption causes decreased synthesis of nicotinic acid
onset usually 3–9 years of age
pellagra-like skin eruption (scaling in sun-exposed areas)
intermittent cerebellar ataxia, nystagmus, and diplopia
psychiatric manifestations (psychosis, emotional lability) are less common
aminoaciduria (excessive indicanuria)

autosomal recessive

> **References**
> **Lee EB:** Metabolic diseases and the skin. Pediatr Clin N Am 1983; 30:597–608.

HASHIMOTO–PRITZKER DISEASE
see HISTIOCYTOSIS

HAXTHAUSEN DISEASE, KERATODERMA CLIMACTERICUM

Manifestations and Major Findings
affects postmenopausal women
painful hyperkeratosis of the palms and soles
thickening of skin over the knees
obesity

> **References**
> **Deschamps P, Leroy D, Pedailles S, Mandard JC:** Keratoderma climactericum (Haxthausen's disease): clinical signs, laboratory findings and etretinate treatment in 10 patients. Dermatologica 1986; 172:258–262.
> **Zultak M, Bedeaux C, Blanc D:** Keratoderma climactericum treatment with topical estrogen. Dermatologica 1988; 176:151–152.

HAY–WELLS SYNDROME
see ANKYLOBLEPHARON–ECTODERMAL DYSPLASIA–CLEFTING SYNDROME

HECK DISEASE, FOCAL EPITHELIAL HYPERPLASIA

Manifestations and Major Findings
virally-induced benign epithelial proliferations
human papillomavirus types 13 and 32 involved
numerous ovoid or round papules (1–2 mm) with smooth or slightly corrugated surface of the oral mucosa
most commonly affects American Indian, Eskimo, and South American children
histology shows numerous binucleate epithelial cells in the midepidermis

> **References**
> **Buchner A, Ramon Y:** Focal epithelial hyperplasia: report of two cases from Israel and review of the literature. Arch Dermatol 1973; 107:97–98.
> **Jaramillo F, Rodríguez G:** Multiple oral papules in a native South American girl. Arch Dermatol 1991; 127:887–892.
> **Starnik TM, Woerdeman MJ:** Focal epithelial hyperplasia of the oral mucosa: report of two cases from the Netherlands and review of the literature. Br J Dermatol 1977; 96:375–380. ▷ ▷ ▷

> Tan KN, Medak H, Cohen L, Burlakow P: Focal epithelial hyperplasia in a Mexican Indian. Arch Dermatol 1969; 100:474–477.

HEERFORDT SYNDROME,
UVEOPAROTID FEVER, HEERFORDT–WALDENSTRÖM SYNDROME

Manifestations and Major Findings
sarcoidosis
enlargement of parotid and lacrimal glands
anterior uveitis
fever
facial and cranial nerve palsies

HELWEG-LARSSEN–LUDWIGSEN SYNDROME, HYPOHIDROSIS WITH NEUROLABYRINTHITIS

Manifestations and Major Findings
congenital anhidrosis or severe hypohidrosis
neurolabyrinthitis developing in fourth or fifth decade
no dental or hair anomalies

autosomal dominant

> **References**
> Reed WB, Stone VM, Boder E, et al.: Hereditary syndromes with auditory and dermatologic manifestations. Arch Dermatol 1967; 95:456–459.

HEMANGIOMA–THROMBOCYTOPENIA SYNDROME see KASABACH–MERRITT SYNDROME

HEMOLYTIC UREMIC SYNDROME

Manifestations and Major Findings
renal cortical necrosis with acute renal insufficiency
microangiopathic hemolytic anemia with burr cells, helmet cells, and schistocytes
purpura caused by leukocytoclastic vasculitis
thrombocytopenia
infants and young children affected
prodrome with coryza and cough
gastrointestinal bleeding and diarrhea
Escherichia coli infection in the stool
central nervous system disturbances
–confusion
–somnolence
–convulsions
–coma

> **References**
> Bell WR, Braine HG, Ness PM, Kickler TS: Improved survival in thrombotic thrombocytopenic purpura-hemolytic-uremic syndrome. N Engl J Med 1991; 325:398–403.
> Martin DL, MacDonald KL, White KE, Soler JT, et al.: The epidemiology and clinical aspects of the hemolytic uremic syndrome in Minnesota. N Engl J Med 1990; 323:1161–1167.
> Piette WW, Stone MS: A cutaneous sign of IgA-associated small dermal vessel leukocytoclastic vasculitis in adults (Henoch–Schönlein purpura). Arch Dermatol 1989; 125:53–56.
> Rowe PC, Orrbine E, Wells GA, McLaine PN, et al.: Epidemiology of hemolytic-uremic syndrome in Canadian children from 1986 to 1988. J Pediatr 1991; 119:218–224.
> Siegler RL, Edwin SS, Christofferson RD, Mitchell MD: Endothelin in the urine of children with the hemolytic uremic syndrome. Pediatrics 1991; 88:1063–1066.
> Siegler RL, Milligan MK, Burningham TH, Christofferson RD, et al.: Long-term outcome and prognostic indicators in the hemolytic-uremic syndrome. J Pediatr 1991; 118:195–200.

HEMOPHAGOCYTIC SYNDROME

Manifestations and Major Findings
panniculitis
purpura
pancytopenia
hepatosplenomegaly
lymphadenopathy
high fever
coagulopathy
histology shows proliferation of mature histiocytes with prominent erythrophagocytosis and cytophagocytosis
associated with viral infection by cytomegalovirus, Epstein–Barr virus, or varicella-zoster virus

References
Danish EH, Dahms BB, Kumar ML: Cytomegalovirus-associated hemophagocytic syndrome. Pediatrics 1985; 75:280–283.
Smith KJ, Skelton HG, Yeager J, Angritt P, et al.: Cutaneous histopathologic, immunohistochemical, and clinical manifestations in patients with hemophagocytic syndrome. Arch Dermatol 1992; 128:193–200.

Olson JC, Kelly KJ, Pan CG, Wortmann DW: Pulmonary disease with hemorrhage in Henoch–Schönlein purpura. Pediatrics 1992; 89:1177–1181.
Piette WW, Stone MS: A cutaneous sign of IgA-associated small dermal vessel leukocytoclastic vasculitis in adults (Henoch–Schönlein purpura). Arch Dermatol 1989; 125:53–56.

HENOCH–SCHÖNLEIN PURPURA, ANAPHYLACTOID PURPURA

Manifestations and Major Findings
prodromal symptoms of headache, anorexia, and fever
gastrointestinal pain and hemorrhage (intussusception)
painful swelling of the joints (polyarthralgia)
localized edema with easy bruising – commonly of face, scalp, and dorsa of the hands
- palpable purpura or erythematous urticarial lesions (Fig. 67)
leukocytoclastic vasculitis with perivascular IgA on direct immunofluorescence
hematuria and/or proteinuria (usually transient)
chronic renal failure (rare)
most often occurs at 4–7 years of age
preceding infection (viral or streptococcal)
elevated serum IgA

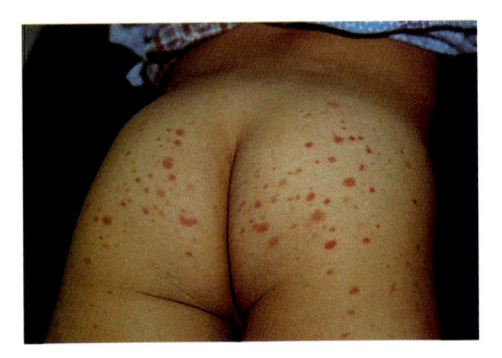

- *Figure 67* Purpuric lesions seen in Henoch–Schönlein purpura, classically below the wrist.

References
Dubin BA, Bronson DM, Eng AM: Acute hemorrhagic edema of childhood: an unusual variant of leukocytoclastic vasculitis. J Am Acad Dermatol 1990; 23:347–350.

HEPARIN NECROSIS

Manifestations and Major Findings
cutaneous necrosis at the site of heparin injections – occasionally at distal sites
burning pain in lesions
most often associated with subcutaneous heparin injection (but may be intravenous)
large vessel thrombosis with epidermal necrosis
thrombocytopenia
occurs most often in obese, middle-aged, diabetic women on the abdomen or thighs
lesions begin 6–13 days after injection

References
Gold JA, Watters AK, O'Brien E: Coumarin versus heparin necrosis. J Am Acad Dermatol 1987; 16:148–150.
Hall JC, McConahay D, Gibson D, Crockett J, et al.: Heparin necrosis. An anticoagulation syndrome. J Am Med Assoc 1980; 244:1831–1832.
Tuneu A, Moreno A, de Moragas JM: Cutaneous reactions secondary to heparin injections. J Am Acad Dermatol 1985; 12:1072–1077.

HEPATOLENTICULAR DEGENERATION SYNDROME
see WILSON DISEASE

HEREDITARY ACROKERATOTIC POIKILODERMA, WEARY SYNDROME, WEARY–KINDLER SYNDROME

Manifestations and Major Findings
acral vesicles and bullae in infancy
eczematous dermatitis in childhood (spares the face)
mottled poikiloderma

reticulated hyperpigmentation (especially flexural areas)
keratotic papules develop in childhood on the hands, feet, knees, and elbows

autosomal dominant

References
Hovnanian A, Blanchet-Bardon C, deProst Y: Poikiloderma of Theresa Kindler: report of a case with ultrastructural study, and review of the literature. Pediatr Dermatol 1989; 6:82–90.
Weary PE, Manley WF, Graham GF: Hereditary acrokeratotic poikiloderma. Arch Dermtol 1971; 103:409–422.

HEREDIATRY ANGIOEDEMA,
ANGIONEUROTIC EDEMA

Manifestations and Major Findings
absent or dysfunctioning C1 esterase inhibitor
usual onset in early childhood
associated with abdominal or urinary symptoms

Cutaneous Manifestations
urticaria or edema in deep subcutaneous tissues
commonly involves lips, eyelids, genitalia, tongue, and larynx
itching absent
lesions often painful
lesions last a few hours to 3 days
may be fatal with laryngeal involvement and obstruction

autosomal dominant

References
Colten HR: Hereditary angioneurotic edema 1887–1987. N Engl J Med 1987; 317:43–45.
Donaldson VH: The challenge of hereditary angioneurotic edema. N Engl J Med 1983; 308:1094–1095.

HEREDITARY HEMORRHAGIC TELANGIECTASIA
see OSLER–WEBER–RENDU SYNDROME

HEREDITARY SCLEROSING POIKILODERMA OF WEARY

Manifestations and Major Findings
generalized poikiloderma beginning in childhood
sclerosis of the palms and soles
- linear and reticulated hyperkeratotic or sclerotic bands in flexural areas (Fig. 68)
clubbing of the fingers
calcinosis of the soft tissues
dental caries
normal hair
normal nails

autosomal dominant

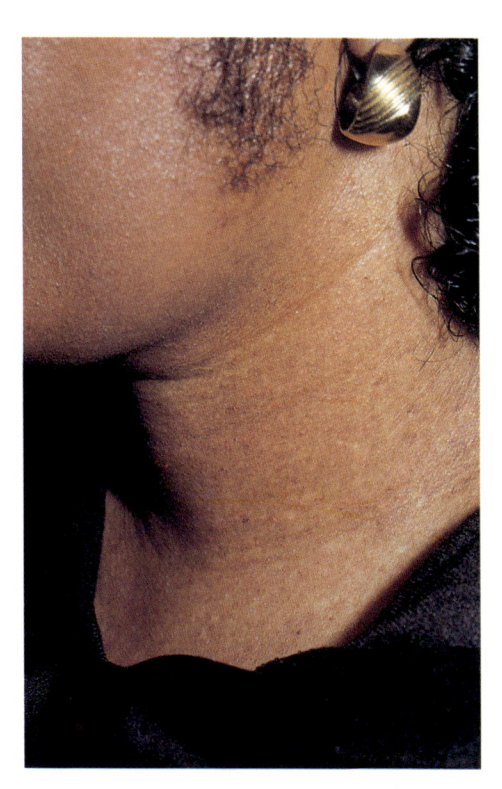

• *Figure 68 Poikiloderma of the neck is a feature of hereditary sclerosing poikiloderma of Weary.*

References
Weary PE, Hsu Y-T, Richardson DR, Caravati CM, et al.: Hereditary sclerosing poikiloderma: report of two families with an unusual and distinctive genodermatosis. Arch Dermatol 1969; 100:413–422.

▷ ▷ ▷

> ▷ ▷ ▷
> Vennos EM, Collins M, James WD: Rothmund–Thomson syndrome: review of the world literature. J Am Acad Dermatol 1992; 27:750–762.

HERLITZ TYPE EPIDERMOLYSIS BULLOSA see EPIDERMOLYSIS BULLOSA; JUNCTIONAL

HERMANSKY–PUDLAK SYNDROME see also ALBINISM

Manifestations and Major Findings
tyrosinase-positive albinism
cream-colored or hypopigmented skin color
yellow, red, or brown hair
blue-gray to brown eyes
nystagmus and photophobia may be present
prolonged bleeding time
abnormal platelet aggregation (absence of dense bodies)
yellow, ultraviolet-fluorescing, ceroid deposits in bone marrow macrophages, reticuloendothelial system, and other organs
fatal bleeding after aspirin ingestion
pulmonary involvement (ceroid deposition)
granulomatous colitis
most common in Puerto Rico and Holland

autosomal recessive

> **References**
> Mahadeo R, Markowitz J, Fisher S, Daum F: Hermansky–Pudlak syndrome with granulomatous colitis in children. J Pediatr 1991; 118:904–906.
> Gregory B, Ho VC: Cutaneous manifestations of gastrointestinal disorders. Part II. J Am Acad Dermatol 1992; 26:371–383.
> Bologna JL, Pawelek JM: Biology of hypopigmentation. J Am Acad Dermatol 1988; 19:217–255.
> Schachne JP, Glaser N, Lee S, Kress Y, et al.: Hermansky–Pudlak syndrome: case report and clinicopathologic review. J Am Acad Dermatol 1990; 22:926–932.

HIDROTIC ECTODERMAL DYSPLASIA SYNDROME
see ECTODERMAL DYSPLASIA; HIDROTIC

HIRSCHSPRUNG DISEASE

Manifestations and Major Findings
agangliosis of gastrointestinal tract
absence of parasympathetic ganglion cells from submucosal and myenteric plexuses of the gut
Hirschsprung disease is associated with Down syndrome, Waardenburg syndrome, neuroblastoma, pheochromocytoma, pyloric stenosis, deafness, and Aarskog syndrome.

> **References**
> Mallory SB, Wiener E, Nordlund JJ: Waardenburg syndrome with Hirschsprung's disease. Pediatr Dermatol 1986; 3:119–124.

HISTIOCYTOSIS, LANGERHANS CELL HISTIOCYTOSIS

Types of Histiocytosis and Features

1 acute disseminated histiocytosis, Letterer–Siwe disease
accumulation of Langerhans cells (monocyte/macrophage cell series) in various tissues
cutaneous findings
– • purpuric seborrheic dermatitis (characteristically of the scalp) (Fig. 69)
– reddish-brown purpuric papules and nodules
– • moist erosions/ulcerations, accentuated in the flexures (Fig. 70)
– lesions mainly in the groin and postauricular areas
– external and middle ear involvement common with crusted petechial scaling or draining
hepatosplenomegaly
generalized lymphadenopathy
fever
malaise
failure to thrive
diarrhea
mastoid involvement (X-ray diagnosis)
oral involvement
– periodontal inflammation
– infiltration of the gums
– loss of teeth
lung involvement
– dyspnea
– pneumothorax
bone involvement – especially calvarium, femur, scapulae, ribs, and vertebrae
– asymptomatic or with swelling, pain, or pathologic fractures

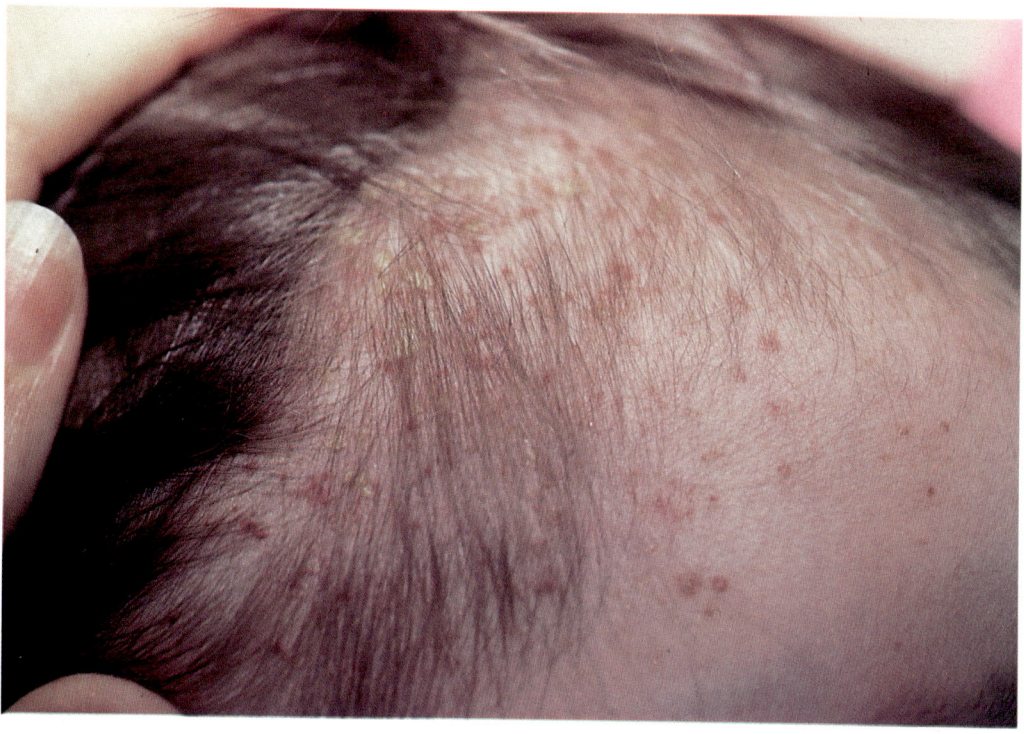

Figure 69 Purpuric seborrheic papules of the scalp in acute disseminated Langerhans cell histiocytosis (Letterer–Siwe disease).

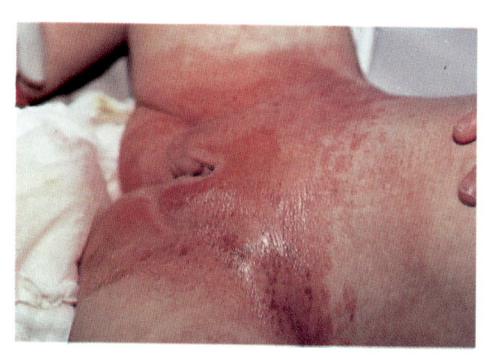

Figure 70 Moist ulcerative erosions of the groin in acute disseminated Langerhans cell histiocytosis (Letterer–Siwe disease).

cutaneous hemorrhagic eczematous or xanthomatous lesions
histiocytic granulomas in liver, spleen, skeletal system, lungs, gastrointestinal tract, central nervous system, lymph nodes, and bone marrow
stomatitis
onset usually before 5 years of age

3 eosinophilic granuloma
chronic localized histiocytosis
lesions most common in the bones – skin or oral mucosa may be involved
usually chronic
tendency toward spontaneous healing

4 congenital self-healing reticulohistiocytosis, Hashimoto–Pritzker disease
- congenital asymptomatic papules and nodules or papulovesicles (Fig. 71)
generalized distribution
lesions regress spontaneously within a few months
no recurrences
lesion number varies from one to numerous
lesions resemble healing varicella
no systemic involvement
electron microscopy shows Birbeck granules and dense bodies in the histiocytes

neuroendocrine involvement
– diabetes insipidus
– growth hormone deficiency
onset usually before 3 years of age

2 chronic multifocal histiocytosis, Hand–Schüller–Christian disease
triad of findings
– osteolytic bone defects (usually the skull)
– exophthalmos (retro-orbital infiltration)
– diabetes insipidus (pituitary stalk involvement)

▷ ▷ ▷

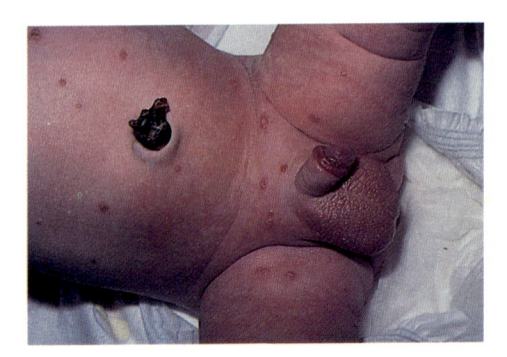

Figure 71 Asymptomatic lesions resembling healing varicella in congenital self-healing reticulohistiocytosis.

▷ ▷ ▷
5 xanthoma disseminatum
histiocytosis of mononuclear phagocytes other than Langerhans cells (non-X histiocytosis)
no lipid abnormalities
disseminated xanthomas (clustering in flexural areas)
visceral involvement possible
pituitary involvement with diabetes insipidus
usual good prognosis, but may have extensive skin involvement

References
Berger TG, Lane AT, Headington JT, Kartmann K, et al.: A solitary variant of congenital self-healing reticulohistiocytosis: solitary Hashimoto–Pritzker disease. Pediatr Dermatol 1985; 3:230–236.
Dolezal JF, Thomson ST: Hand–Schüller–Christian disease in a septuagenarian. Arch Dermatol 1978; 114:85–87.
Knobler RM, Neumann RA, Gebhart W, Radaskiewicz T, et al.: Xanthoma disseminatum with progressive involvement of the central nervous and hepatobiliary systems. J Am Acad Dermatol 1990; 23:341–346.
Moschella SL, Cropley TG: Mononuclear phagocytic and dendritic cell systems. J Am Acad Dermatol 1990; 22:1091–1097.
Parker F: Xanthomas and hyperlipidemias. J Am Acad Dermatol 1985; 13:1–30.
Roper SS, Spraker MK: Cutaneous histiocytosis syndromes. Pediatr Dermatol 1985; 3:19–30.
Varotti C, Bettoli V, Berti E, Cavicchini S, et al.: Xanthoma disseminatum: a case with extensive mucous membrane involvement. J Am Acad Dermatol 1991; 25:433–436.
Wood GS, Haber RS: Novel histiocytoses considered in the context of histiocyte subset differentiation. Arch Dermatol 1993; 129:210–214.

HODGKIN DISEASE

Manifestations and Major Findings
malignant disorder arising in lymph nodes
Reed–Sternberg cells (large bizarre nuclei in reticulum cells) are pathognomonic
adenopathy – usually in neck, axillae, or groin
fever
night sweats
fatigue
weight loss
localized or generalized pruritus
pulmonary involvement
superior vena caval obstruction
spinal cord compression
bone involvement – usually painful
hepatic involvement
infectious complications
immunologic abnormalities

Cutaneous Manifestations
small dermal nodules on the scalp
nonspecific skin lesions more common
hyperpigmentation (may resemble Addison disease)
prurigo nodularis
ichthyosiform atrophy – initially on the legs, may become universal
alopecia
exfoliative dermatitis
herpes zoster
erythema nodosum

References
Hayes TG, Rabin VR, Rosen T, Zubler MA: Hodgkin's disease presenting in the skin: case report and review of the literature. J Am Acad Dermatol 1990; 22:944–947.

HOLOCARBOXYLASE DEFICIENCY
see BIOTIN DEFICIENCY

HOLT–ORAM SYNDROME,
HEART–HAND SYNDROME

Manifestations and Major Findings
upper limb defects (may be asymmetric)
- thumb hypoplasia
- phocomelia
- upper limb bone defects
cardiac anomalies
- atrial septal defect
- ventricular septal defect

OCCASIONAL FINDINGS
hypertelorism
absent pectoralis major muscle
vertebral anomalies

autosomal dominant

HOMOCYSTINURIA

Manifestations and Major Findings
deficiency of cystathionine β-synthase or methyltetrahydrofolate homocysteine methyltransferase
dolichostenomelia
marfanoid appearance
ocular abnormalities
- myopia
- ectopia lentis
increased platelet adhesiveness
arterial and venous thromboses
premature arteriosclerotic vascular disease
central nervous system involvement
- low intelligence
- seizures
- psychiatric abnormalities
joint hyperextensibility
hepatomegaly
tall stature
arachnodactyly
osteoporosis
scoliosis
'codfish' vertebrae with vertebral collapse
homocysteine in the urine
positive urine cyanide-nitroprusside test

Cutaneous Manifestations
malar flush
large facial pores
livedo reticularis of the legs
tissue-paper scars on the hands
pigmentary dilution of the skin and hair
fine, sparse, and brittle hair

autosomal recessive

> **References**
> Carson NAJ, Dent CE, Field CMB, Gaull GE: Homocystinuria: clinical and pathological review of ten cases. J Pediatr 1965; 66:565–583.
> Clarke R, Daly L, Robinson K, Naughten E, Cahalane S, et al.: Hyperhomocysteinemia: an independent risk factor for vascular disease. N Engl J Med 1991; 324:1149–1155.
> Lee EB: Metabolic disease and the skin. Pediatr Clin N Am 1983; 30:597–608.

HOWEL–EVANS SYNDROME,
HOWEL–EVANS–CLARK SYNDROME

Manifestations and Major Findings
palmoplantar keratoderma (late onset)
carcinoma of esophagus
oral leukoplakia

autosomal dominant or sporadic transmission

> **References**
> Gregory B, Ho VC: Cutaneous manifestations of gastrointestinal disorders. Part I. J Am Acad Dermatol 1992; 26:153–166.
> Khanna SK, Agnone FA, Leibowitz AI, Raschke RA, et al.: Nonfamilial diffuse palmoplantar keratoderma associated with bronchial carcinoma. J Am Acad Dermatol 1993; 28:295–297.
> Parnell DD, Johnson SAM: Tylosis palmaris et plantaris: its occurrence with internal malignancy. Arch Dermatol 1969; 100:7–9

HUNTER SYNDROME
see MUCOPOLYSACCHARIDOSES; TYPE II

HUNZIKER–LAUGIER SYNDROME
see LAUGIER–HUNZIKER SYNDROME

HURIEZ SYNDROME

Manifestations and Major Findings
present at birth or in early childhood
internal malignancy
affects Belgian families

Cutaneous Manifestations
diffuse scleroatrophy of the hands
sclerodactyly
nail changes with aplasia, ridging, and clubbing
keratoderma of the palms
hypohidrosis
squamous cell carcinoma may develop in atrophic skin

autosomal dominant

> **References**
> Griffiths WAD, Leigh IM, Marks R 1992. Disorders of keratinization. In Rook/Wilkinson/Ebling (eds.) Textbook of Dermatology, 5th edition, p.1382. (London: Blackwell Scientific Publications).
> Patrizi A, DiLernia V, Patrone P: Palmoplantar keratoderma with sclerodactyly (Huriez syndrome). J Am Acad Dermatol 1992; 26:855–857.

HURLER SYNDROME
see MUCOPOLYSACCHARIDOSES; TYPE I

HUTCHINSON–GILFORD SYNDROME see PROGERIA

HUTCHINSON SUMMER PRURIGO, ACTINIC PRURIGO

Manifestations and Major Findings
childhood onset
delayed papular eczematous eruption on UVA/UVB exposure
accentuated in photodistribution
most common in American Indians

HYDANTOIN SYNDROME,
PSEUDOLYMPHOMA SYNDROME, DILANTIN SYNDROME, PHENYTOIN SYNDROME

Manifestations and Major Findings
caused by phenytoin
- morbilliform, scarlatiniform, urticarial or exfoliative dermatitis (Fig. 72)

fever
malaise
arthralgia
lymphadenopathy (particularly cervical)
hepatic abnormalities
eosinophilia

Lymph node biopsy may reveal certain features suggestive of lymphoma.

> **References**
> Silverman AK, Fairley J, Wong RC: Cutaneous and immunologic reactions to phenytoin. J Am Acad Dermatol 1988; 18:721–741.
> Tomsick RS: The phenytoin syndrome. Cutis 1983; 32:535–541.

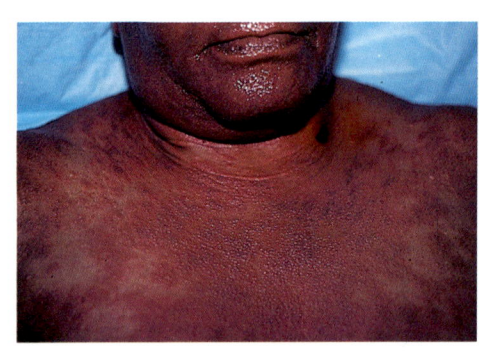

• *Figure 72 Dermatitis caused by phenytoin hypersensitivity in hydantoin syndrome.*

HYPEREOSINOPHILIC SYNDROME

Manifestations and Major Findings
persistent blood eosinophilia (>1500/mm^3 for >6 months)
no apparent cause (e.g. parasites, allergies, drugs)
prominent organ involvement (heart, lungs, liver, spleen, hematopoietic) with eosinophilia
fever

weight loss
malaise
diarrhea
arthralgia
affects middle-aged males
Hypereosinophilic syndrome is associated with lymphomatoid papulosis and aquagenic pruritus.

Cutaneous Manifestations
urticaria
angioedema
nonspecific pruritic maculopapular eruption
dermatographism

> **References**
> **Chusid MJ, Dale DC, West BC, et al.:** The hypereosinophilic syndrome. Medicine 1975; 54:1–27.
> **Kazmierowski JA, Chusid MJ, Parrillo JE, Fauci AS:** Dermatologic manifestations of the hypereosinophilic syndrome. Arch Dermatol 1978; 114:531–535.
> **Newton JA, Singh AK, Greaves MW, Spry CJF:** Aquagenic pruritus associated with the idiopathic hypereosinophilic syndrome. Br J Dermatol 1990; 122:103–106.
> **Wolf C, Pehamberger H, Breyer S, Leiferman KM, et al.:** Episodic angioedema with eosinophilia. J Am Acad Dermatol 1989; 20:21–27.

HYPERIMMUNOGLOBULIN E SYNDROME, HYPER IgE SYNDROME, BUCKLEY SYNDROME. HILL–QUIE SYNDROME, JOB SYNDROME

Manifestations and Major Findings
markedly elevated serum IgE (over ten times upper normal limit)
recurrent infections
– skin
– nasal sinuses
– respiratory tract
– ears
– nails
infective organisms
– • *Staphylococcus aureus*, creating cold abscesses (Fig. 73)
– *Candida* (especially nails)
– *Haemophilus influenzae*
– pneumococci
– group A streptococci
– *Aspergillus*

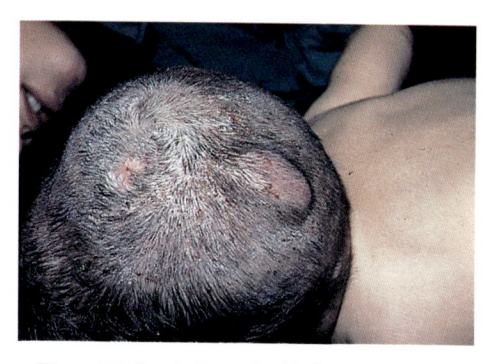

• **Figure 73** Staphylococcal cold abscesses are common infections in hyperimmunoglobulin E syndrome.

infections of ears, sinuses, joints and viscera
recurrent bronchitis and pneumonia
pneumatoceles
lung empyemas
intermittent chemotactic defects
eosinophilia
inconsistent, abnormal cell-mediated immunity
growth failure
coarse facial features
osteoporosis with fractures
craniosynostosis
A subgroup of patients with hyperimmunoglobulin E syndrome who are females with fair skin, red hair, and hyperextensible joints are called Job syndrome patients.

Cutaneous Manifestations
excoriated, papular and pustular eruption (resembling atopic eczema)
eruption favors the scalp and flexures
dystrophic nail changes

> **References**
> **Hill HR:** The syndrome of hyperimmunoglobulinemia E and recurrent infections. Am J Dis Child 1982; 136:767–771.
> **Jeppson JD, Jaffe HS, Hill HR:** Use of recombinant human interferon gamma to enhance neutrophil chemotactic responses in Job syndrome of hyperimmunoglobulinemia E and recurrent infections. J Pediatr 1991; 118:383–387.
> **Kamei R, Honig PJ:** Neonatal Job's syndrome featuring a vesicular eruption. Pediatr Dermatol 1988; 5:75–82.

HYPERLIPIDEMIAS

Hyperlipidemias and their Features

type I; Bürger–Grütz hyperchylomicronemia
rarest form of hyperlipidemia
chylomicron pattern on ultracentrifugation
slightly raised cholesterol
highly raised triglycerides
caused by absence of lipoprotein lipase
onset in early childhood
eruptive xanthomas (66%)
lipemia retinalis
hepatosplenomegaly
abdominal pain
pancreatitis
diabetes
autosomal recessive

type IIA; hyperbetalipoproteinemia, familial hypercholesterolemia
LDL pattern on ultracentrifugation
raised cholesterol
normal/slightly raised triglycerides
caused by nonfunctioning LDL receptors
tuberous, intertriginous and tendon xanthomas
xanthelasma
atherosclerosis
onset in 1st or 2nd decade
hypothyroidism
nephrotic syndrome
autosomal dominant

type IIB; combined hyperlipoproteinemia
LDL/VLDL pattern on ultracentrifugation
raised cholesterol
normal/slightly raised triglycerides
same clinical features as type IIA
adult onset
abnormal glucose tolerance test
hepatic disease
autosomal dominant

type III; broad betalipoproteinemia, familial dysbetalipoproteinemia
chylomicron remnant/VLDL remnant pattern on ultracentrifugation
moderately raised cholesterol (variable)
moderately raised triglycerides
caused by homozygous apo E2-induced decreased remnant clearance combined with VLDL overproduction
adult onset
• planar xanthomas (palmar creases) (Fig. 74)
tuberoeruptive and tuberous xanthomas
xanthelasma
premature atherosclerosis

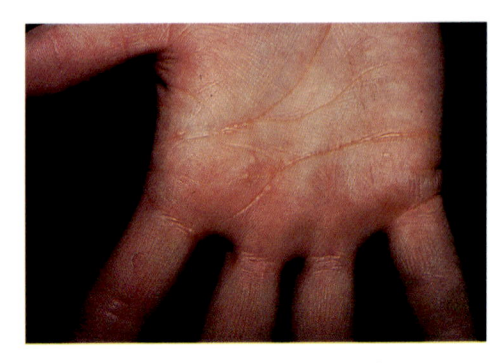

• *Figure 74 Palmar xanthomas are pathognomonic for type III familial dysbetalipoproteinemia.*

type IV; hyperprebetalipoproteinemia
most common form of hyperlipidemia
VLDL pattern on ultracentrifugation
slightly raised cholesterol
moderately raised triglycerides
carbohydrate induced
adult onset
atherosclerosis
abnormal glucose tolerance test
tuberoeruptive xanthomas
hypothyroidism
diabetes
pancreatitis
glycogen storage disease
nephrotic syndrome
multiple myeloma
autosomal dominant

type V; mixed hyperprebetalipoproteinemia and chylomicronemia
chylomicron/VLDL pattern on ultracentrifugation
slightly raised cholesterol
moderately raised triglycerides
caused by VLDL overproduction or defective VLDL catabolism
eruptive xanthomas
abdominal pain
pancreatitis
associated with diabetes mellitus, hypertension, hyperuricemia, and polyneuropathy

Disorders Characterized by the Accumulation of Unusual Sterols

1 cerebrotendinous xanthomatosis
tuberous and tendonous xanthomas
xanthelasma
neurologic dysfunction
cataracts
atherosclerosis

respiratory insufficiency
cholelithiasis
endocrine abnormalities
caused by abnormal bile acid synthesis and cholestanol accumulation
laboratory features
– plasma cholestanol > 1mg/dl
– plasma cholesterol normal or low
– elevated biliary cholestanol and bile acid precursors
– lowered chenodeoxycholic acid
– elevated cholestanol content of xanthomas

2 β-sitosterolemia
tuberous and tendonous xanthomas
xanthelasma
atherosclerosis
hemolysis
platelet disorders
hypersplenism
arthritis
probably caused by intestinal mucosal cell inability to esterify plant sterols resulting in increased absorption
laboratory features
– elevated plasma sitosterol, campesterol, and stigmasterol
– plasma cholesterol normal or slightly elevated
– elevated plant sterol content of xanthomas

Types of Xanthomas, Features, and Associated Diseases

1 eruptive xanthomas
small, yellow papules with reddish base
occur in crops
occasionally coalesce
common sites are buttocks, shoulders, and extensor surfaces of the extremities
pruritus
caused by elevated triglycerides
major associations
– lipoprotein lipase deficiency
– type I familial hyperlipoproteinemia
– type V (mixed hyperprebetalipoproteinemia and chylomicronemia)
– diabetes mellitus
– alcohol ingestion
– estrogen ingestion
– type 1 glycogen-storage disease (von Gierke disease)

2 tendonous xanthomas
slowly enlarging subcutaneous nodules
nodules attached to tendons, ligaments, fascia, and periosteum
asymptomatic
most common on extensor tendons of the hands and feet, and Achilles tendon
causes
– elevated cholesterol
– elevated or altered LDL
major associations
– type IIA familial hypercholesterolemia
– cerebrotendinous xanthomatosis
– β-sitosterolemia
– hyperapobetalipoproteinemia

3 palmar crease xanthomas
planar xanthomas in palmar creases
causes
– elevated chylomicron remnants
– elevated VLDL remnants
major associations
– type III familial dysbetalipoproteinemia (pathognomonic)

4 planar xanthomas
yellow/orange macules
generalized occurence
causes
– elevated cholesterol
major associations
– cirrhosis
– biliary atresia
– type III broad betalipoproteinemia

5 intertriginous xanthomas
slightly raised yellow/orange plaques
cobblestone surface
arise in interdigital webs, axillae, and antecubital and popliteal fossae
causes
– elevated cholesterol
– elevated LDL
major association
– type IIA homozygous familial hypercholesterolemia (pathognomonic)

6 tuberoeruptive/tuberous xanthomas
small papules to lobulated tumors
firm, yellow lesions with erythematous halos
usually painless
seen over pressure areas or extensor surfaces of the limbs, especially knees and elbows
causes
– elevated chylomicron remnants
– elevated VLDL/VLDL remnants
– elevated LDL
major associations
– type III familial dysbetalipoproteinemia
– type IIA homozygous familial hypercholesterolemia (rarely in heterozygote)

▷ ▷ ▷
- cerebrotendinous xanthomatosis
- β-sitosterolemia
- hypothyroidism
- hepatic cholestasis

7 diffuse plane xanthomas (generalized plane xanthomatosis)
diffuse planar xanthomas
occur anywhere
major associations
- dysglobulinemias
- paraproteinemias

8 xanthoma palpebratum (xanthelasmas)
bilateral, symmetrical, soft, velvety plaques
occur around eyelids (usually around inner canthus)
major associations
- many hyperlipidemic states (elevated cholesterol)
- normolipemia
- subtle lipoprotein defects

References
Cruz PD, East C, Bergstresser PR: Dermal, subcutaneous, and tendon xanthomas: diagnostic markers for specific lipoprotein disorders. J Am Acad Dermatol 1988; 19:95–111.
Maher-Wiese VL, Marmer EL, Grant-Kels JM: Xanthomas and the inherited hyperlipoproteinemias in children and adolescents. Pediatr Dermatol 1990; 7:166–173.
Varotti C, Bettoli V, Berti E, Cavicchini S, Caputo R: Xanthomas disseminatum: a case with extensive mucous membrane involvement. J Am Acad Dermatol 1991; 25:433–436.

HYPOCHONDROPLASIA

Manifestations and Major Findings
mild to moderate short limbs
short stature
short, broad hands and feet
near-normal craniofacies
caudal narrowing of the spine
mild bowing of the legs
X-ray features qualitatively similar to achondroplasia but less severe

autosomal dominant

HYPOMELANOSIS OF ITO,
INCONTINENTIA PIGMENTI ACHROMIANS

Manifestations and Major Findings
• asymmetric, hypopigmented whorls and streaks (Fig. 75)
'marble cake' appearance of lesions
lesions follow Blaschko lines to varying extent
usually present at birth
progressive but may repigment

NEUROLOGIC ABNORMALITIES
seizures
mental retardation
EEG abnormalities
developmental delay

OCULAR ABNORMALITIES
strabismus
nystagmus
heterochromia
microphthalmia
hypertelorism

SKELETAL ABNORMALITIES
macrocephaly
scoliosis
limb defects
hypotonia
hemihypertrophy

Dermatologic Syndromes 113

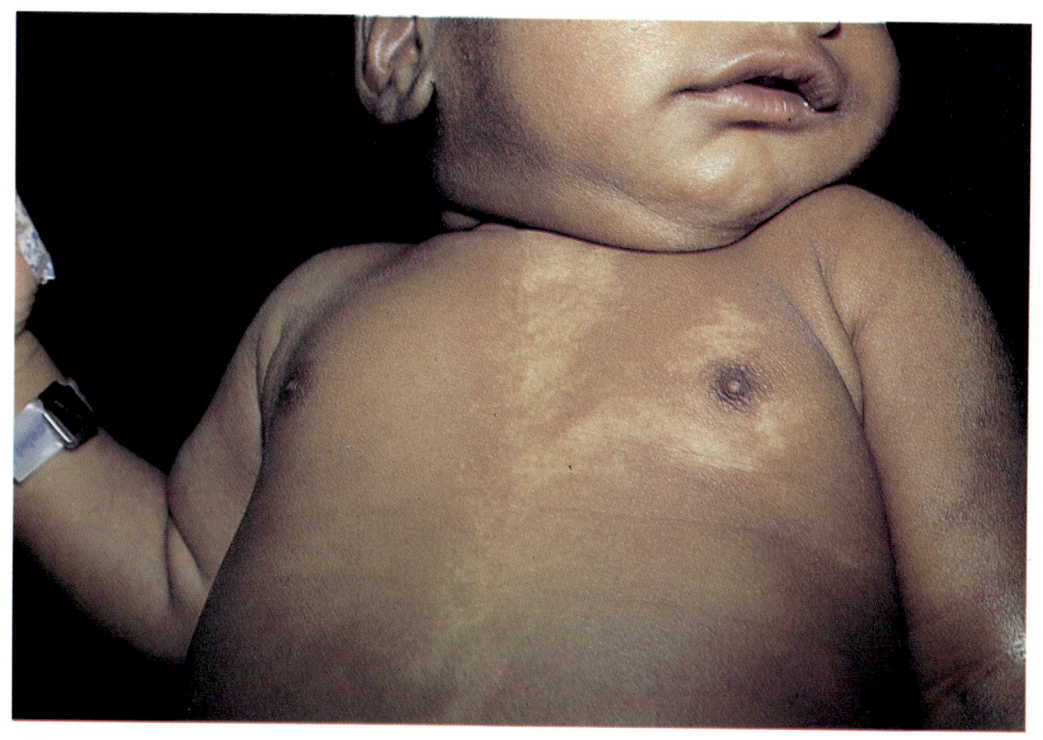

• **Figure 75** *Hypomelanosis of Ito causes asymmetric, hypopigmented whorls and streaks.*

OTHER FINDINGS
diffuse alopecia
ridging of the nails
dental anomalies
deafness

autosomal dominant or sporadic (female predominance)

References
Bolognia JL, Pawelek JM: Biology of hypopigmentation. J Am Acad Dermatol 1988; 19:217–255.

▷ ▷ ▷
Glover MT, Brett EM, Atherton DJ: Hypomelanosis of Ito: spectrum of the disease. J Pediatr 1989; 115: 75–80.
Ruiz-Maldonado R, Toussaint S, Tamayo L, Laterza A, et al.: Hypomelanosis of Ito: diagnostic criteria and report of 41 cases. Pediatr Dermatol 1992; 9:1–10.
Sybert VP: Hypomelanosis of Ito. Pediatr Dermatol 1990; 7:74–76.

I

IBIDS SYNDROME
see TRICHOTHIODYSTROPHY

I-CELL DISEASE see MUCOLIPIDOSIS II

ICHTHYOSES see DISORDERS OF CORNIFICATION

INCONTINENTIA PIGMENTI,
BLOCH–SULZBERGER SYNDROME, BLOCH–SIEMENS SYNDROME

Manifestations and Major Findings
four stages which may overlap
- • vesicles (often in linear groups) in infancy (Fig. 76)
- verrucous lesions usually on extremities
- • irregular marbled pigmentation (blue-gray to brown) usually on the trunk, following Blaschko lines (Fig. 77)

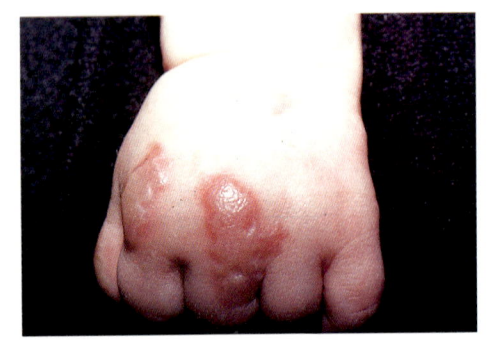

• *Figure 76* Linearly grouped vesicles in the early bullous stage of incontinentia pigmenti.

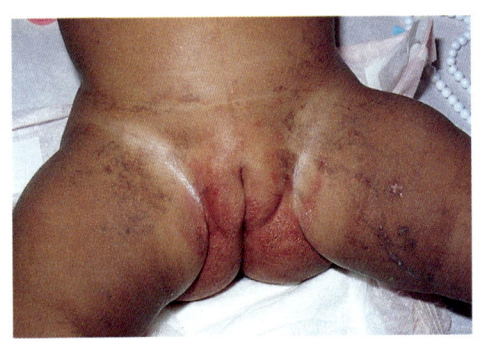

• *Figure 77* Irregular blue-gray/brown hyperpigmented macules sworling along Blaschko lines seen in incontinentia pigmenti. Some keratotic papules are also present.

- hypopigmented streaks
skeletal abnormalities, especially skull
peripheral blood eosinophilia during the blistering stage (up to 50% eosinophils)
mild nail dystrophy
scarring alopecia in patches
hypoplasia of the eyebrows and eyelashes

DENTAL ABNORMALITIES
anodontia
peg-shaped teeth
delayed dentition
caries

NEUROLOGIC ABNORMALITIES
mental retardation
seizures
developmental delay
motor abnormalities
spastic tetraplegia or diplegia

OCULAR ABNORMALITIES
strabismus
cataracts
uveitis
optic atrophy
retinal anomalies

X-linked dominant (short arm of X chromosome); lethal in hemizygous males

> **References**
> **Bessems PJMJ, Jagtman BA, van de Staak WJBM, Hulsmans RFHJ:** Progressive, persistent, hyperkeratotic lesions in incontinentia pigmenti. Arch Dermatol 1988; 124:29–30.
> **Cannizzaro LA, Hecht F:** Gene for incontinentia pigmenti maps to band Xp11 with an (X;10) (p11;q22) translocation. Clin Genet 1987; 32:66–69.
> **Carney RG:** Incontinentia pigmenti: a world statistical analysis. Arch Dermatol 1976; 112:535–542.
> **Cohen BA:** Incontinentia pigmenti. Neurol Clin 1987; 5:361–377.
> **Kegel MF:** Dominant disorders with multiple organ involvement. Dermatol Clin 1987; 5:205–219.
> ▷ ▷ ▷
> **Menni S, Piccinno R, Biolochini A, Plebani A:** Immunologic investigations in eight patients with incontinentia pigmenti. Pediatr Dermatol 1990; 7:275–277.
> **Moss C, Ince P:** Anhidrotic and achromians lesions in incontinentia pigmenti. Br J Dermatol 1987; 116:839–849.
> **Person JR:** Incontinentia pigmenti: a failure of immune tolerance? J Am Acad Dermatol 1985; 13:120–123.
> **Prendiville JS, Gorski JL, Stein CK, Esterly NB:** Incontinentia pigmenti in a male infant with Klinefelter syndrome. J Am Acad Dermatol 1989; 20:937–940.
> **Sommer A, Liu PH:** Incontinentia pigmenti in a father and his daughter. Am J Med Genet 1984; 17:655–659.
> **Wickland DA, Weston WL:** Incontinentia pigmenti: a four generation study. Arch Dermatol 1980; 116:701–703.

INCONTINENTIA PIGMENTI ACHROMIANS
see HYPOMELANOSIS OF ITO

J

JACQUET ULCERS, JACQUET EROSIVE DIAPER DERMATITIS

Manifestations and Major Findings
- 'punched-out' ulcers in diaper area with raised crater-like edges (Fig. 78)
due to infrequent diaper changes

References
Hara M, Watanabe M, Tagami H: Jacquet erosive diaper dermatitis in a young girl with urinary incontinence. Pediatr Dermatol 1991; 8:160–161.

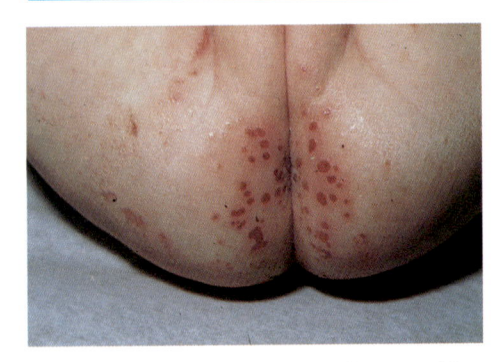

- *Figure 78* 'Punched-out' Jacquet ulcers caused by infrequent diaper changes.

JADASSOHN–LEWANDOWSKY SYNDROME *see* PACHYONYCHIA CONGENITA

JADASSOHN NEVUS *see* NEVUS SEBACEUS OF JADASSOHN

JADASSOHN–PELLIZZARI ANETODERMA

Manifestations and Major Findings
small, discrete, erythematous, dome-shaped papules or localized depressions of the skin
post-inflammatory occurrence
loss of normal elastic fibers
herniation of fatty tissue
elastolysis preceded by erythema or urticaria

References
Hodak E, Shamai-Lubovitz O, David M, Hazaz B, et al.: Primary anetoderma associated with a wide spectrum of autoimmune abnormalities. J Am Acad Dermatol 1991; 25:415–418.
Hodak E, Shamai-Lubovitz O, David M, Hazaz B, et al.: Immunologic abnormalities associated with primary anetoderma. Arch Dermatol 1992; 128:799–803.
Venencie PY, Winkelmann RK: Histopathologic findings in anetoderma. Arch Dermatol 1984; 120:1040–1044.
Venencie PY, Winkelmann RK: Monoclonal antibody studies in the skin lesions of patients with anetoderma. Arch Dermatol 1985; 121:747–749.

JESSNER LYMPHOCYTIC INFILTRATE, JESSNER–KANOF BENIGN LYMPHOCYTIC INFILTRATION, LYMPHOCYTIC INFILTRATION OF THE SKIN

Manifestations and Major Findings
raised erythematous papules or plaques
asymptomatic
lesions usually on the face and upper trunk

histology shows perivascular lymphocytic infiltration
lesions persist or spontaneously involute
relapsing course

> **References**
> Mullen RH, Jacobs AH: Jessner's lymphocytic infiltrate in two girls. Arch Dermatol 1988; 124: 1091–1093.
> Toonstra J, Wildschut A, Boer J, Smeenk G, et al.: Jessner's lymphocytic infiltration of the skin. Arch Dermatol 1989; 125:1525–1530.

JOB SYNDROME
see HYPERIMMUNOGLOBULIN E SYNDROME

JOHANSON–BLIZZARD SYNDROME

Manifestations and Major Findings
ectodermal dysplasia
deafness (bilateral sensorineural)
severe growth retardation
short stature
failure to thrive
normal mentation to severe retardation
malabsorption due to pancreatic insufficiency causing generalized edema
hypotonia with hyperextensible joints
hypothyroidism (primary)
genitourinary abnormalities
cardiac defects

Cutaneous Manifestations
aplasia cutis of the scalp
café au lait macules
hypoplastic nipples and areolae
cutaneous midline dimples

Characteristic Facies
sparse, coarse hair
frontal upsweep of hair
extension of lateral hairline onto forehead
absent permanent teeth or peg-shaped teeth
microcephaly
hypoplastic nasal alae (beak-like nose)
aplasia of lacrimal puncta

autosomal recessive

> **References**
> Baraitser M, Hodgson SV: The Johanson–Blizzard syndrome. J Med Genet 1982; 19:302–303.
> Johanson A, Blizzard R: A syndrome of congenital aplasia of the alae nasi, deafness, hypothyroidism, dwarfism, absent permanent teeth and malabsorption. J Pediatr 1971; 79:982–987.
> Solomon LM, Cook B, Klipfel W: The ectodermal dysplasias. Dermatol Clin 1987; 5:231–237.

JUVENILE RHEUMATOID ARTHRITIS *see* STILL DISEASE

K

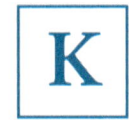

KALLIN SYNDROME
see EPIDERMOLYSIS BULLOSA; SIMPLEX

KALLMANN SYNDROME

Manifestations and Major Findings
hypogonadism due to gonadotropin-releasing hormone deficiency
cryptorchidism
micropenis
anosmia

OTHER FINDINGS
eunuchoid habitus with abnormally wide arm span
decreased sexual hair
cleft lip and palate
craniofacial asymmetry
skeletal abnormalities
ophthalmic abnormalities
urogenital abnormalities – renal hypo- or agenesis
cardiovascular abnormalities
neurologic deficits

> **References**
> Bick D, Curry CJR, McGill JR, Schorderet DF, et al.: Male infant with ichthyosis, Kallmann syndrome, chondrodysplasia punctata, and an Xp chromosome deletion. Am J Med Genet 1989; 33:100–107.
> Bick D, Franco B, Sherins RJ, Heye B, et al.: Brief report: intragenic deletion of the KALIG-1 gene in Kallmann's syndrome. N Engl J Med 1992; 326:1752–1755.
> Caviness VS: Kallmann's syndrome – beyond "migration". N Engl J Med 1992; 326:1775–1777.
> Dimitrovski C, Plaseski A, Bogoev M, Sadikaro S: Kallmann's syndrome associated with atrial septal defect. J Am Med Assoc 1982; 248:1358–1359.

KAPOSI SARCOMA, IDIOPATHIC HEMORRHAGIC SARCOMA

Types of Kaposi Sarcoma and Features

1 classic type (sporadic)
- reddish-brown/purple macules, nodules, and plaques (Fig. 79)
common on lower extremities
multifocal neoplastic process arising from vascular and lymphatic endothelium (predominantly in the dermis)
telangiectasias
indolent course beginning around the ankle and spreading up the leg
edema in the lower limbs
affects elderly males of Mediterranean origin
sporadic inheritance

2 endemic type
nodules or infiltrative purplish-red lesions
edema
possible lymphadenopathy, bony or visceral involvement
indolent course
occurs in tropical Africa (Zaïre, Uganda, Rwanda)

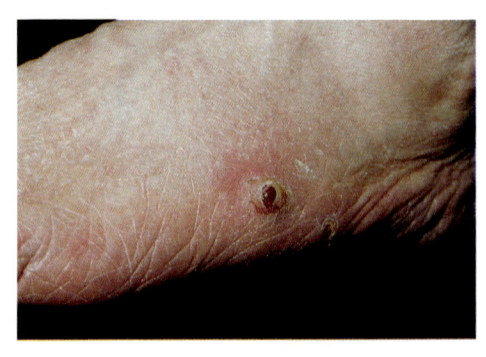

• *Figure 79* Kaposi sarcoma; a reddish-brown nodule on the foot.

3 epidemic type
reddish/salmon-colored macules or purplish nodules
nodules often on the face and mucous membranes
widely dispersed lesions – common on the feet
mucosal surface involvement common
lymph node involvement
associated with human immunodeficiency virus (HIV) infection

4 non-HIV immunosuppression type
seen in transplant patients undergoing chemotherapy
both cutaneous and systemic involvement
lesions may be aggressive and fatal

> **References**
> Cooper JS, Sacco J, Newall J: The duration of local control of classic (non-AIDS associated) Kaposi's sarcoma by radiotherapy. J Am Acad Dermatol 1988; 19:59–66.

KAPOSI VARICELLIFORM ERUPTION, ECZEMA HERPETICUM

Manifestations and Major Findings
disseminated cutaneous infection
causes
- herpesvirus type 1 (eczema herpeticum) (Fig. 80)
- vaccinia virus (eczema vaccinatum)
- other viruses (e.g. Coxsackie A16)

occurs in patients with pre-existing skin diseases
- atopic dermatitis
- seborrheic dermatitis
- Darier disease

lesions may be confined to abnormal skin or disseminated
high fever often present

> **References**
> Atherton DJ, Harper JI: Management of eczema herpeticum (letter). J Am Acad Dermatol 1988; 18:757–758.
> Fivenson DP, Breneman DL, Wander AH: Kaposi's varicelliform eruption. Arch Dermatol 1990; 126: 1037–1039.
> Masessa JM, Grossman ME, Knobler EH, Bank DE: Kaposi's varicelliform eruption in cutaneous T cell lymphoma. J Am Acad Dermatol 1989; 21:133–135.

KASABACH–MERRITT SYNDROME,
HEMANGIOMA–THROMBOCYTOPENIA SYNDROME

Manifestations and Major Findings
- hemangioma – usually large and rapidly growing (Fig. 81)
thrombocytopenia with petechiae and/or purpura
consumptive coagulopathy and anemia
usually occurs in infancy

> **References**
> Esterly NB: Kasabach–Merritt syndrome in infants. J Am Acad Dermatol 1983; 8:504–513.
> Larsen EC, Zinkham WH, Eggleston JC, Zitelli BJ: Kasabach–Merritt syndrome: therapeutic considerations. Pediatrics 1987; 79:971–980.
> Maceyko RF, Camisa C: Kasabach–Merritt syndrome. Pediatr Dermatol 1991; 8:133–136.

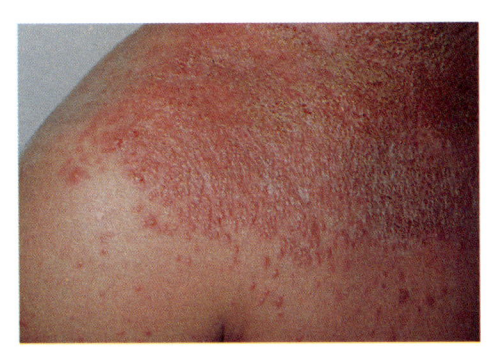

• *Figure 80* Kaposi varicelliform eruption caused by herpesvirus type 1 infection.

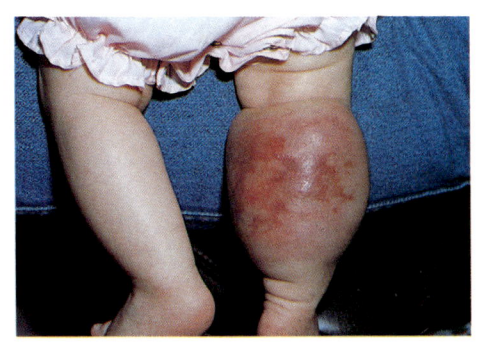

• *Figure 81* A large, rapidly growing hemangioma of the leg in an infant with Kasabach–Merritt syndrome.

▷ ▷ ▷
2 keratoderma associated with carcinoma of esophagus
see Howel–Evans syndrome

3 keratoderma associated with arsenic ingestion

4 keratoderma associated with myxedema

5 secondary hypertrophic pulmonary osteoarthropathy

6 keratodermas associated with other dermatoses
psoriasis
Reiter disease
pityriasis rubra pilaris
atopic dermatitis/lichen simplex chronicus
lupus erythematosus
lichen planus
Darier disease
dermatophytosis
syphilis
yaws
drugs (arsenic, gold, quinacrine)
acanthosis nigricans
Sezary syndrome
pachydermoperiostosis

References
Wevers A, Kuhn A, Mahrle G: Palmoplantar keratoderma with tonotubular keratin. J Am Acad Dermatol 1991; 24:638–642.

KERATOSIS FOLLICULARIS
see DARIER DISEASE

KERATOSIS LICHENOIDES CHRONICA see NÉKAM DISEASE

KETRON–GOODMAN DISEASE,
GENERALIZED PAGETOID RETICULOSIS

Manifestations and Major Findings
disseminated, hyperkeratotic, erythematous nodular plaques
epidermis infiltrated with cells having pagetoid appearance
variant of mycosis fungoides (cutaneous T cell lymphoma) with pronounced epidermotropism of infiltrating cells
no Pautrier microabscesses
variable course

References
Ketron LW, Goodman MH: Multiple lesions of the skin apparently of epithelial origin resembling clinically mycosis fungoides. Report of a case. Arch Dermatol Syphilol 1931; 24:758–777.
Mielke V, Wolff HH, Winzer M, Sterry W: Localized and disseminated pagetoid reticulosis. Arch Dermatol 1989; 125:402–406.

KID SYNDROME, KERATITIS ICHTHYOSIS DEAFNESS SYNDROME, SENTER SYNDROME
see also DISORDERS OF CORNIFICATION; DOC 15

Manifestations and Major Findings
*k*eratitis (may lead to blindness)
*i*chthyosiform erythroderma (usually present at birth)
*d*eafness – nonprogressive, neurosensory

OTHER FINDINGS
verrucous, well-marginated, plaques
prominent follicular keratoses
palmoplantar hyperkeratosis – pebbly quality
perioral furrowing
increased susceptibility to cutaneous infections
hypotrichosis of eyebrows, eyelashes, and scalp
nail dystrophy
small, carious teeth
impaired sweating
breast hypoplasia
cryptorchidism
susceptibility to mucosal neoplasms in later life

autosomal dominant or recessive

References
Grob JJ, Breton A, Bonafe JL, Sauvan-Ferdani M, et al.: Keratitis, ichthyosis, and deafness (KID) syndrome. Arch Dermatol 1987; 123:777–782.
Langer K, Konrad K, Wolff K: Keratitis, ichthyosis and deafness (KID) syndrome: report of three cases and a review of the literature. Br J Dermatol 1990; 122:689–697.
▷ ▷ ▷

▷ ▷ ▷
Nazzaro V, Blanchet-Bardon C, Lorette G, Civatte J: Familial occurrence of KID (keratitis, ichthyosis, deafness) syndrome. Case reports of a mother and daughter. J Am Acad Dermatol 1990; 23:385–388.
Senter TP, Jones KL, Sakati N, Nyhan WL: Atypical ichthyosiform erythroderma and congenital neurosensory deafness – a distinct syndrome. J Pediatr 1978; 92:68–72.
Skinner BA, Greist MC, Norins AL: The keratitis, ichthyosis, and deafness (KID) syndrome. Arch Dermatol 1981; 117:285–289.
Williams ML: The ichthyoses – pathogenesis and prenatal diagnosis: a review of recent advances. Pediatr Dermatol 1984; 2:1–24.

KIMURA DISEASE

Manifestations and Major Findings
subcutaneous nodules and tumors
localized to the head and neck regions
lymphadenopathy
peripheral eosinophilia
elevated serum IgE
occurs mainly in Asian males
histopathology shows lymphoid follicles in the dermis with many eosinophils
Kimura disease can be associated with renal disease, asthma, or Loeffler syndrome.

KINDLER SYNDROME,
KINDLER–WEARY SYNDROME

Manifestations and Major Findings
blistering from birth
improves or ceases with age
• progressive sclerotic poikiloderma with atrophy (Fig. 85)
acrokeratotic papules on the palms and soles
photosensitivity
dental abnormalities – periodontosis

References
Bordas X, Palou J, Capdevila JM, Mascaro JM: Kindler's syndrome. J Am Acad Dermatol 1982; 6:263–265. ▷ ▷ ▷

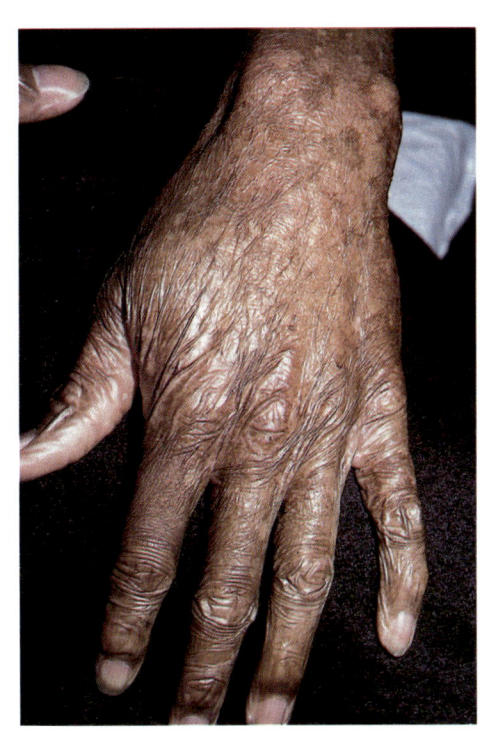

• *Figure 85 Sclerotic poikiloderma with atrophy of a hand in a patient with Kindler syndrome.*

▷ ▷ ▷
Forman AB, Prendiville JS, Esterly NB, Hebert AA, et al.: Kindler syndrome: report of two cases and review of the literature. Pediatr Dermatol 1989; 6:91–101.
Hovnanian A, Blanchet-Bardon C, de Prost Y: Poikiloderma of Theresa Kindler: report of a case with ultrastructural study, and review of the literature. Pediatr Dermatol 1989; 6:82–90.

KINKY HAIR SYNDROME
see MENKES SYNDROME

KITAMURA RETICULATE ACROPIGMENTATION,
RETICULATE ACROPIGMENTATION OF KITAMURA

Manifestations and Major Findings
• reticulated, hyperpigmented, slightly atrophic, polygonal macules (Fig. 86)

usually affects extensor surfaces of distal extremities
may involve entire body
characteristic pits and breaks on palmar epidermal ridge patterns
onset before 20 years of age
most common in Japanese females

autosomal dominant or sporadic inheritance

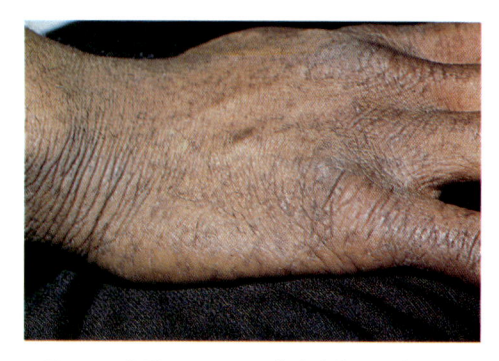

• *Figure 86* Hyperpigmented, slightly atrophic, polygonal macules on the extensor surface of the hand in Kitamura reticulate acropigmentation.

References
Fulk CS: Primary disorders of hyperpigmentation. J Am Acad Dermatol 1984; 10:1–16.
Griffiths WAD: Reticulate acropigmentation of Kitamura. Br J Dermatol 1976; 95:437–443.
Kameyama K, Morita M, Sugaya K, Nishiyama S, et al.: Treatment of reticulate acropigmentation of Kitamura with azelaic acid. J Am Acad Dermatol 1992; 26:817–820.
Wallis MS, Mallory SB: Reticulate acropigmentation of Kitamura with localized alopecia. J Am Acad Dermatol 1991; 25:114–116.

KLEIN–WAARDENBURG SYNDROME *see* WAARDENBURG SYNDROME

KLINEFELTER SYNDROME,
XXY SYNDROME

Manifestations and Major Findings
occurs in XXY males (47 chromosomes)
tall stature
long limbs
infertility
small testicles with decreased testosterone
varicose veins
scoliosis
clinodactyly

NEUROLOGIC ABNORMALITIES
language disabilities
dyslexia
mental retardation (mild)
psychiatric disorders
behavioral problems

Cutaneous Manifestations
cystic acne
scant body hair
leg ulcers

References
Graham JM, Bashir AS, Stark RE, Silbert A, Walzer S: Oral and written language abilities of XXY boys: implications for anticipatory guidance. Pediatrics 1988; 81:795–806.
Misra RS, Mukherjee A, Nath I, Jain RK, Sharma AK: Extensive verrucosis, squamous cell carcinoma, and immunologic abnormality in Klinefelter's syndrome. Int J Dermatol 1986; 25:529–530.

KLIPPEL–FEIL SYNDROME

Manifestations and Major Findings
fused cervical vertebrae
short neck
limitation of head movement
hair growth low down on neck

OTHER FINDINGS
ear abnormalities
hearing impairment
genitourinary abnormalities
cardiac defects (ventricular septal defect)
diverse abnormalities of the extremities

KLIPPEL–TRENAUNAY SYNDROME,
ANGIO-OSTEOHYPERTROPHY SYNDROME,
OSTEOHYPERTROPHIC ANGIOECTASIA

Manifestations and Major Findings
- congenital vascular malformation (port-wine stain) of one or more extremities (Fig. 87)

hypertrophy of underlying bone and soft tissue (present at birth or later) with or without bony overgrowth

varicose veins

OTHER FINDINGS
syndactyly
polydactyly
scoliosis
visceral vascular malformations
recurrent cellulitis in affected limbs
pain common

References
Mahmoud SF, El-Benhawi MO, El-Tonsy MH, Kalantar SM: Klippel–Trenaunay syndrome. J Am Acad Dermatol 1988; 18:1169–1172.
Mullins FJ, Naylor D, Redetski H: The Klippel–Trenaunay–Weber syndrome. Arch Dermatol 1962; 86:202–206.
Ring DS, Mallory SB: Klippel–Trenaunay syndrome. Pediatr Dermatol 1992; 9:80–82.
Young AE 1988. Combined vascular malformations. In Mulliken JB, Young AE (eds.) Vascular Birthmarks: Hemangiomas and Malformations, p.246–274. (Philadelphia: WB Saunders).

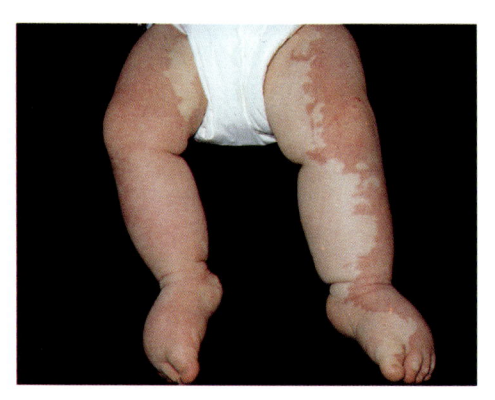

- *Figure 87* Congenital vascular malformation (port-wine stain) of the legs in Klippel–Trenaunay syndrome.

KÖBNER SYNDROME
see EPIDERMOLYSIS BULLOSA; SIMPLEX

KUSKE–PORTUGAL SYNDROME
see EPIDERMOLYSIS BULLOSA; DYSTROPHIC

KWASHIORKOR

Manifestations and Major Findings
protein malnutrition (severe) with relative carbohydrate excess
failure to thrive
- edema (Fig. 88)

xerophthalmia
hypoalbuminemia (<2.5 g/100 ml)
fatty infiltration of the liver
mental disturbances
more common in children

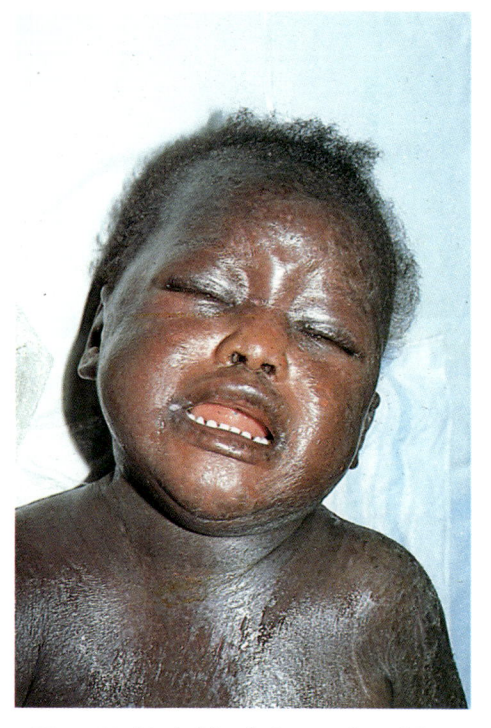

- *Figure 88* Marked facial edema, scaling of the skin, and loss of hair in a child with kwashiorkor.

Cutaneous Manifestations
depigmentation of the hair and skin
flag sign – alternate bands of color on hair indicating periods of malnutrition and good nutrition
'flaky paint' thickening of hyperkeratotic plaques on pressure points (knees, elbows)
cheilosis
hair loss (Fig. 88)

> **References**
> **Jelliffe DB, Jelliffe EFP:** Causation of Kwashiorkor: toward a multifactorial consensus. Pediatrics 1992; 90:110–113.
> **McLaren DS:** Skin in protein energy malnutrition. Arch Dermatol 1987; 123:1674a–1676a.
> **Miller SJ:** Nutritional deficiency and the skin. J Am Acad Dermatol 1989; 21:1–30.

KYRLE DISEASE, HYPERKERATOSIS FOLLICULARIS ET PARAFOLLICULARIS

Manifestations and Major Findings
perforating dermatosis
transepidermal elimination of basophilic debris
keratotic papules (2–8 mm) with crateriform depressions or horny plugs
lesions usually on the extremities
may be localized or generalized
onset at 50–70 years of age

Kyrle disease can be associated with diabetes mellitus or renal failure.

> **References**
> **Chang P, Fernandez V:** Acquired perforating disease associated with chronic renal failure. Int J Dermatol 1992; 31:117–118.
> **Cohen RW, Auerbach R:** Acquired reactive perforating collagenosis. J Am Acad Dermatol 1989; 20:287–289.
> **Patterson J:** The perforating disorders. J Am Acad Dermatol 1984; 10:561–581.

L

LAFORA DISEASE

Manifestations and Major Findings
hereditary neurometabolic disease
progressive myoclonic seizures
dementia
histology shows Lafora bodies (PAS-positive intracytoplasmic inclusions) in eccrine duct cells and peripheral nerves

autosomal recessive

> **References**
> Berkovic SF, Andermann F, Carpenter S, Wolfe LS: Progressive myoclonus epilepsies: specific causes and diagnosis. N Engl J Med 1986; 315:296–305.
> Carpenter S: Skin biopsy for diagnosis of hereditary neurologic metabolic disease. Arch Dermatol 1987; 123:1618–1621.
> Newton GA, Sanchez RL, Swedo J, Smith EB: Lafora's disease. Arch Dermatol 1987; 123: 1667–1669.
> Samlaska CP, McBurney J, Sau P, James WD: Lafora's disease: what is the best site for skin biopsy? J Am Acad Dermatol 1989; 21:791–792.

LAMB SYNDROME
see CARNEY SYNDROME

LAMBERT–EATON MYASTHENIC SYNDROME

Manifestations and Major Findings
acquired autoimmune disease
muscle weakness
usually affects males over 40 years of age
Associated with other autoimmune disorders and carcinoma (usually small cell carcinoma of the lung). Weakness may predate tumors by 3 years.

AUTONOMIC MANIFESTATIONS
dry mouth
impotence
decreased sweating
orthostatic hypotension
altered pupillary reflexes

LANGER–GIEDION SYNDROME,
see TRICHORHINOPHALANGEAL SYNDROME; TYPE II

LAUGIER–HUNZIKER SYNDROME

Manifestations and Major Findings
benign, acquired, lentiginous pigmentation of labial and buccal mucosa and nails
not associated with systemic abnormalities (e.g. gastrointestinal polyps)

> **References**
> Koch SE, LeBoit PE, Odom RB: Laugier–Hunziker syndrome. J Am Acad Dermatol 1987; 16:431–434.
> Sterling GB, Libow LF, Grossman ME: Pigmented nail streaks may indicate Laugier–Hunziker syndrome. Cutis 1988; 42:325–326.

LAUNOIS–BENSAUDE SYNDROME

Manifestations and Major Findings
widespread lipomatosis
symmetric deposition of subcutaneous fat

usually involves upper back, shoulders, and arms but can be more widespread
similar to Madelung disease but more widespread

> **References**
> Carlin MC, Ratz JL: Multiple symmetric lipomatosis: treatment with liposuction. J Am Acad Dermatol 1988; 18:359–362.
> Enzi G: Multiple symmetric lipomatosis an updated clinical report. Medicine 1984; 63:56–64.
> Ross M, Goodman MM: Multiple symmetric lipomatosis (Launois–Bensaude Syndrome). Int J Dermatol 1992; 31:80–82.
> Ruzicka T, Vieluf D, Landthaler M, Braun-Falco O: Benign symmetric lipomatosis of Launois–Bensaude. J Am Acad Dermatol 1987; 17:663–674.

LAURENCE–MOON SYNDROME

Manifestations and Major Findings
mental retardation
retinitis pigmentosa leading to blindness
hypogenitalism
spastic paraplegia

OTHER FINDINGS
ataxia
slow development
renal abnormalities

autosomal recessive

> **References**
> Green JS, Parfrey PS, Harnett JD, Farid NR, et al.: The cardinal manifestations of Bardet–Biedl syndrome, a form of Laurence–Moon–Biedl syndrome. N Engl J Med 1989; 321:1002–1009.

LAWRENCE–SEIP SYNDROME
see LIPOATROPHIC DIABETES SYNDROME

LEINER DISEASE, ERYTHRODERMIA DESQUAMATIVA

Manifestations and Major Findings
erythroderma and generalized scaling develops in first weeks of life
usually follows weaning from the breast
diarrhea
weight loss, emaciation, and failure to thrive
anemia
secondary bacterial infection (often severe) with Gram-negative bacteria and *Staphylococcus aureus*

Leiner disease may be associated with complement component (C5) functional abnormality, defective polymorphonuclear leukocyte phagocytosis, hypogammaglobulinemia, chemotactic dysfunction, hyperimmunoglobulin E syndrome, or other nonspecific immunodeficiencies.

> **References**
> Evans DIK, Holzel A, MacFarlane H: Yeast opsonization defect and immunoglobulin deficiency in severe infantile dermatitis (Leiner's disease). Arch Dis Child 1977; 52:691–695.
> Glover MT, Atherton DJ, Levinsky RJ: Syndrome of erythroderma, failure to thrive, and diarrhea in infancy: a manifestation of immunodeficiency. Pediatrics 1988; 81:66–72.

LEOPARD SYNDROME, MULTIPLE LENTIGINES SYNDROME, CARDIOCUTANEOUS SYNDROME, LENTIGINOSIS PROFUSA SYNDROME

Manifestations and Major Findings
*l*entigines – primarily face and upper trunk
*e*lectrocardiographic abnormalities – especially conduction defects
*o*cular hypertelorism
*p*ulmonary stenosis
*a*bnormal genitalia (undescended testes, hypospadias, gonadal hypoplasia)
*r*etardation of growth
*d*eafness of sensorineural type

OTHER FINDINGS
low-set ears
abnormal dermatoglyphics
dental defects
webbing of fingers
renal aplasia
mandibular prognathism

autosomal dominant with variable expressivity

References
Fulk CS: Primary disorders of hyperpigmentation. J Am Acad Dermatol 1984; 10:1–16.
Gorlin RJ, Anderson RC, Blaw M: Multiple lentigenes syndrome. Am J Dis Child 1969; 112:652–662.
Nordlund JJ, Lerner AB, Braverman IM, McGuire JS: The multiple lentigines syndrome. Arch Dermatol 1973; 107:259–261.
Selmanowitz VJ, Orentreich N, Felsenstein JM: Lentiginosis profusa syndrome. Arch Dermatol 1971; 104:393–401.
Uhle P, Norvell SS: Generalized lentiginosis. J Am Acad Dermatol 1988; 18:444–447.

LEPRECHAUNISM
see DONAHUE SYNDROME

LEPROSY
see HANSEN DISEASE

LESCH–NYHAN SYNDROME

Manifestations and Major Findings
hypoxanthine guanine phosphoribosyl transferase (HGPRT) deficiency
normal at birth
developmental abnormalities apparent by 6 months of age
self-mutilation – particularly biting of lower lip
severe mental retardation
choreoathetosis
spasticity
tophi on the pinnae
gouty arthritis in partial deficiency
hyperuricemia with urate deposits in kidney

X-linked recessive

References
Lloyd KG, Hornykiewicz O, Davidson L, Shannak K, et al.: Biochemical evidence of dysfunction of brain neurotransmitters in the Lesch–Nyhan syndrome. N Engl J Med 1981; 305:1106–1111.
Reed WB, Fish CH: Hyperuricemia with self-mutilation and choreoathetosis: Lesch–Nyhan syndrome. Arch Dermatol 1966; 94:194–195.

LESER–TRÉLAT SIGN

Manifestations and Major Findings
numerous eruptive seborrheic keratoses
pruritus in some cases
May be associated with internal malignancy.

References
Halevy S, Feuerman EJ: The sign of Leser–Trélat. A cutaneous marker for internal malignancy. Int J Dermatol 1985; 24:359–361.
Holdiness MR: On the classification of the sign of Leser–Trélat. J Am Acad Dermatol 1988; 19:754–757.
Lindelöf B, Sigurgeirsson B, Melander S: Seborrheic keratoses and cancer. J Am Acad Dermatol 1992; 26:947–950.
Rampen FHJ, Schwengle LEM: The sign of Leser–Trélat: does it exist? J Am Acad Dermatol 1989; 21:50–55.
Venencie PY, Perry HO: Sign of Leser–Trélat: report of two cases and review of the literature. J Am Acad Dermatol 1984; 10:83–88.

LETTERER–SIWE DISEASE
see HISTIOCYTOSIS

LEWANDOWSKY–LUTZ SYNDROME
see EPIDERMODYSPLASIA VERRUCIFORMIS

LICHEN MYXEDEMATOSUS
see SCLEROMYXEDEMA

LIPOATROPHIC DIABETES SYNDROME, LAWRENCE–SEIP SYNDROME, BERARDINELLI–SEIP SYNDROME

Manifestations and Major Findings
generalized and marked wasting of subcutaneous fat
insulin-resistant diabetes without ketoacidosis
hepatosplenomegaly
generalized muscular hypertrophy
prominent ears
acanthosis nigricans
hypertrichosis
thick, curly scalp hair

hypertension
corneal opacities
elevated metabolic rate
hyperlipidemia
cutaneous xanthomas

probable autosomal recessive

> **References**
> Roth DE, Schikler KN, Callen JP: Annular atrophic connective tissue panniculitis of the ankles. J Am Acad Dermatol 1989; 21:1152–1156.

LIPODYSTROPHY (PARTIAL),
BARRAQUER–SIMONS DISEASE

Manifestations and Major Findings
progressive lipodystrophy
symmetrical loss of fat – typically from face, arms, and trunk
complete loss of adipose tissue over affected areas
subcutaneous fat retention in lower half of body
progressive membranous mesangiocapillary glomerulonephritis
low complement component (C3)
diabetes mellitus
retinitis pigmentosa
chronic leukocytoclastic vasculitis
onset in childhood or young adulthood
more common in females

> **References**
> Sissons JGP, West RJ, Fallows J, et al.: The complement abnormalities of lipodystrophy. N Engl J Med 1976; 294:461–465.

LIPOID PROTEINOSIS, URBACH–WIETHE DISEASE, HYALINOSIS CUTIS ET MUCOSAE, LIPOGLYCOPROTEINOSIS

Manifestations and Major Findings
infiltration of hyaline material into skin, oral cavity, larynx, and internal organs
hoarseness (beginning in infancy)
nodules on the vocal cords/larynx
respiratory obstruction by nodules
thick, firm tongue
coarse facies
parotitis
neurologic findings
 –seizures
 –sickle-shaped intracranial calcifications lateral to and above sella turcica

Cutaneous Manifestations
hemorrhagic crusts, crops of bullae, and pustules (early)
yellow papules on face, eyelids, neck, and hands
beaded papules on eyelid margins
occasional vesicles, ulcers, and pitted scars
diffuse thickening of the skin
hyperkeratotic, dark lesions over fingers, elbows, knees, and buttocks (later)
alopecia due to scalp papules

autosomal recessive

> **References**
> Aubin F, Blanc D, Badet JM, Chobaut J-C: Lipoid proteinosis. Pediatr Dermatol 1989; 6:109–113.
> Bauer EA, Santa-Cruz DJ, Eisen AZ: Lipoid proteinosis: in vivo and in vitro evidence for a lysosomal storage disease. J Invest Dermatol 1981; 76:119–125.
> Konstantinov K, Kabakchiev P, Karchev T, Kobayasi T, et al.: Lipoid proteinosis. J Am Acad Dermatol 1992; 27:293–297.
> Moy LS, Moy RL, Matsuoka LY, et al.: Lipoid proteinosis: ultrastructural and biochemical studies. J Am Acad Dermatol 1987; 16:1193–1201.
> Rook A: Lipoid proteinosis: Urbach–Wiethe disease. Br J Dermatol 1976; 94:341–342.

LIP-TIP SYNDROME

Manifestations and Major Findings
vitiligo with depigmentation of distal digits and lips

LISON SYNDROME

Manifestations and Major Findings
spastic paraparesis
hypopigmented macules from birth

hyperpigmentation of exposed areas
diffuse lentigines
canities (premature graying of hair)
small, thin face with 'sharp' facial features
scoliosis

> **References**
> Lison M, Kornbrut B, Feinstein A, Hiss Y, et al.: Progressive spastic paraparesis, vitiligo, premature graying, and distinct facial appearance. Am J Med Genet 1981; 9:351–357.

LOBO DISEASE, LOBOMYCOSIS, KELOIDAL BLASTOMYCOSIS

Manifestations and Major Findings
infection with *Paracoccidioides (Glenosporella) loboi* also called *Loboa loboi*
skin involvement
no internal organ or mucous membrane involvement
lesions resemble keloids
occur on earlobes, distal extremities, and buttocks
most common in South and Central America
acquired through trauma and spread by autoinoculation

> **References**
> Fuchs J, Milbradt R, Pecher SA: Lobomycosis (keloidal blastomycosis): case reports and overview. Cutis 1990; 46:227–234.
> Talhari S, Cunha MdGS, Schettini APM, Talhari AC: Deep mycoses in Amazon region. Int J Dermatol 1988; 27:481–484.
> Rodriguez-Toro G: Lobomycosis. Int J Dermatol 1993; 32:324–332.

LÖFGREN SYNDROME

Manifestations and Major Findings
erythema nodosum
bilateral hilar lymphadenopathy
fever
acute iridocyclitis
arthritis/arthralgia
usually self-limiting
Associated with sarcoidosis, psitticosis, and Hodgkin disease.

LOOSE ANAGEN HAIR SYNDROME

Manifestations and Major Findings
anagen hairs loosely anchored
trichograms show 98–100% anagen hairs
hair easily pulled from the scalp
thin, patchy, often blonde hair
premature keratinization of inner root sheaths
cuticle resembles a rumpled sock
usually affects girls aged 2–9 years

> **References**
> Baden HP, Kvedar JC, Magro CM: Loose anagen hair as a cause of hereditary hair loss in children. Arch Dermatol 1992; 128:1349–1353.
> Hamm H, Traupe H: Loose anagen hair of childhood: the phenomenon of easily pluckable hair. J Am Acad Dermatol 1989; 20:242–248.
> O'Donnell BP, Sperling LC, James WD: Loose anagen hair syndrome. Int J Dermatol 1992;31: 107–109.
> Price VH, Gummer CL: Loose anagen syndrome. J Am Acad Dermatol 1989; 20:249–256.

LOUIS-BAR SYNDROME
see ATAXIA TELANGIECTASIA

LOWE SYNDROME
see OCULOCEREBRORENAL SYNDROME

LUCIO PHENOMENON
see HANSEN DISEASE

LUPUS ERYTHEMATOSUS

Criteria for Systemic Lupus Erythematosus

Patients should have at least four of the following eleven symptoms before being diagnosed as having systemic lupus erythematosus:

1 malar rash
fixed erythema (flat or raised) over malar eminences with tendency to spare nasolabial folds

2 •discoid rash (Fig. 89)
erythematous raised patches with adherent keratotic scaling and follicular plugging – atrophic scarring may occur in older lesions

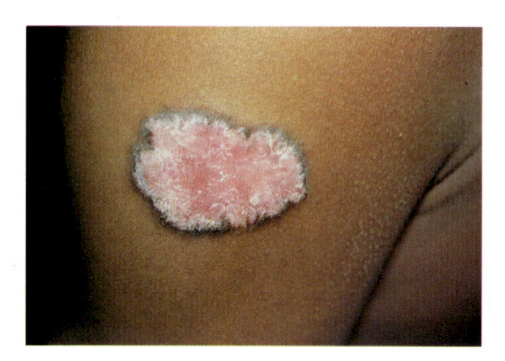

Figure 89 Discoid lupus erythematosus showing scarring and atrophy, and rimmed by hyperpigmentation.

3 photosensitivity
rash resulting from unusual reaction to sunlight

4 oral (or nasopharyngeal) ulcers
usually painless

5 arthritis
nonerosive arthritis involving two or more peripheral joints – characterized by tenderness, swelling, or effusion

6 serositis
pleuritis; convincing history of pleuritic pain, 'rub' heard by physician, or evidence of pleural effusion
or pericarditis; documented by electrocardiogram, audible 'rub', or evidence of pericardial effusion

7 renal disorder
persistent proteinuria; 0.5 g/day (three positive tests if quantitation not performed)
or cellular casts; red blood cells, hemoglobin, granular or tubular cells
or a combination

8 neurologic disorder
seizures; in the absence of offending drugs or known metabolic derangement (uremia, ketoacidosis, or electrolyte imbalance)
or psychosis; in the absence of offending drugs or known metabolic derangement (uremia, ketoacidosis, or electrolyte imbalance)

9 hematologic disorder
hemolytic anemia; with reticulocytosis
or leukopenia; $< 4.0 \times 10^9$/L (< 4000/mm^3) total on more than two 0occasions
or lymphopenia; $< 1.5 \times 10^9$/L (< 1500/mm^3) on more than two occasions
or thrombocytopenia; $< 100 \times 10^9$/L ($\times 10^3$/mm^3) in the absence of offending drugs

10 immunologic disorder
positive lupus erythematosus cell preparation
or anti-DNA antibody to native DNA in abnormal titre
or anti-Sm antibody (Sm nuclear antigen)
or false-positive serological test for syphilis known to be positive for at least 6 months and confirmed by negative *Treponema pallidum* immobilization or fluorescent treponemal antibody-absorption test

11 antinuclear antibody-positive

> **References**
> Condemi JJ: The autoimmune diseases. J Am Med Assoc 1992; 268:2882-2892.
> Kaneko F, Tanji O, Hasegawa T, Ohto H, et al.: Neonatal lupus erythematosus in Japan. J Am Acad Dermatol 1992; 26:397–403.
> Tan EM, Cohen AS, Fries JF, Masi AT, et al.: The 1982 revised criteria for the classification of systemic lupus erythematosus. Arthritis Rheum 1982; 25: 1271–1277.

LUTZ–SPLENDORE–ALMEIDA DISEASE, PARACOCCIDIOIDAL GRANULOMA, PARACOCCIDIOIDOMYCOSIS

Manifestations and Major Findings
chronic granulomatous disease
caused by *Paracoccidioides brasiliensis* (dimorphic fungus)
occurs in South and Central America (mainly Brazil)
usually seen in 20–50 year old males
begins with primary pulmonary infection
hematogenous spread
skin lesions follow – papules, pustules, and ulcerating nodules
mucous membranes involved (oropharynx, gingiva) – papules and ulcerating nodules
lymphadenopathy
visceral and skeletal involvement
dissemination leading to death

> **References**
> Londero AT, Ramos CD: Paracoccidioidomycosis. Am J Med 1972; 52:771–775.
> Murray HW, Littman ML, Roberts RB: Disseminated paracoccidioidomycosis (South American blastomycosis). Am J Med 1974; 56:209–220.

LYELL SYNDROME
see TOXIC EPIDERMAL NECROLYSIS

LYME DISEASE, LYME ARTHRITIS

Etiology
Borrelia burgdorferi (spirochete) infection
B. burgdorferi is carried by *Ixodes* tick
– *I. dammini* or *I. pacificus* (USA)
– *I. ricinus* (Europe)
also carried by *Amblyomma* tick
– *A. americanum*

Stages of Lyme Disease and Features

1 stage I
- erythema chronicum migrans (Fig. 90)
  – annular expanding erythematous plaque >5cm
  – usually starts 4–20 days after tick bite
  – duration of 3 weeks
  – resolves leaving a bluish hue
- headache
- arthralgias/arthritis
- malaise
- fever

2 stage II
- recurrent erythema chronicum migrans
- meningitis
- neuritis
- carditis

3 stage III
- acrodermatitis chronica atrophicans (progressive erythema, atrophy, and pigmentation of one extremity)
- chronic neurologic symptoms – cranial nerve palsies
- myositis
- arthritis
- cardiomyopathy

> **References**
> **Gellis SE, Stadecker MJ, Steere AC:** Spirochetes in atrophic skin lesions accompanied by minimal host response in a child with Lyme disease. J Am Acad Dermatol 1991; 25:395–397.
> **Steere AC:** Lyme Disease. N Engl J Med 1989; 586–596.
> **Stechenberg BW:** Lyme disease: the latest great imitator. Pediatr Infect Dis J 1988; 7:402–409.
> **Szer IS, Taylor E, Steere AC:** The long-term course of Lyme arthritis in children. N Engl J Med 1991; 325:159–163.

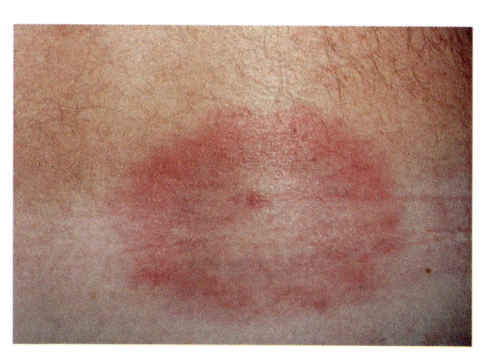

- *Figure 90* Erythema chronicum migrans (an expanding, annular, erythematous plaque) in Lyme disease.

LYMPHOCYTIC INFILTRATION OF THE SKIN
see JESSNER LYMPHOCYTIC INFILTRATE

LYMPHOCYTIC MENINGORADICULITIS
see BANNWARTH SYNDROME

LYMPHOCYTOMA CUTIS
see SPIEGLER–FENDT PSEUDOLYMPHOMA

M

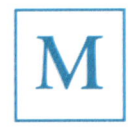

MACROCEPHALY WITH MULTIPLE LIPOMATA AND HEMANGIOMAS
see BANNAYAN–ZONANA SYNDROME

MADELUNG DISEASE, MULTIPLE SYMMETRIC LIPOMATOSIS, BENIGN SYMMETRIC LIPOMATOSIS (LAUNOIS–BENSAUDE), MADELUNG–LAUNOIS–BENSAUDE SYNDROME
see also LAUNOIS–BENSAUDE SYNDROME

Manifestations and Major Findings
multiple massive lipomas are symmetrical around neck and upper trunk – 'horse collar distribution'
symmetric and disproportionate accumulation of unencapsulated, mature fatty tissue
mediastinal compression
peripheral and autonomic neuropathy
Madelung disease is associated with alcoholism, liver disease, diabetes, malignant tumors of upper airways, hyperuricemia, and hyperlipidemia.

References
Carlin MC, Ratz JL: Multiple symmetric lipomatosis: treatment with liposuction. J Am Acad Dermatol 1988; 18:359-362.
Enzi G: Multiple symmetric lipomatosis: an updated clinical report. Medicine 1984; 63:56–64.
Lamb AS, Guill MA: Multiple symmetrical lipomatosis. Cutis 1992; 49:246–248.
Requena L, Hasson A, Arias D, Martín L, et al.: Acquired symmetric lipomatosis of the soles. J Am Acad Dermatol 1992; 26:860–862.
Ruzicka T, Vieluf D, Landthaler M, Braun-Falco O: Benign symmetric lipomatosis Launois–Bensaude. J Am Acad Dermatol 1987; 17:663–674.

MADURA FOOT, MYCETOMA, MADUROMYCOSIS

Manifestations and Major Findings
usually follows traumatic inoculation of organisms
–fungi (*Exophiala, Madurella*)
–actinomycetes (*Nocardia, Actinomadura*)
localized chronic skin infection
severe damage to skin and subcutaneous tissues
osteomyelitis of affected feet or hands
most common in Central and South America, Africa, and India
earliest stage is a firm painless nodule which later drains and discharges pus and granules
Granules are formed by organisms (representing microcolonies) within abscesses and discharged through draining sinuses; granules are of varying size, shape, and color – depending on genus and species.

References
Tomecki KJ, Steck WD, Hall GS, Dijkstra JWE: Subcutaneous mycoses. J Am Acad Dermatol 1989; 21:785–790.
Wortman PD: Treatment of a Nocardia brasiliensis mycetoma with sulfamethoxazole and trimethoprim, amikacin, and amoxicillin and clavulanate. Arch Dermatol 1993;129:564–567.

MAFFUCCI SYNDROME, DYSCHONDROPLASIA WITH HEMANGIOMATA SYNDROME, KAST–MAFFUCCI SYNDROME, KAST SYNDROME

Manifestations and Major Findings
multiple vascular and lymphatic malformations affecting skin, mucosae, and internal organs

radiologically translucent enchondromata (usually asymmetrical) – primarily of the hands, feet and tubular long bones
marked bony deformities
usually normal at birth
nodules appear later
café au lait macules
increased incidence of malignant, mesodermally-derived tumors (chondrosarcoma, sarcoma)

> **References**
> Lewis RJ, Ketcham AS: Maffucci's Syndrome: functional and neoplastic significance. J Bone Joint Surg Am 1973; 55:1465–1479.
> Tilsley DA, Burden PW: A case of Maffucci's syndrome. Br J Dermatol 1981; 105:331–336.

MAGIC SYNDROME

Manifestations and Major Findings
*m*outh *a*nd *g*enital ulcers
*i*nflamed *c*artilage (polychondritis)
possible variant (overlap) of Behçet disease and relapsing polychondritis
cutaneous lesions may be vesiculopustular with extensive crusting and necrotic ulcerations
keratitis

> **References**
> Firestein GS, Gruber HE, Weisman MH, et al.: Mouth and genital ulcers with inflamed cartilage: MAGIC Syndrome. Am J Med 1985; 79:69–72.
> Orme RL, Nordlund JJ, Barich L, Brown T: The MAGIC syndrome (mouth and genital ulcers with inflamed cartilage). Arch Dermatol 1990; 126: 940–944.

MAJOCCHI DISEASE
see PURPURA PIGMENTOSA CHRONICA

MAJOCCHI GRANULOMA

Manifestations and Major Findings
hair follicle involvement of dermatophyte infection
infection produces granuloma

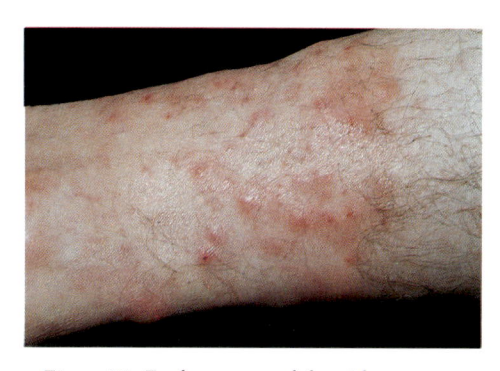

• *Figure 91 Erythematous nodules with inflammation in Majocchi granuloma.*

erythematous nodules with inflammation and scaling (Fig. 91)
usually occurs on shaved legs of women, beards of men, and scalps of children

MAKAI SUBCUTANEOUS LIPOGRANULOMATOSIS
ROTHMAN–MAKAI SYNDROME

MAL DE MELEDA, KERATODERMA PALMOPLANTARIS TRANSGREDIENS, MELEDA DISEASE, ACROERYTHROKERATODERMA

Manifestations and Major Findings
slowly progressive palmoplantar keratoderma
hyperkeratosis on wrists and extremities (transgrediens)
hyperhidrosis
psoriasiform plaques in groin, axillae, angles of the mouth, and on the extremities
atopic dermatitis with secondary infection
koilonychia
onychogryphosis
onset before 3 years of age
resembles Greither syndrome
named after Balkan island in Adriatic Sea with inbred population

OTHER FINDINGS
lingua plicata (scrotal tongue)
syndactyly
hair on palms and soles

autosomal recessive

> **References**
> Lestringant GG, Halawani NA, Zagzouk F: Mal de Meleda (letter). Int J Dermatol 1989; 28:277–278.
> Sybert VP, Dale BA, Holbrook KA: Palmar-plantar keratoderma. J Am Acad Dermatol 1988; 18:75–86.

MALHERBE CALCIFYING EPITHELIOMA
see PILOMATRIXOMA OF MALHERBE

MALIGNANT ATROPHIC PAPULOSIS see DEGOS DISEASE

MANDIBULOFACIAL DYSOSTOSIS
see TREACHER COLLINS SYNDROME

MAPLE SYRUP URINE DISEASE

Manifestations and Major Findings
inborn error of metabolism
impaired degradation of branched-chain amino acids
elevated leucine, isoleucine, and valine concentrations in blood, urine, and tissues
onset in neonatal period
poor feeding
vomiting
respiratory problems
hypotonia
seizures
urine has maple syrup odor in untreated patients
recurrent episodes of eruptive dermatitis when dietary restriction of protein intake causes low isoleucine/leucine levels

> **References**
> Koch SE, Packman S, Koch TK, Williams ML: Dermatitis in treated maple syrup urine disease. J Am Acad Dermatol 1993; 28:289–292.

MARASMUS

Manifestations and Major Findings
severe and prolonged protein/calorie malnutrition
dry, wrinkled, loose skin
subcutaneous fat loss – especially buccal
follicular hyperkeratosis
lanugo hair over the entire body
poor hair and nail growth
no peripheral edema

> **References**
> McLaren DS: Skin in protein energy malnutrition. Arch Dermatol 1987; 123:1674a–1676a.
> Miller SJ: Nutritional deficiency and the skin. J Am Acad Dermatol 1989; 21:1–30.

MARFAN SYNDROME

Cutaneous Manifestations
striae atrophicae
elastosis perforans serpiginosa
deficiency of subcutaneous fat
wide sideburns

SKELETAL ABNORMALITIES
long extremities
tall stature
joint laxity
- thumb sign (Fig. 92) – thumb (interphalangeal joint) projects beyond ulnar border when hand is clenched

wrist sign – thumb (interphalangeal joint) and fifth fingertip overlap when opposite wrist is grasped at narrowest circumference
high-arched palate
dolichocephaly
arachnodactyly
kyphoscoliosis
pectus excavatum/carinatum
abnormal skeletal proportions

OCULAR FINDINGS
ectopia lentis
myopia
retinal detachment

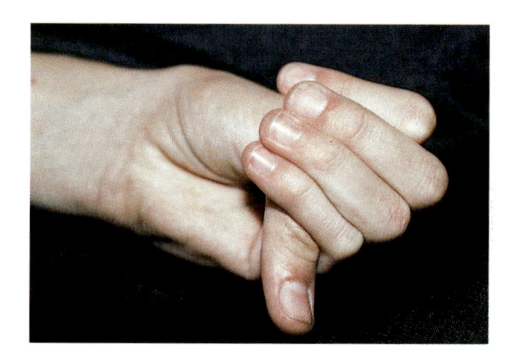

Figure 92 The 'thumb sign', seen in Marfan syndrome.

OTHER FINDINGS
normal intelligence
deafness
pulmonary malformations with spontaneous pneumothorax
cardiovascular disease
– aortic dilatation leading to aneurysm
– mitral or aortic valvular incompetence or prolapse

autosomal dominant with variable expression

References
Cohen PR, Schneiderman P: Clinical manifestations of the Marfan Syndrome. Int J Dermatol 1989; 28:291–299.
Gross DM, Robinson LK, Smith LT, Glass N, et al.: Severe perinatal Marfan syndrome. Pediatrics 1989; 84:83–89.
Morse RP, Rockenmacher S, Pyeritz RE, Sanders SP, et al.: Diagnosis and management of infantile Marfan Syndrome. Pediatrics 1990; 86:888–895.
Tsipouras P, Del Mastro R, Sarfarazi M, Lee B, et al.: Genetic linkage of the Marfan Syndrome, ectopia lentis, and congenital contractural arachnodactyly to the fibrillin genes on chromosomes 15 and 5. N Engl J Med 1992; 326:905–909.

MARGOLIS SYNDROME
see ZIPRKOWSKI–MARGOLIS SYNDROME

MARIE UNNA HYPOTRICHOSIS,
HEREDITARY TRICHODYSPLASIA

Manifestations and Major Findings
congenital hypotrichosis with progression
longitudinal grooving of the hair shafts
irregular twisting of the hair shafts
short, sparse body and scalp hair
androgenic alopecia (adolescence) – wiry hair and scarring alopecia
widespread facial milia
normal mentation

autosomal dominant

References
Frieden IJ 1991. Genetic Hair Disorders. In Alper JC (ed.) Genetic Disorders of the Skin, p.209–220. (St Louis: Mosby–Year Book).
Solomon LM, Esterly NB, Medenica M: Hereditary trichodysplasia: Marie Unna's hypotrichosis. J Invest Dermatol 1971; 57:389–400.

MARINESCO–SJÖGREN SYNDROME *see also* TRICHOTHIODYSTROPHY

Manifestations and Major Findings
cerebellar ataxia
nystagmus
mental retardation
growth retardation
hypotonia
congenital cataracts
abnormal teeth – absent lateral incisors
may be severe form of trichothiodystrophy

Cutaneous Manifestations
thin, brittle fingernails
fine, sparse, short scalp hair
deficient hair pigment
sulfur-deficient hair
trichoschisis (clean transverse hair fractures)
banding or irregular birefringence of hair shafts on polarized microscopy

autosomal recessive

References
Norwood WF: The Marinesco–Sjögren syndrome. J Pediatr 1964; 65:431–437.
Price VH, Odom RB, Ward WH, Jones FT: Trichothiodystrophy. Arch Dermatol 1980; 116: 1375–1384.
Whiting DA: Structural abnormalities of the hair shaft. J Am Acad Dermatol 1987; 16:1–25.

MARJOLIN ULCER

Manifestations and Major Findings

- squamous cell or basal cell carcinoma (Fig. 93)

arise in areas of chronic ulceration (burn scars)

References
Phillips TJ, Salman SM, Rogers GS: Nonhealing leg ulcers: a manifestation of basal cell carcinoma. J Am Acad Dermatol 1991; 25:47–49.

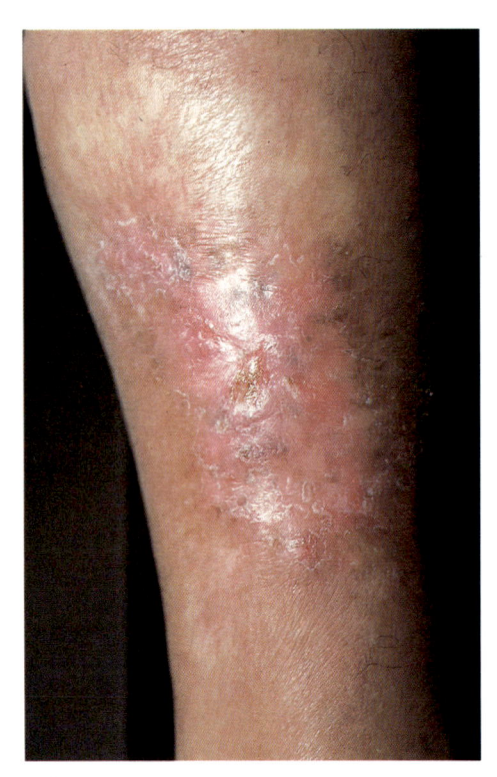

- *Figure 93 Developing squamous cell carcinoma in Marjolin ulcer.*

MAROTEAUX–LAMY SYNDROME
see MUCOPOLYSACCHARIDOSES; TYPE VI

MARSHALL SYNDROME
see CUTIS LAXA; ACQUIRED

MARSHALL–SMITH SYNDROME

Manifestations and Major Findings
accelerated growth and maturation (prenatal onset)
underweight for length
mental and motor retardation
respiratory problems
broad middle phalanges
hypotonia
hypertrichosis

Characteristic Facies
shallow orbits
low nasal bridge
proptosis
micrognathia
prominent forehead

sporadic inheritance

References
Fitch N: The Syndromes of Marshall and Weaver. J Med Genet 1980; 17:174–178.
Johnson JP, Carey JC, Glassy FJ, et al.: Marshall–Smith Syndrome: two case reports and a review of pulmonary manifestations. Pediatrics 1983; 71: 219–223.

MARTIN–BELL SYNDROME
see FRAGILE X SYNDROME

MASTOCYTOSIS

Manifestations and Major Findings
reddish-brown macules, papules, or nodules on the skin
histology shows numerous mast cells
flushing

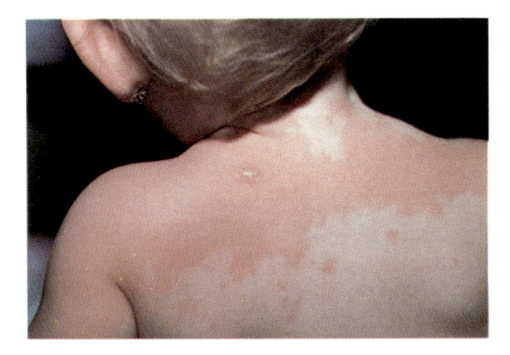

Figure 94 Darier sign (local urtication upon stroking) is a feature of mastocytosis. This patient also had generalized flushing from a solitary mastocytoma.

- Darier sign (Fig. 94) – local urtication (wheal and flare) of lesion after stroking
pruritus
gastrointestinal symptoms
hepatosplenomegaly
headache
tachycardia
malaise
hypotension
dyspnea
syncope
shock

Clinical Forms of Mastocytosis

1 **solitary mastocytoma**
  yellow/brownish nodule (*peau d'orange* sign)

2 **urticaria pigmentosa**
  - numerous reddish-brown macules and papules (Fig. 95)

3 **telangiectasia macularis eruptiva perstans**
  telangiectatic, hyperpigmented, diffuse macules

4 **diffuse infiltrative mastocytosis**
  thickened doughy skin
  blisters

5 **systemic mastocytosis**
  bone, gastrointestinal, hematopoietic, reticuloendothelial, and skin involvement

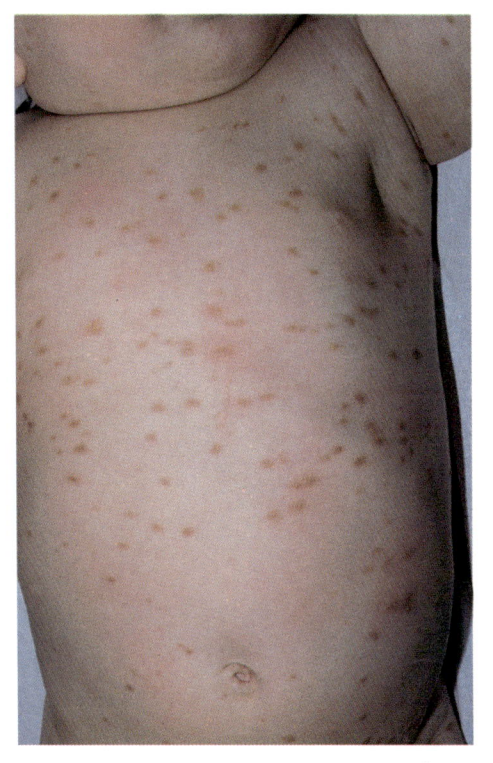

Figure 95 Numerous reddish-brown macules and papules are clinical manifestations of urticaria pigmentosa.

McCUNE–ALBRIGHT SYNDROME,
ALBRIGHT SYNDROME, POLYOSTOTIC FIBROUS DYSPLASIA, OSTEITIS FIBROSA CYSTICA

Manifestations and Major Findings
triad of findings
– polyostotic fibrous dysplasia (cystic lesions in long bones and pelvis most common) – progressive worsening
– • *café au lait* macules (usually large) on trunk (Fig. 96)
– sexual precocity (predominantly females)

OTHER FINDINGS
endocrine abnormalities
– acromegaly
– hyperthyroidism
ovarian cysts
malignancy risk (low) in fibrous dysplasia
intramuscular myxomas

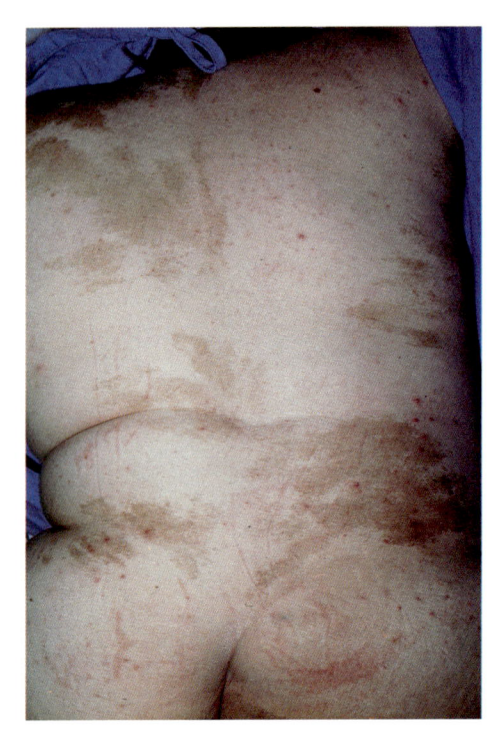

Figure 96 Large café au lait macules on the trunk in McCune–Albright syndrome.

lymphoid or myeloid metaplasia
facial asymmetry

sporadic inheritance

> **References**
> Albright F, Scoville B, Sulkowitch H: Syndrome characterized by osteitis fibrosa disseminata, areas of pigmentation, and gonadal dysfunction. Endocrinology 1938; 22:411–421.
> Feingold KR, Elias PM: Endocrine–skin interactions. J Am Acad Dermatol 1987; 17:933.
> Riccardi VM: Neurofibromatosis and Albright's syndrome. Dermatol Clin 1987; 5:193–203
> Roth JG, Esterly NB: McCune–Albright syndrome with multiple bilateral café au lait spots. Pediatr Dermatol 1991; 8:35–39.
> Shenker A, Weinstein LS, Moran A, et al.: Severe endocrine and nonendocrine manifestations of the McCune–Albright syndrome associated with activating mutations of stimulatory G protein Gs. J Pediatr 1993; 123:509–518.
> Weinstein LS, Shenker A, Gejman PV, Merino MJ, et al.: Activating mutations of the stimulatory G protein in the McCune–Albright syndrome. N Engl J Med 1991; 325:1688–1695.

McKUSICK SYNDROME
see CARTILAGE–HAIR HYPOPLASIA

MEDIAN CLEFT FACE SYNDROME
see FRONTONASAL DYSPLASIA SEQUENCE

MELENEY ULCER, BACTERIAL SYNERGISTIC GANGRENE

Manifestations and Major Findings
progressive, synergistic, bacterial infection
aerobic streptococcus and *Staphylococcus aureus* or Gram-negative bacillus
leads to gangrene
often postoperative
ulcer has burrowing, bluish, undermined edge
extends rapidly

> **References**
> Feingold DS, Hirschmann JV, Leyden JJ: Bacterial infections of the skin. J Am Acad Dermatol 1989; 20:469–475.

MELKERSSON–ROSENTHAL SYNDROME, GRANULOMATOUS CHEILITIS

Manifestations and Major Findings
recurrent edema of the lips and face simulating angioedema (upper lip most common)
attacks may be accompanied by fever and malaise
lingua plicata (scrotal tongue)
recurrent facial paralysis
other cranial nerves may be affected
– olfactory nerve
– auditory nerve
– glossopharyngeal nerve
– hypoglossal nerve
histology shows granulomatous inflammation

> **References**
> Allen CM, Camisa C, Hamzeh S, Stephens L: Cheilitis granulomatosa: report of six cases and review of the literature. J Am Acad Dermatol 1990; 23:444–450. ▷ ▷ ▷

▷ ▷ ▷
Fisher AA: Chronic lip edema with particular reference to the Melkersson–Rosenthal syndrome. Cutis 1990; 45:144–146.
Greene RM, Rogers RS: Melkersson–Rosenthal syndrome: a review of 36 patients. J Am Acad Dermatol 1989; 21:1263–1270.

MENDES DACOSTA SYNDROME
see ERYTHROKERATODERMIA VARIABILIS and EPIDERMOLYSIS BULLOSA; SIMPLEX

MENKES SYNDROME, KINKY HAIR SYNDROME, MENKES KINKY HAIR SYNDROME

Manifestations and Major Findings
abnormal absorption, distribution, and metabolism of copper-binding proteins and metallothionein
low serum copper and ceruloplasmin
decreased activity of lysyl oxidase
coarse facies
growth retardation
progressive cerebral deterioration
severe mental retardation
seizures
impaired temperature regulation
susceptible to infection – especially pneumonia
tortuous vessels due to degenerated elastic tissue
bladder diverticula
inconsistent aminoaciduria
usually fatal by 3–4 years of age

HAIR ABNORMALITIES
pili torti (180° twists to hair shafts)
hair appears kinky
trichorrhexis nodosa
pale hair color

SKELETAL ABNORMALITIES
osteoporosis
scalloped vertebrae
metaphyseal spurring
wormian skull bones

X-linked recessive

References
Danks DM, Campbell PE, Stevens BJ, Mayne V, et al.: Menkes's kinky hair syndrome. Pediatrics 1972; 50:188–201.
Menkes JH: Kinky hair disease: 25 years later. Brain Dev 1988; 10:77–79.
Menkes JH, Alter M, Steigleder KK, Weakley DR, Sung JH: A sex-linked recessive disorder with retardation of growth, peculiar hair, and focal cerebral and cerebellar degeneration. Pediatrics 1962; 29:764–779.
Price VH: Disorders of the hair in children. Pediatr Clin N Am 1978; 25:305–320.

MERCURY POISONING
see PINK DISEASE

METAGERIA, PREMATURE AGING SYNDROME

Manifestations and Major Findings
loss of subcutaneous fat
bird-like facies
early atherosclerosis
early diabetes mellitus
tall and thin habitus

Cutaneous Manifestations
generalized poikiloderma
skin atrophy – most marked on the limbs
sparse, fine hair
sclerodermatous skin on the hands and feet

autosomal recessive

References
Beauregard S, Gilchrest BA: Syndromes of premature aging. Dermatol Clin 1987; 5:109–121.
Gilkes JJH, Sharvill DE, Wells RS: The premature ageing syndromes. Report of eight cases and description of a new entity named metageria. Br J Dermatol 1974; 91:243–262.

MIBELLI, ANGIOKERATOMA OF
see ANGIOKERATOMAS; MIBELLI

MICHELIN TIRE BABY SYNDROME

Manifestations and Major Findings
generalized folded skin
caused by diffuse, underlying, lipomatous or smooth muscle hamartomas
symmetric ringed creases around extremities
resembles Michelin tire advertising logo
Michelin tire baby syndrome may be related to; hemihypertrophy; limb abnormalities (valgus deformities, overlapping toes, lax joints); facial abnormalities (cleft palate, lateral clefting of lip, microcephaly); abnormal dentition; neurologic abnormalities (developmental delay, seizures); hypertrichosis; obesity.

> **References**
> Collins MRL, James WD, Rodman OG: The Michelin tire baby syndrome. J Assoc Military Dermatol 1989; 15:10.
> Gardner EW, Miller HM, Lowney ED: Folded skin associated with underlying nevus lipomatosus. Arch Dermatol 1979; 115:978–979.
> Ross CM: Generalized folded skin with an underlying lipomatous nevus: 'The Michelin tire baby'. Arch Dermatol 1969; 100:320–323.
> Schnur RE, Herzberg AJ, Spinner N, Kant JA, et. al.: Variability in the Michelin tire syndrome. J Am Acad Dermatol 1993; 28:364–370.

MIESCHER GRANULOMATOSIS,
CHEILITIS GRANULOMATOSA, MIESCHER CHEILITIS

Manifestations and Major Findings
diffuse, nontender, soft to firm swelling of one or both lips
histology shows non-necrotizing granulomas with edema, lymphangiectasia, and perivascular inflammation.

> **References**
> Allen CM, Camisa C, Hamzeh S, Stephens L: Cheilitis granulomatosa: report of six cases and review of the literature. J Am Acad Dermatol 1990; 23: 444–450.

MIKULICZ DISEASE

Manifestations and Major Findings
parotitis
bilateral or unilateral painless enlargement of salivary and lacrimal glands
xerostomia
decreased/absent lacrimation
may be caused by sarcoidosis

MILROY DISEASE

Manifestations and Major Findings
• primary congenital lymphedema (Fig. 97)
affects legs and/or hands and arms
appears at birth or infancy

autosomal dominant

> **References**
> Smeltzer DM, Stickler GB, Schirger A: Primary lymphedema in children and adolescents: a follow-up study and review. Pediatrics 1985; 76:206–218.

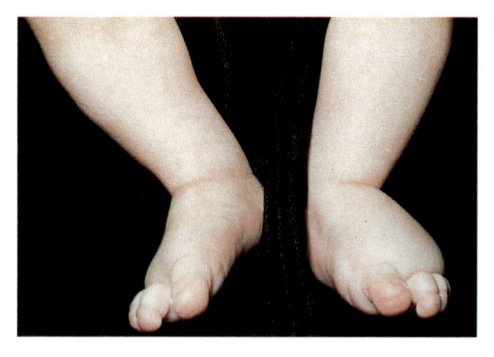

• *Figure 97 Primary congenital lymphedema of the foot in Milroy disease.*

MÖBIUS SYNDROME, MÖBIUS SEQUENCE

Manifestations and Major Findings
6th and 7th cranial nerve palsies
usually bilateral
mask-like facies
dysphagia

micrognathia
ptosis
Möbius syndrome may be associated with limb anomalies (talipes equinovarus).

MOHR SYNDROME
see OROFACIODIGITAL SYNDROME

MONDOR DISEASE, SCLEROSING PERIPHLEBITIS OF THE CHEST WALL

Manifestations and Major Findings
thrombophlebitis of the superficial veins or lymphatics of the anterior chest wall
tender or nontender cord in pectoral region
history of trauma
association with breast cancer
more common in women
can also be seen on the penis

> **References**
> Aloi FG, Tomasini CF, Molinero A: Railway track-like dermatitis: an atypical Mondor's disease? J Am Acad Dermatol 1989; 20:920–923.
> Samlaska CP, James WD: Superficial thrombophlebitis II. Secondary hypercoagulable states. J Am Acad Dermatol 1990; 23:1–18.

MONGOLIAN SPOT

Manifestations and Major Findings
congenital dermal melanocytosis
macular, blue/gray pigmentation present at birth
most common over the sacral area
mainly occurs in Orientals and Blacks
histology shows spindle-shaped melanocytes in reticular dermis

> **References**
> Hidano A: Persistent Mongolian spot in the adult. Arch Dermatol 1971; 103:680–681.
> Jacobs AH, Walton RG: The incidence of birthmarks in the neonate. Pediatrics 1976; 58:218–222.

MONILETHRIX SYNDROME
see also HAIR SHAFT ANOMALIES

Manifestations and Major Findings
• beaded hair (microscopically) (Fig. 98)
hair breaks easily
involved hair mainly on the scalp
may also affect eyebrows, eyelashes, and pubic hair
follicular keratosis on nape of neck and scalp
variable age of onset (usually early)

OTHER FINDINGS
koilonychia
dental abnormalities
mild mental retardation
juvenile cataracts

autosomal dominant or recessive

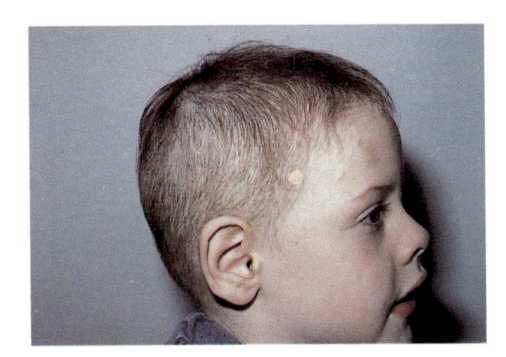

• *Figure 98 Short, broken-off hairs in monilethrix syndrome. This child's hair was never cut.*

> **References**
> de Berker D, Dawber RPR: Variations in the beading configuration in monilethrix. Pediatr Dermatol 1991; 9:19–21.
> Price VH: Disorders of the hair in children. Pediatr Clin N Am 1978; 25:305–320.
> Whiting DA: Structural abnormalities of the hair shaft J Am Acad Dermatol 1987; 16:1–25.

MORGAGNI–STEWART–MOREL SYNDROME, HYPEROSTOSIS FRONTALIS INTERNA

Manifestations and Major Findings
symmetrical benign thickening of the inner table of frontal or frontoparietal skull bones
progressive visual failure
primarily affects middle-aged or elderly women

ENDOCRINE ABNORMALITIES
obesity
gonadal disturbances
hirsutism and other signs of virilization

NEUROLOGIC ABNORMALITIES
headache
epilepsy
psychosis

> **References**
> Gegick CG, Danowski TS, Khurana RC, Vidalon C, et al.: Hyperostosis frontalis interna and hyperphosphatasemia. Ann Intern Med 1973; 79:71–75.

MORQUIO SYNDROME
see MUCOPOLYSACCHARIDOSES; TYPE IV

MORVAN SYNDROME

Manifestations and Major Findings
progressive sensory loss
recurrent painless infection around the nails
perforating ulcers
- loss of soft tissue (Fig. 99)
- resorption of phalanges (Fig. 99)
muscular atrophy
Morvan syndrome is associated with syringomyelia (progressive myelopathy with cavitation of central spinal cord) and leprosy.

> **References**
> Tashiro K, Fukazawa T, Moriwaka F, Hamada T, et al.: Syringomyelic syndrome: Clinical features in 31 cases confirmed by CT myelography or magnetic resonance imaging. J Neurol 1987; 235:26–30.

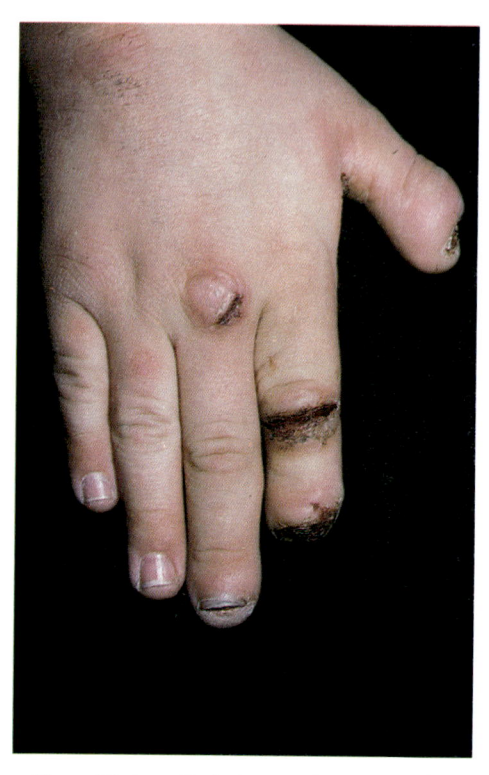

• *Figure 99 Loss of soft tisssue and resorption of phalanges in Morvan syndrome.*

MOSCHCOWITZ SYNDROME
see THROMBOTIC THROMBOCYTOPENIC PURPURA

MOYNAHAN SYNDROME, XERODERMA-TALIPES-ENAMEL DEFECT

Manifestations and Major Findings
ectodermal dysplasia
– xeroderma with red, dry, flaky skin
– slow hair growth (dry, poor texture)
– enamel defects (poorly formed teeth)
– hypohidrosis
– nail dystrophy
blistering of the skin
talipes equinovarus
photophobia
cleft palate
mild mental retardation

autosomal dominant

References
Moynahan EJ: XTE syndrome (xeroderma, talipes, and enamel defect): a new heredo-familial syndrome. Two cases. Homozygous inheritance of a dominant gene. Proc R Soc Med 1970; 63:447–448.

References
Gelmetti C, Rigoni C, Alessi E, Ermacora E, et al.: Pityriasis lichenoides in children: a long-term follow-up of eighty-nine cases. J Am Acad Dermatol 1990; 23:473–478.
Longley J, Demar J, Feinstein RP, Milelr RL, et. al.: Clinical and histological features of pityriasis lichenoides et varioliformis acuta in children. Arch Dermatol 1987; 123:1335–1339.

MUCHA–HABERMANN SYNDROME, PITYRIASIS LICHENOIDES ET VARIOLIFORMIS ACUTA (PLEVA)

Manifestations and Major Findings
- macules, vesicles, and papulonecrotic lesions develop in crops (Fig. 100)
lesions leave varioliform scarring

OTHER FINDINGS
mild fever
malaise
lymphadenopathy
arthralgias/arthritis
more common in men
variable course

MUCKLE–WELLS SYNDROME

Manifestations and Major Findings
urticaria, fever, and limb pain
periodic recurrent attacks (24–48 h)
progressive deafness
amyloidosis (renal, cutaneous)
usually begins in childhood
progressive course

autosomal dominant

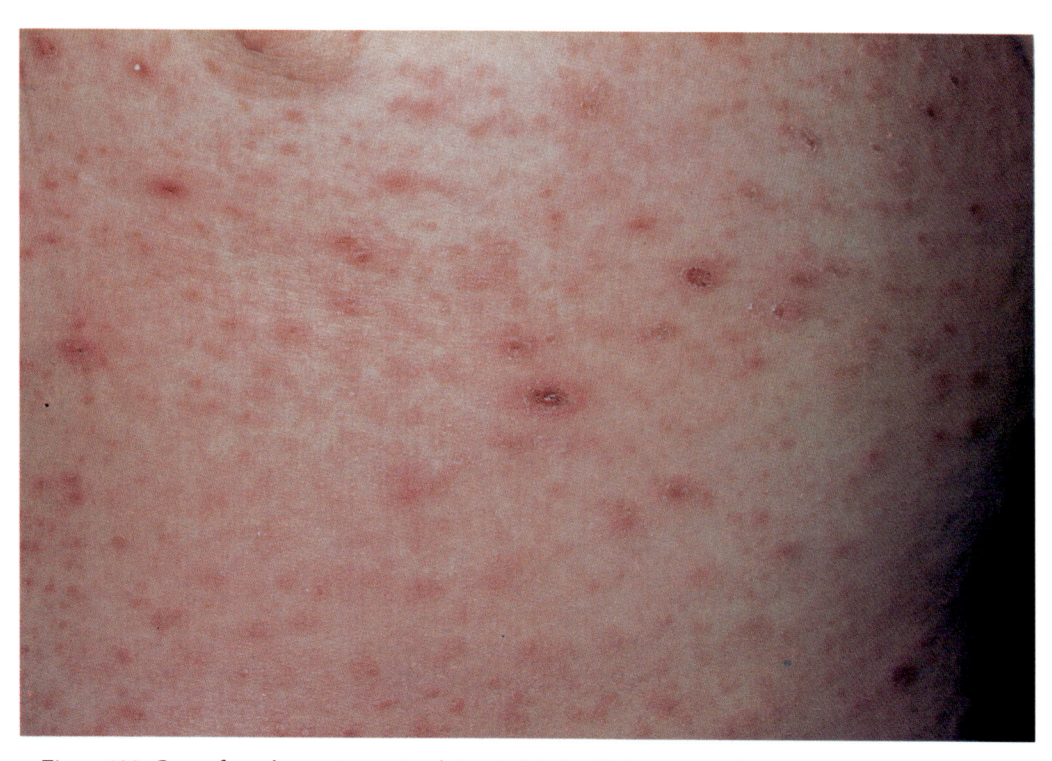

• *Figure 100* Crops of papulonecrotic, scarring lesions in Mucha–Habermann syndrome.

> **References**
> Breathnach SM: Amyloid and amyloidosis. J Am Acad Dermatol 1988; 18:1–16.
> Muckle TJ: The 'Muckle Wells' syndrome. Br J Dermatol 1979; 100:87–92.

MUCOCUTANEOUS LYMPH NODE SYNDROME see KAWASAKI DISEASE

MUCOLIPIDOSIS II, I-CELL DISEASE

Manifestations and Major Findings
N-acetylglucosaminyl phosphotransferase deficiency
radiologic findings of dysostosis multiplex
restricted joint movement
symptoms begin in first year
usually fatal before 6 years of age due to congestive heart failure

Characteristic Facies
coarse Hurler-like features
– puffy eyelids
– gingival hyperplasia
– thick tongue

Cutaneous Manifestations
thickened skin during early infancy
skin becomes less tight with age
hemangiomas

autosomal recessive

MUCOLIPIDOSIS III, PSEUDO-HURLER POLYDYSTROPHY

Manifestations and Major Findings
N-acetylglucosaminyl phosphotransferase deficiency
milder symptoms than mucolipidosis II
symptoms begin at 2–4 years of age
coarse Hurler-like features
corneal opacities on slit lamp examination
growth retardation
progressive joint stiffness with joint contractures
clawhand deformity by 6 years of age
radiographic findings of dysostosis multiplex
synophrys (growing together of eyebrows)
mild mental retardation/learning disabilities

autosomal recessive

MUCOPOLYSACCHARIDOSES

Types of Mucopolysaccharidosis (MPS) and Features

type I-H mucopolysaccharidosis, Hurler syndrome
α-L-iduronidase deficiency
urinary dermatan sulfate and heparan sulfate
corneal clouding
hepatosplenomegaly
skeletal deformities – dysostosis multiplex
severe short stature
stiff joints
coarse facial features
large tongue
prominent forehead
thickening of the skin
hypertrichosis
progressive mental retardation
deafness
fatal by 10 years of age
autosomal recessive

type I-H/S mucopolysaccharidosis, Hurler/Scheie syndrome
α-L-iduronidase deficiency
urinary dermatan sulfate and heparan sulfate
• type I-H/I-S MPS intermediate phenotype (Fig. 101)
onset at 3–8 years of age
normal intelligence or mild retardation
progressive visceral involvement
fatal by third decade
autosomal recessive

type I-S mucopolysaccharidosis, Scheie syndrome
α-L-iduronidase deficiency
urinary dermatan sulfate and heparan sulfate
less severe than type I-H MPS
onset by 5 years of age
corneal opacities
joint stiffness
aortic valve disease
normal intelligence
normal stature

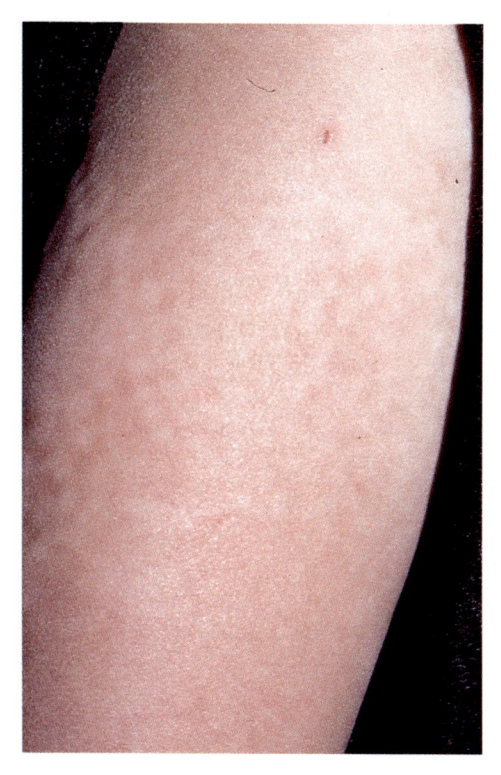

Figure 101 Skin-colored papules I-H/S mucopolysaccharidosis (Hurler/Scheie), also seen in type II mucopolysaccharidosis (Hunter).

carpal tunnel syndrome
broad mouth with full lips
autosomal recessive

**type II-A mucopolysaccharidosis,
severe Hunter syndrome**
iduronate sulfate sulfatase deficiency
urinary dermatan sulfate and heparan sulfate
similar to type I-H MPS except
– no corneal clouding
– milder course
onset at 2–4 years of age
central nervous system degeneration
slow progression
mental retardation
hepatosplenomegaly
coarse facial features
hypertrichosis
deafness
no gibbus deformity of the spine
papular plaques
skin lesions (papules over scapular area)
fatal by 10–15 years of age
X-linked recessive

**type II-B mucopolysaccharidosis,
mild Hunter syndrome**
iduronate sulfate sulfatase deficiency
urinary dermatan sulfate and heparan sulfate
somatic involvement greater than type II-A MPS
normal intelligence
survival to 50–60 years of age
X-linked recessive

**type III-A mucopolysaccharidosis,
Sanfilippo syndrome A**
heparan-*N*-sulfatase deficiency
urinary heparan-*N*-sulfate
central nervous system involvement
lesser somatic involvement
normal development up to 3–4 years of age
later loss of developmental 'milestones'
hyperactivity
behavioral problems
coarse blonde hair
hypertrichosis
mild hepatosplenomegaly
macrocephaly
mild dysostosis multiplex
normal survival
autosomal recessive

**type III-B mucopolysaccharidosis,
Sanfilippo syndrome B**
α-*N*-acetylglucosaminidase deficiency
urinary heparan sulfate
phenotype similar to type III-A MPS
autosomal recessive

**type III-C mucopolysaccharidosis,
Sanfilippo syndrome C**
acetyl-CoA: α-glucosaminide-*N*-acetyltransferase deficiency
urinary heparan sulfate
phenotype similar to type III-A MPS
autosomal recessive

**type III-D mucopolysaccharidosis,
Sanfilippo syndrome D**
N-acetylglucosaminide-6-sulfatase deficiency
urinary heparan sulfate
phenotype similar to type III-A MPS
autosomal recessive

**type IV-A mucopolysaccharidosis,
Morquio syndrome A**
N-acetylgalactosamine-6-sulfate sulfatase deficiency
urinary keratan sulfate
corneal clouding
spondyloepiphyseal dysplasia
– severe kyphosis
– genu valgum (knock-knee)
short stature   ▷ ▷ ▷

▷ ▷ ▷
sternal protrusion
aortic regurgitation
cutaneous findings
– telangiectasias – especially on the face and limbs
– thickened skin
– *café au lait* macules
ligamentous laxity
normal or slightly impaired intelligence
fatal due to complications of cervical spine instability

autosomal recessive

type IV-B mucopolysaccharidosis, Morquio syndrome B
β-galactosidase deficiency
urinary keratan sulfate
phenotype similar to type IV-A MPS

autosomal recessive

type V mucopolysaccharidosis
name no longer used

type VI mucopolysaccharidosis, Maroteaux–Lamy syndrome
N-acetylgalactosamine-4-sulfate sulfatase (arylsulphatase B) deficiency
urinary dermatan sulfate
phenotype may be severe, like type I-H MPS, except with normal intelligence
or may be mild with short stature
or intermediate
corneal changes (mild)
severe osseous changes with stiffness – especially hands, elbows, shoulders, and knees
valvular heart disease
neutrophil inclusions
survival to 20 years of age

autosomal recessive

type VII mucopolysaccharidosis, Sly syndrome
β-glucuronidase deficiency
urinary dermatan sulfate and heparan sulfate
phenotype similar to type I-H MPS with central nervous system and visceral involvement
recognizable in neonatal period

autosomal recessive

type VIII mucopolysaccharidosis, DiFerrante syndrome
glucosamine-6-sulfate sulfatase deficiency
urinary keratan sulfate and heparan sulfate
short stature
mild dysostosis multiplex
ring-shaped metachromasia of lymphocytes

autosomal recessive

References
Finlayson LA: Hunter syndrome (Mucopolysaccharidosis II). Pediatr Dermatol 1990; 7:150–152.
Spranger J: Mini Review: Inborn errors of complex carbohydrate metabolism. Am J Med Genet 1987; 28:489–499.
Warkentin PI, Dixon MS, Schafer I, Strandjord SE, Coccia PF: Bone marrow transplantation in Hunter syndrome: a preliminary report. Birth Defects 1986; 22 (1):31–39.
Whitley CB, Ramsay NKC, Kersey JH, Krivit W: Bone marrow transplantation for Hurler Syndrome: assessment of metabolic correction. Birth Defects 1986; 22 (1):7–24.

MUCOSAL NEUROMA SYNDROME,

MULTIPLE ENDOCRINE NEOPLASIA SYNDROMES;
TYPE 2B (3)

Manifestations and Major Findings

neuromata extending from the lips to the rectum
large prominent lips with a bumpy surface
medullary carcinoma of thyroid (>85%)
– usually in adolescence
– bilateral and multicentric
pheochromocytoma (50%) – often bilateral
neuromas of the conjunctiva with thickened margins displacing the cilia
everted eyelid sign (spontaneous)

OTHER FINDINGS
asthenic body-build with muscle wasting (marfanoid habitus)
early fatality (20–30 years) due to thyroid carcinoma
parathyroid disorders (rare)
laxity of joints
café au lait macules
kyphoscoliosis
medullated corneal nerves

autosomal dominant or sporadic

References
Feingold KR, Elias PM: Endocrine–skin interactions. J Am Acad Dermatol 1988; 19:1–20.   ▷ ▷ ▷

> > >
Kaufman FR, Roe TF, Isaacs H, Weitzman JJ: Metastic medullary thyroid carcinoma in young children with mucosal neuroma syndrome. Pediatrics 1982; 70:263–267.
Kirk JF, Flowers FP, Ramos-Caro FA, Browder JF: Multiple endocrine neoplasia type III: case report and review. Pediatr Dermatol 1991; 8:124–128.

MUIR–TORRE SYNDROME
see TORRE–MUIR SYNDROME

MULIBREY NANISM SYNDROME,
PERHEENTUPA SYNDROME, MULIBREY TYPE DWARFISM

Manifestations and Major Findings
frequent multiple organ involvement
– *mu*scle (hypotonia)
– *li*ver (hepatomegaly)
– *br*ain (J-shaped sella turcica, dolichocephaly)
– *ey*e (yellow dots in fundus)
severe short stature (nanism)
hypotonia
pericardial constriction – infantile onset
fibrous dysplasia of the long bones
high-pitched voice
triangular facies with prominent forehead
cutaneous hemangiomas – particularly on limbs
delayed onset of puberty in females
normal intelligence
syndrome of Finnish ethnic origin

autosomal recessive

References
Voorhess ML, Husson GS, Blackman MS: Growth failure with pericardial constriction. Am J Dis Child 1976; 130:1146–1148.

MULTIPLE CARBOXYLASE DEFICIENCY *see* BIOTIN DEFICIENCY AND BIOTIN-RESPONSIVE DISORDERS

MULTIPLE ENDOCRINE NEOPLASIA SYNDROMES

Manifestations and Major Findings
neoplasia of cell lines of APUD (*a*mine *p*recursor *u*ptake and *d*ecarboxylation) system

Types of Multiple Endocrine Neoplasia and Features

1 **multiple endocrine neoplasia type 1, Wermer syndrome**
parathyroid hyperplasia or tumors
pancreatic tumors – secrete gastrin, insulin, pancreatic polypeptides or glucagon
pituitary adenomas – usually secrete prolactin
adrenal adenomas
thymomas
thyroid abnormalities
carcinoid tumors
lipomas
gastric polyps
schwannomas

autosomal dominant; chromosome 11

2 **multiple endocrine neoplasia type 2A, Sipple syndrome**
parathyroid hyperplasia or adenoma
medullary thyroid carcinoma or C cell hyperplasia
pheochromocytoma – usually bilateral
scapular pruritic skin lesions (childhood onset) – macules later becoming hyperkeratotic

autosomal dominant

3 **multiple endocrine neoplasia type 3 (also called 2B)**
see mucosal neuroma syndrome

References
Alberts WM, McMeekin JO, George JM: Mixed multiple endocrine neoplasia syndromes. J Am Med Assoc 1980; 244:1236–1237.
Bugalho MJGM, Limbert E, Sobrinho LG, Clode AL, et al.: A kindred with multiple endocrine neoplasia Type 2A associated with pruritic skin lesions. Cancer 1992; 70:2664-2667.
Feingold KR, Elias PM: Endocrine–skin interactions. J Am Acad Dermatol 1988; 19:1–20.
Friedman E, Sakaguchi K, Bale AE, Falchetti A, et al.: Clonality of parathyroid tumors in familial multiple endocrine neoplasia type I. N Engl J Med 1989; 321: 213–218. > > >

> > >
Kirk JF, Flowers FP, Ramos-Caro FA, Browder JF: Multiple endocrine neoplasia type III: case report and review. Pediatr Dermatol 1991; 8:124–128.
Nunziata V: Hereditary localized pruritus in affected members of a kindred with multiple endocrine neoplasia type 2A (Sipple's syndrome). Clin Endocrinol 1989; 30:57–63.
Thakker RV, Bouloux P, Wooding C, Chotai K, et al.: Association of parathyroid tumors in multiple endocrine neoplasia type I with loss of alleles on chromosome 11. N Engl J Med 1989; 321:218–224.

MULTIPLE HAMARTOMA SYNDROME see COWDEN DISEASE

MULTIPLE LENTIGINES SYNDROME see LEOPARD SYNDROME

MULTIPLE PTERYGIUM SYNDROME, ESCOBAR SYNDROME

Manifestations and Major Findings
congenital joint contractures (arthrogryposis)
pterygium (multiple) across major joints
–sides of neck
–popliteal fossa
–axillae
–antecubital fossa
–interdigital area (syndactyly)
–intercrural area
–chin to sternum
–clubfoot deformity
–scoliosis (with or without vertebral anomalies)
–camptodactyly (flexural contraction of fingers)
short stature
normal intelligence

Characteristic Facies
ptosis of the eyelids
downslanting eyes
epicanthal folds
cleft palate
high-arched palate
multiple minor facial anomalies
sad, emotionless face

autosomal recessive

References
Hall JG, Reed SD, Rosenbaum J, et al.: Limb pterygium syndromes: A review and report of eleven cases. Am J Med Genet 1982; 12:377–409.
Ramer JC, Ladda RL, Demuth WW: Multiple pterygium syndrome. An overview. Am J Dis Child 1988; 142:794–798.

MULTIPLE SULFATASE DEFICIENCY SYNDROME see also DISORDERS OF CORNIFICATION; DOC 13

Manifestations and Major Findings
impaired activity of all known lysosomal sulfatases including steroid sulfatase
ichthyosis resembling X-linked ichthyosis (see DOC 2)
neurodegenerative disease
coarse facies (Hurler-like features)
hepatosplenomegaly
skeletal changes with dysostosis multiplex
mental retardation
storage granules in neutrophils

autosomal recessive

MULTIPLE TRICHOEPITHELIOMAS
see BROOKE SYNDROME

MÜNCHAUSEN SYNDROME

Manifestations and Major Findings
persons seek medical care by feigning illness
absence of any organic medical or surgical disease
false medical histories
fabricated physical signs and laboratory findings
needless medical evaluations, operations, and treatment
psychiatric illness

Cutaneous Manifestations
dermatitis artefacta
dermatological pathomimickry
• neurotic excoriations (Fig. 102)
ulcerations of the skin

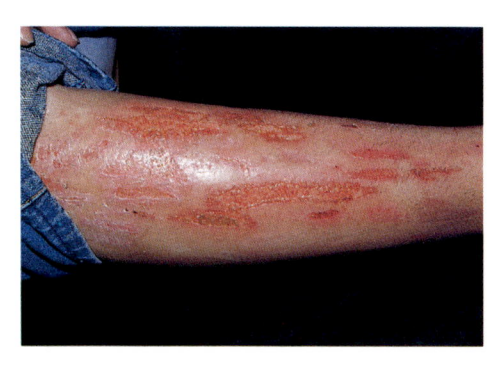

Figure 102 Neurotic excoriations; one of many factitial symptoms found in Münchausen syndrome.

References
Ifudu O, Kolasinski SL, Friedman EA: Brief report: kidney-related Munchausen's syndrome. N Engl J Med 1992; 327:388–389.

MÜNCHAUSEN SYNDROME BY PROXY

Manifestations and Major Findings
a form of child abuse
illness in child is fabricated by the parent
numerous hospitalizations
persistent or recurrent illnesses
cause of illnesses cannot be found
discrepancies between history and clinical findings

References
Jones JG, Butler HL, Hamilton B, Perdue JD, et al.: Munchausen syndrome by proxy. Child Abuse Negl 1986; 10:33–40.
Makar AF, Squier PJ: Munchausen syndrome by proxy: father as a perpetrator. Pediatrics 1990; 85: 370–373.
McGuire TL, Feldman KW: Psychologic morbidity of children subjected to Munchausen syndrome by proxy. Pediatrics 1989; 83:289–292.
McNeese MC, Hebeler JR: The abused child. CIBA Clinical Symposia 1977; 29:1–36.

MYOTONIC DYSTROPHY,
STEINERT SYNDROME

Manifestations and Major Findings
tonic spasms of muscles (myotonia)
atrophy of skin, fat, and muscles
hypotonia in infancy
premature frontal hair recession – especially males
myopathic facies (immobile)
hypogonadism
cataracts
premature aging
scoliosis
heart conduction defects
variable time of onset

autosomal dominant with variable expression

N

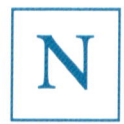

NAEGELI–FRANCESCHETTI–JADASSOHN SYNDROME

see FRANCESCHETTI–JADASSOHN SYNDROME

NAIL ABNORMALITIES

Summary of Nail Abnormality Definitions

1. **agnail**
   hang nail
   hard spicules at the edge of the nail

2. **anonychia**
   absence of a nail from birth
   associated with
   – nail-patella syndrome
   – ectodermal dysplasias
   – maternal hydantoin ingestion
   – Coffin–Siris syndrome

3. **Beau's lines**
   transverse depressions in all nails
   caused by any condition temporarily interfering with the rate of nail growth
   – severe infections
   – stress
   – hyperthyroidism
   – surgery

4. **blue lunulae**
   associated with Wilson disease

5. **blue nails**
   associated with
   – antimalarial drugs
   – argyria
   – bleomycin
   – congenital pernicious anemia
   – minocycline, phenolphthalein, and phenothiazines
   – Wilson disease

6. **brachyonychia**
   short nails
   nail width greater than the length
   associated with
   – Rubinstein–Taybi syndrome
   – Down syndrome
   – hyperparathyroidism

7. **clubbing**
   bulbous, fusiform enlargement of distal fingers/toes
   Lovibond's angle over 180°
   associated with
   – lung carcinoma or lung disease
   – cyanotic cardiovascular diseases
   – idiopathic causes

8. **fragilitas unguium**
   brittle nails
   may be associated with
   – malnutrition
   – trauma (particularly from constant wetting of the hands)

9. **half-and-half nails (Lindsay's nails)**
   seen in renal failure
   proximal nail is white
   distal 20–50% of nail is red, pink, or brown

10. **hapalonychia**
    soft nails

11. **Hutchinson's sign**
    periungual spread of pigment into proximal and lateral nail folds
    important indicator of subungual melanoma (not pathognomonic)

12. **koilonychia**
    spoon-shaped or flat nails
    associated with
    – iron deficiency anemia
    – Plummer–Vinson syndrome (idiopathic or familial)

13 leukonychia
white nails
congenital or acquired
may be associated with
- alopecia areata
- hypoalbuminemia
- cirrhosis
- exfoliative dermatitis
- Darier disease
- acrokeratosis verruciformis
- pellagra
- zinc deficiency

14 macronychia
large but otherwise normal nails
associated with
- neurofibromatosis
- tuberous sclerosis

15 median nail dystrophy of Heller
split or canal in the nail plate
split runs from cuticle to free edge
usually found just off-center
caused by trauma or idiopathic
most common on the thumb

16 Mee's lines
white bands in the nail plate
lines move with the plate as it grows
may be associated with
- arsenic or thallium ingestion
- cardiac insufficiency
- Hodgkin disease
- Hansen disease
- malaria
- pellagra
- renal failure
- sickle cell anemia

17 micronychia
small but otherwise normal nails
associated with
- ectodermal dysplasia
- dyskeratosis congenita
- nail-patella syndrome

18 Muehrcke's lines
paired, white, parallel bands on all nails
bands do not move
seen with hypoalbuminemia

19 onychalgia nervosa
exquisitely sensitive nails

20 onychauxis
thick nails

21 onychia
inflammation of the nail
post-traumatic or with paronychia

22 onychocryptosis (unguis incarnatus)
ingrown nails
associated with
- diabetes
- aging
- newborns
- narrow shoes
- trauma

23 onychogryphosis
acquired nail thickening
caused by trauma, aging or unknown etiology

24 onychoheterotropia
misplaced nails

25 onycholysis
separation of the nail plate from the nail bed
separation at the distal and lateral attachments
caused by
- hypo- or hyperthyroidism
- trauma
- psoriasis
- candidal infections
- diabetes
- phototoxic reactions to drugs
  (tetracycline, thorazine)
- idiopathic causes

26 onychomadesis
separation of the entire nail plate from the bed

27 onychomycosis
fungal infection of the nails

28 onychophagia
nail-biting

29 onychoschizia (lamellar dystrophy)
splitting of the nails into layers parallel to the surface
small pieces may flake
usually caused by minor injury or water

30 onychorrhexis
excess longitudinal ridging

31 onychotillomania
habitual picking at nails
associated with median nail dystrophy of Heller

32 pachyonychia
thickening of the nails
usually increasing thickness from base to tip
associated with pachyonychia congenita

▷ ▷ ▷

33 panaritium (whitlow)
abscess at the side or base of a nail

34 paronychia
inflammation of a nail fold
usually caused by infection (bacteria, fungi, yeast)

35 pincer nail dystrophy
overcurvature of a nail
pain
partial strangulation of the soft tissues

36 platyonychia
increased nail curvature along the long axis

37 Plummer's nails
upwardly curved end of the nails
caused by thyrotoxicosis or other onycholysis

38 polyonychia
two or more separate nails on one digit

39 pterygium inversum unguis
distal nail bed remains adherent to ventral nail plate

40 pterygium
wing-shaped destruction of the nail matrix
overgrowth of the cuticle onto the nail
eventual destruction of the nail
scarring
associated with
– cicatricial pemphigoid
– dyskeratosis congenita
– graft versus host disease
– Raynaud disease
– systemic sclerosis

41 racket nail
congenital abnormality of a nail
broad, short nail
most common on the thumb

42 red lunulae
associated with
– collagen vascular disease
– alopecia areata
– alcoholism
– congestive heart failure
– chronic obstructive pulmonary disease
– other disorders

43 splinter hemorrhages
associated with
– subacute bacterial endocarditis
– trauma
– vasculitis
– cirrhosis
– trichinosis
– scurvy
– psoriasis
– chronic glomerulonephritis
– Darier disease

44 Terry's nails
1–2 mm of distal nail is pink
white proximal nail
associated with
– hypoalbuminemia
– hepatic cirrhosis

45 trachyonychia
uniform roughness of the nail plate surface
associated with
– ichthyosis vulgaris
– ectodermal dysplasia
– IgA deficiency
– amyloidosis
– alopecia areata

46 twenty nail dystrophy
acquired excess ridging of all nails
with or without pitting
seen in childhood

47 V-shaped lunulae
associated with nail-patella syndrome

48 whitlow
recurring vesicles around the distal finger or nail
painful
caused by herpes inoculation

49 yellow nails (see also yellow nail syndrome)
thickened yellow nails
associated with
– chronic lymphedema
– pleural effusion
– bronchiectasis
– chronic bronchitis
– carcinoma of the larynx
– rheumatoid arthritis
– sinusitis
– thyroid disease
– psoriasis
– pachyonychia congenita
– jaundice
– drugs (tetracycline, penicillamine)

References
Baran R: Pincer and trumpet nails. Arch Dermatol 1974; 110:639–640.   ▷ ▷ ▷

▷ ▷ ▷
Baran R, Kechijian P: Longitudinal melanonychia (melanonychia striata): diagnosis and management. J Am Acad Dermatol 1989; 21:1165–1175.
Barth JH, Dawber RPR: Diseases of the nails in children. Pediatr Dermatol 1987; 4:275–290.
Cohen PR: Red lunulae: case report and literature review. J Am Acad Dermatol 1992; 26:292–294.
Feldman SR, Gammon WR: Unilateral Muehrcke's lines following trauma. Arch Dermatol 1989;125: 133–134.
Jerasutus S, Suvanprakorn P, Kitchawengkul O: Twenty nail dystrophy. Arch Dermatol 1990; 126: 1068–1070.
Lindsay PG: The half-and-half nail. Arch Intern Med 1967; 119:583–587.
Muehrcke HC: The fingernails in chronic hypoalbuminemia. Br Med J 1956; I:1327–1338.
Telfer NR, Barth JH, Dawber RPR: Congenital and hereditary nail dystrophies – an embryological approach to classification. Clin Exp Dermatol 1988; 13:160–163.
Terry R: White nails in hepatic cirrhosis. Lancet 1954; I:756–759.
Wilkerson MG, Wilkin JK: Red lunulae revisited: a clinical and histopathologic examination. J Am Acad Dermatol 1989; 20:453–457

NAIL–PATELLA SYNDROME,
NAIL–PATELLA–ELBOW SYNDROME, CONGENITAL ILIAC HORNS SYNDROME, HEREDITARY OSTEO-ONYCHODYSPLASIA SYNDROME

Manifestations and Major Findings
onychodystrophy – hypoplasia and splitting
medial thumbnail most commonly involved
usual sparing of toenails
triangular lunulae
absent or rudimentary patellae
unstable knees
elbow dysplasia
subluxation of head of radius
iliac horns (calcifications from posterior aspect of ilium)

OTHER FINDINGS
renal abnormalities
– glomerulonephritis
– renal dysplasia
– Goodpasture syndrome
hypoplasia of the scapulae
scoliosis
cloverleaf pigmentation of irides (Lester's iris)
laxity of the skin
hyperhidrosis

autosomal dominant

References
Lucas GL, Opitz JM: The nail-patella syndrome. J Pediatr 1966; 68:273–288.
Kucirka SJ, Scher RK: Heritable nail disorders. Dermatol Clin 1987; 5:179–191.
Sabnis SG, Antonovych TT, Argy WP, Rakowski TA, et al.: Nail-patella syndrome. Clin Nephrol 1980; 14:148–153.

NAME SYNDROME, LAMB SYNDROME, CARNEY SYNDROME, see also CARNEY SYNDROME

Manifestations and Major Findings
*n*evi (blue)
*a*trial myxomas
*m*yxoid neurofibromas
*e*phelides

autosomal dominant

References
Atherton DJ, Pitcher DW, Wells RS, MacDonald DM: A syndrome of various cutaneous pigmented lesions, myxoid neurofibromata and atrial myxoma: the NAME syndrome. Br J Dermatol 1980; 103: 421–429.
Carney JA, Headington JT, Su WPD: Cutaneous myxomas. Arch Dermatol 1986; 122:790–798.
Rhodes AR, Silverman RA, Harrist TJ, Perez-Atayde AR: Mucocutaneous lentigines, cardiomucocutaneous myxomas, and multiple blue nevi: The 'LAMB' syndrome. J Am Acad Dermatol 1984; 10:72–82.

NECROLYTIC MIGRATORY ERYTHEMA
see GLUCAGONOMA SYNDROME

NÉKAM DISEASE, KERATOSIS LICHENOIDES CHRONICA, POROKERATOSIS STRIATA LICHENOIDES

Manifestations and Major Findings
violaceous, papular and nodular lesions
linear and reticulate patterns
most marked on the hands and feet
facial seborrheic dermatitis
chronic and progressive course

> **References**
> David M, Filhaber A, Rotem A, et al.: Keratosis lichenoides chronica with prominent telangiectasia: response to etretinate. J Am Acad Dermatol 1989; 21:1112–1114.
> Margolis MH, Cooper GA, Johnson SAM: Keratosis lichenoides chronica. Arch Dermatol 1972; 105: 739–743.
> Ryatt KS, Greenwood R, Cotterill JA: Keratosis lichenoides chronica. Br J Dermatol 1982; 106: 223–225.

NEONATAL LUPUS ERYTHEMATOSUS

Manifestations and Major Findings
congenital heart block caused by fibrosis of the conducting pathway
Ro (SSA) antibody usually always present in neonate and mother, sometimes with La (SSB) and RNP antibodies
hepatosplenomegaly
lymphadenopathy
hematologic abnormalities
thrombocytopenia
mothers may have vague symptoms (arthralgia, malaise) or be asymptomatic

Cutaneous Manifestations
scaly, annular, erythematous, photosensitive eruption
central atrophy of lesions in first months of life
lesions may be purpuric
rash improves in 4–6 months

> **References**
> Watson R, Kang JE, May M, Hudak M, et al.: Thrombocytopenia in the neonatal lupus syndrome. Arch Dermatol 1988; 124:560–563.

NETHERTON SYNDROME, COMEL–NETHERTON SYNDROME, see also DISORDERS OF CORNIFICATION; DOC 9 and HAIR SHAFT ANOMALIES

Manifestations and Major Findings
'bamboo' hairs (trichorrhexis invaginata)
- ichthyosis linearis circumflexa (double-edged scale) (Fig. 103)

OTHER FINDINGS
generalized erythema and scaling begins at birth or in first few months of life
diffusely red and scaly face
atopy
other hair shaft defects
– trichorrhexis nodosa
– pili torti
inconstant aminoaciduria
mild developmental delay
short stature
anaphylactic reactions to foods
impaired cellular immunity
elevated serum IgE levels

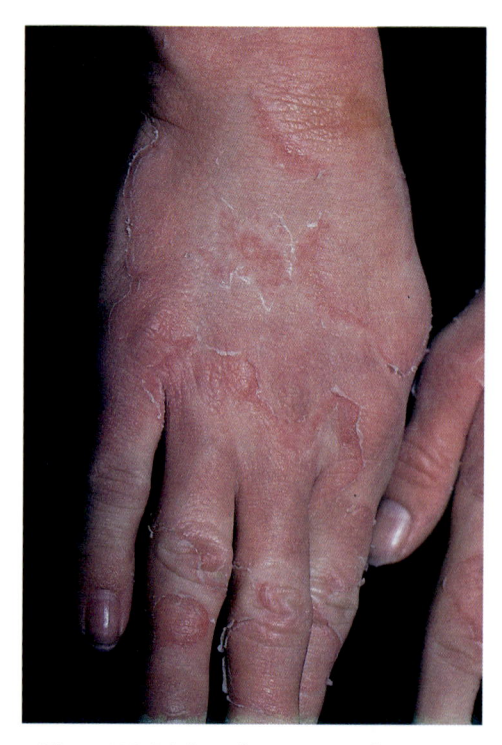

- *Figure 103* Ichthyosis linearis circumflexa seen in Netherton syndrome.

autosomal recessive

> **References**
> Caputo R, Vanotti P, Bertani E: Netherton's syndrome in two adult brothers. Arch Dermatol 1984; 120:220–222.
> Greene SL, Muller SA: Netherton's syndrome. J Am Acad Dermatol 1985; 13:329–337.
> Krafchik BR: Netherton Syndrome. Pediatr Dermatol 1992; 9:157–160.
> Manabe M, Yoshiike T, Negi M, Ogawa H: Successful therapy of ichthyosis linearis circumflexa with PUVA. J Am Acad Dermatol 1983; 8:905–906.
> Price VH: Disorders of the hair in children. Pediatr Clin N Am 1978; 25:305–320.
> Wehr RF, Hickman J, Drochmal L: Effective treatment of Netherton's syndrome with 12% lactate lotion. J Am Acad Dermatol 1988; 19:140–142.
> Wilkinson RD, Curtis GH, Hawk WA: Netherton's disease. Arch Dermatol 1964; 89:46–54.

NEUMANN TYPE PEMPHIGUS VEGETANS

Manifestations and Major Findings

early stages identical to pemphigus vulgaris with bullae and erosions
eroded areas develop hypertrophic granulation tissue
lesions studded with pustules

> **References**
> Lever WF: Pemphigus and pemphigoid: a review of the advances made since 1964. J Am Acad Dermatol 1979; 1:2–31.

NEUROCUTANEOUS MELANOSIS,
TOURAINE SYNDROME

Manifestations and Major Findings

large congenital melanocytic nevus or multiple congenital nevi
most commonly on the head and neck
especially involving posterior midline
benign or malignant pigment cell proliferation of the leptomeninges
poor prognosis

NEUROLOGIC ABNORMALITIES
usually develop in first 2 years of life
increased intracranial pressure or hydrocephalus
leptomeningeal melanosis or melanoma
spinal cord compression

Neurocutaneous melanosis is associated with malformations of the spinal column or central nervous system, Meckel diverticulum, and renal malformations.

> **References**
> Kadonaga JN, Frieden IJ: Neurocutaneous melanosis: definition and review of the literature. J Am Acad Dermatol 1991; 24:747–755.
> Marghoob AA, Orlow SJ, Kopf AW: Syndromes associated with melanocytic nevi. J Am Acad Dermatol 1993; 29:373–388.

NEUROFIBROMATOSIS

Types of Neurofibromatosis, Symptoms, and Diagnostic Criteria

1 classic type (NF-1), von Recklinghausen disease
- multiple *café au lait* macules (Fig. 104) ▷ ▷ ▷

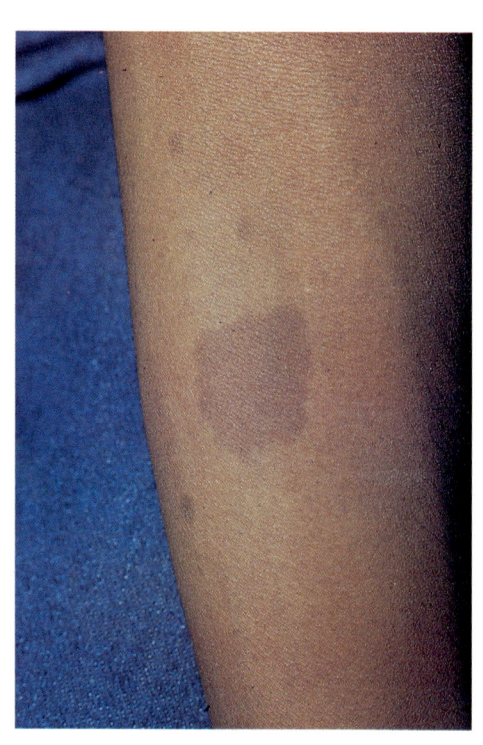

• *Figure 104 Multiple café au lait macules are one of several diagnostic criteria for classic type neurofibromatosis.*

▷ ▷ ▷
macules may vary in size (0.5–50 cm)
axillary or inguinal freckling (Crowe sign)
iris hamartomas (Lisch nodules)
• often diffuse neurofibromas (Fig. 105)
plexiform neurofibromas
optic gliomas
distinctive osseous lesions
– sphenoid dysplasia
– thinning of the long-bone cortex (with or without pseudarthrosis)
kyphoscoliosis
tibial bowing
short stature
macrocephaly
learning disabilities
pruritus
oral cavity tumors
macroglossia
endocrine disturbances
– precocious puberty
– acromegaly
– pheochromocytoma
– hyperparathyroidism
– Addison disease
sarcomatous change in neurofibromas (rare)
brainstem and cerebellar tumors

increased risk for
– rhabdomyosarcoma
– Wilms tumor,
– leukemia
– malignant schwannomas

autosomal dominant; chromosome 17 (proximal long arm)

diagnosis requires two or more of the following:
– *café au lait* macules; six or more, >5 mm in greatest diameter (prepubertal), >15 mm (postpubertal)
– neurofibromas (two or more of any type) or one plexiform neurofibroma
– axillary or inguinal freckling
– optic glioma
– iris hamartomas (two or more)
– distinctive osseous lesions (sphenoid dysplasia or thinning of the long-bone cortex, with or without pseudarthrosis)
– first-degree relative with NF-1 by these criteria

2 central type (NF-2), bilateral acoustic neurofibromatosis
acoustic neuromas of the seventh cranial nerve (90% bilateral)
multiple central nervous system tumors (various types)
few *café au lait* macules or neurofibromas
no axillary freckling
no iris hamartomas (Lisch nodules)
cataracts common

autosomal dominant; chromosome 22 (long arm)

diagnosis requires:
bilateral acoustic neuromas
or
first degree relative with NF-2
plus unilateral acoustic neuroma
or plus two of the following:
– neurofibromas (dermal or subcutaneous)
– plexiform neurofibroma
– schwannoma
– glioma
– meningioma
– lens opacities (posterior, subcapsular)

3 segmental type
café au lait macules
neurofibromas
unilateral segmental distribution
no iris hamartomas (Lisch nodules)

4 other neurofibromatoses

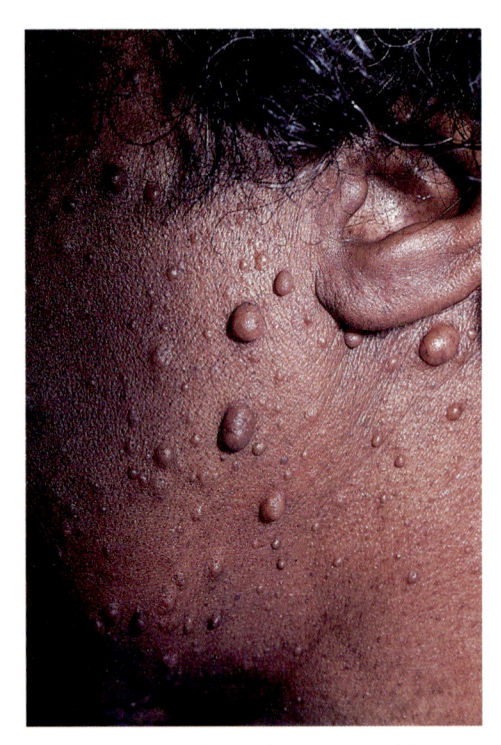

• *Figure 105 Facial neurofibromas; one of the many lesions seen in neurofibromatosis.*

References

Goldberg NS: What is segmental neurofibromatosis? J Am Acad Dermatol 1992; 26:638–640.
Listernick R, Charrow J: Neurofibromatosis type I in childhood. J Pediatr 1990; 116:845–853.
Obringer AC, Meadows AT, Zackai EH: The diagnosis of neurofibromatosis-1 in the child under the age of 6 years. Am J Dis Child 1989; 143:717–719.
Neurofibromatosis Conference Statement. Arch Neurol 1988; 45:575–578.
Sloan JB, Fretzin DF, Bovenmyer DA: Genetic counseling in segmental neurofibromatosis. J Am Acad Dermatol 1990; 22:461–467.
Trattner A, David M, Hodak E, Ben-David E, Sandbank M: Segmental neurofibromatosis. J Am Acad Dermatol 1990; 23:866–869.
Wertelecki W, Rouleau GA, Superneau DW, Forehand LW, et al.: Neurofibromatosis 2: clinical and DNA linkage studies of a large kindred. N Engl J Med 1988; 319:278–283.

NEUTRAL LIPID STORAGE DISEASE

see CHANARIN–DORFMAN SYNDROME

NEVOID BASAL CELL CARCINOMA SYNDROME

see BASAL CELL NEVUS SYNDROME

NEVUS ANELASTICUS OF LEWANDOWSKY, NAEVUS ELASTICUS REGIONIS MAMMARIAE

Manifestations and Major Findings

congenital perifollicular papules on anterior chest
degeneration and absence of elastic fibers
represents a type of connective tissue nevus
may be disseminated

References

Crivellato E: Disseminated nevus anelasticus. Int J Dermatol 1986; 25:171–173.
Sears JK, Stone MS, Argenyi Z: Papular elastorrhexis: a variant of connective tissue nevus. J Am Acad Dermatol 1988; 19:409–414.

NEVUS OF ITO

Manifestations and Major Findings

blue-gray patchy hyperpigmentation
affects the area supplied by the supraclavicular and lateral brachial nerves
common in Orientals
histology identical to nevus of Ota

References

Fulk CS: Primary disorders of hyperpigmentation. J Am Acad Dermatol 1984; 10:1–16.
Vélez A, Fuente C, Belinchón I, Martín N, et al.: Congenital segmental dermal melanocytosis in an adult. Arch Dermatol 1992; 128:521–525.

NEVUS OF OTA, OCULODERMAL MELANOSIS, NEVUS FUSCOCAERULEUS OPHTHALMOMAXILLARIS

Manifestations and Major Findings

- blue-gray patchy pigmentation (Fig. 106)
affects one side of the face and sclera supplied by the ophthalmic and maxillary division of the trigeminal nerve
occasionally bilateral
pigmentation may include eyelids, bulbar and palpebral conjunctiva, sclera, and cheeks
histology shows fusiform or wavy dermal melanocytes with melanin granules and melanophages
present at birth (usually) or puberty
becomes progressively darker with age
common in Orientals

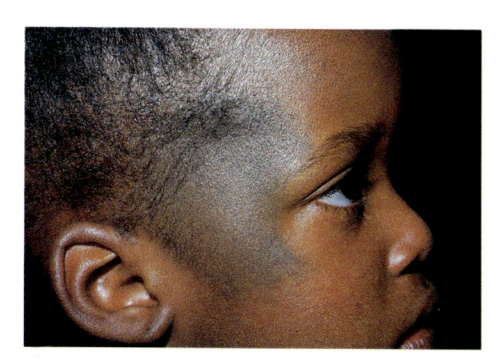

• *Figure 106* Blue-gray patchy pigmentation on one side of the face is seen in nevus of Ota.

Rare associations of nevus of Ota include glaucoma and malignant melanoma.

References
Fulk CS: Primary disorders of hyperpigmentation. J Am Acad Dermatol 1984; 10:1–16.
Kobayashi T: Microsurgical treatment of nevus of Ota. J Dermatol Surg Oncol 1991; 17:936-941.
Vélez A, Fuente C, Belinchón I, Martín N, et al.: Congenital segmental dermal melanocytosis in an adult. Arch Dermatol 1992; 128:521–525.

NEVUS SEBACEUS OF JADASSOHN, SEBACEOUS NEVUS

Manifestations and Major Findings
circumscribed hamartoma with predominantly sebaceous glands
- raised, pinkish-yellow or tan plaque (Fig. 107)

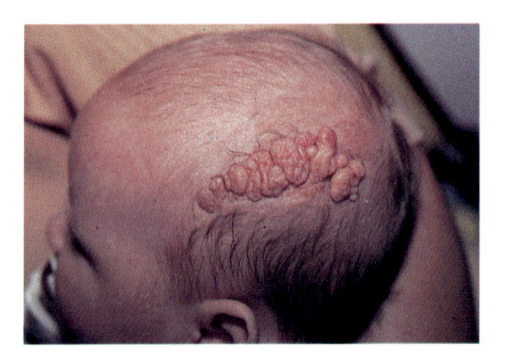

- **Figure 107** Nevus sebaceus of Jadassohn commonly appears as a circumscribed, raised, pinkish-yellow plaque on the head.

velvety surface
most common on the head and neck as a solitary lesion
devoid of hair
lesions thicken and elevate at puberty
may develop appendageal tumors or basal cell carcinomas

References
Sahl WJ: Familial nevus sebaceus of Jadassohn: occurrence in three generations. J Am Acad Dermatol 1990; 22:853–854.

NEVUS SEBACEUS SYNDROME

Manifestations and Major Findings
- linear nevus sebaceus (Fig. 108)
usually extensive with facial involvement
skeletal defects

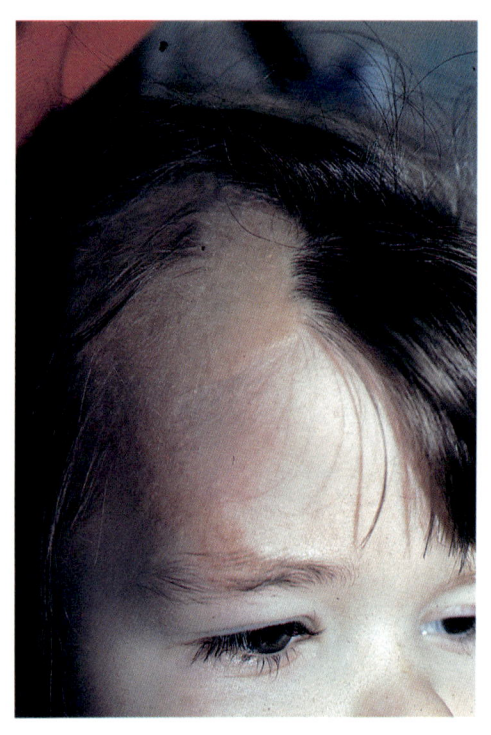

- **Figure 108** Extensive nevus sebaceus in a child with seizures and mental retardation in nevus sebaceus syndrome.

NEUROLOGIC ABNORMALITIES
seizures
mental retardation

OCULAR ABNORMALITIES
esotropia
coloboma
corneal clouding
conjunctival dermoids

References
Happle R: Lethal genes surviving by mosaicism: a possible explanation for sporadic birth defects involving the skin. J Am Acad Dermatol 1987; 16:899–906.

NIEMANN–PICK DISEASE

Manifestations and Major Findings
sphingomyelinase deficiency
leads to sphingomyelin accumulation
emaciation – onset at 2–3 months of age
hepatosplenomegaly
lymphadenopathy
cherry-red macula retinae
mental retardation
ataxia
usually fatal in early childhood

Cutaneous Manifestations
diffuse brown pigmentation of the skin
most marked on the face
xanthomas
waxy induration of the skin
indurated discolored patches
jaundice in the first 6 months of life
suppurative lesions
purpuric lesions
café au lait macules
mongolian spots

autosomal recessive

> **References**
> Mardini MK, Gergan P, Akltar M, et al.:
> Niemann–Pick disease: report of a case with skin involvement. Am J Dis Child 1982; 136:650–651.

NODULAR VASCULITIS see BAZIN DISEASE

NOONAN SYNDROME

Manifestations and Major Findings
phenotype similar to Turner syndrome
normal karyotype (can affect either sex)
short stature (postnatal)
cryptorchidism in males
pulmonary stenosis
other congenital heart defects
lymphedema of the feet and legs
cubitus valgus
halo iris (blue/green) with sparse trabeculae and crypts in iris
normal mentation or mild retardation

Cutaneous Manifestations
pigmented nevi
dystrophic, short, wide nails
hypertrichosis
coarse, light-colored, curly hair
low posterior hairline on the neck
• ulerythema ophryogenes (Fig. 109)

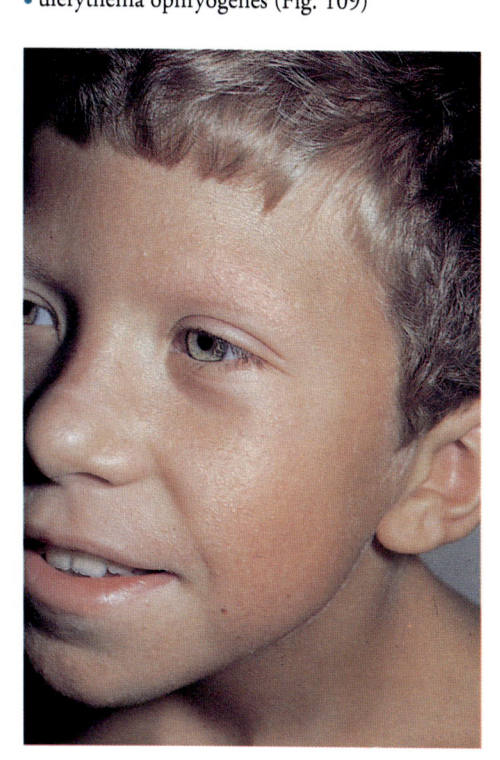

• *Figure 109* Ulerythema ophryogenes seen in Noonan syndrome. Also note the thick curly hair and light green eyes.

Characteristic Facies
hypertelorism
abnormal ears – low-set with thick helix
ptosis
downward sloping palpebral fissures
micrognathia
webbed neck

autosomal dominant or sporadic

> **References**
> Allanson JE, Hall JG, Hughes HE, Preus M, Witt RD: Noonan syndrome: the changing phenotype. Am J Med Genet 1985; 21:507–514. ▷ ▷ ▷

> > > **Burnett JW, Schwartz MF, Berberian BJ:** Ulerythema ophryogenes with multiple congenital anomalies. J Am Acad Dermatol 1988; 18:437–440.
Collins E, Turner G: The Noonan syndrome – a review of the clinical and genetic features of 27 cases. J Pediatr 1973; 83:941–950.
Pierini DO, Pierini AM: Keratosis pilaris atrophicans faciei (ulerythema ophryogenes): a cutaneous marker in the Noonan Syndrome. Br J Dermatol 1979; 100:409–416.
Snell JA, Mallory SB: Ulerythema ophryogenes in Noonan syndrome. Pediatr Dermatol 1990; 7:77–78.
Wyre HW: Cutaneous manifestations of Noonan's syndrome. Arch Dermatol 1978; 114:929–930.

hyperpigmented or purpuric patches on the back where scratched

References
Comings DE, Comings SN: Hereditary localized pruritus. Arch Dermatol 1965; 92:236–237.
Springall DR, Karanth SS, Kirkham N, Darley CR, et al.: Symptoms of notalagia paresthetica may be explained by increased dermal innervation. J Invest Dermatol 1991; 97:555–561.
Weber PJ, Poulos EG: Notalgia paresthetica. J Am Acad Dermatol 1988; 18:25–30.

NOTALGIA PARESTHETICA

Manifestations and Major Findings
abnormal sensation on the back – tingling, burning, hyperalgesia, and tenderness
isolated, predominantly sensory neuropathy of T2–T6 (infrascapular) area

O

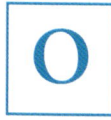

OCHRONOSIS *see* ALKAPTONURIA

OCULOAURICULOVERTEBRAL DYSPLASIA *see* GOLDENHAR SYNDROME

OCULOCEREBRAL SYNDROME WITH HYPOPIGMENTATION
see CROSS SYNDROME

OCULOCEREBROCUTANEOUS SYNDROME
see DELLEMAN–OORTHUYS SYNDROME

OCULOCEREBRORENAL SYNDROME, LOWE SYNDROME

Manifestations and Major Findings
hypotonia
congenital cataracts and/or glaucoma
renal tubular dysfunction (Fanconi syndrome) develops in late infancy
generalized aminoaciduria
mental retardation
growth retardation
failure to thrive
noninflammatory joint swelling with effusion
joint contracture or hypermobility
thin, sparse hair
cryptorchidism

Characteristic Facies
prominent forehead
protruding ears

X-linked recessive

> **References**
> Athreya BH, Schumacher HR, Getz HD, Norman ME, et al.: Arthropathy of Lowe's (oculo-cerebrorenal syndrome). Arthritis Rheum 1983; 26:728–735.
> Charnas LR, Bernardini I, Rader D, Hoeg JM, Gahl WA: Clinical and laboratory findings in the oculocerebrorenal syndrome of Lowe, with special reference to growth and renal function. N Engl J Med 1991; 324:1318–1325.
> Richards W, Donnell GN, Wilson WA, Stowens D, et al.: The oculo-cerebro-renal syndrome of Lowe. Am J Dis Child 1965; 109:185–203.

OCULOCUTANEOUS ALBINISM
see ALBINISM

OCULODENTODIGITAL SYNDROME, OCULODENTODIGITAL DYSPLASIA, OCULODENTOOSSEOUS DYSPLASIA

Manifestations and Major Findings
ocular defects
–microphthalmos and/or microcornea
–malformations of the iris
dental abnormalities
–enamel hypoplasia
–yellowing of the teeth
digital defects
–camptodactyly of the fifth digit
–syndactyly of the fourth and fifth fingers

OTHER FINDINGS
small mouth
thin nose
hypoplastic alae nasi

narrow nostrils
fine, sparse, and dry hair, eyebrows, and eyelashes
neurologic abnormalities

autosomal dominant

> **References**
> Kucirka SJ, Scher RK: Heritable nail disorders. Dermatol Clin 1987; 5:179–191.
> Reisner SH, Kott E, Bornstein B, Salinger H, et al.: Oculodentodigital dysplasia. Am J Dis Child 1969; 118:600–607.

OCULOGLANDULAR SYNDROME
see PARINAUD OCULOGLANDULAR SYNDROME

OCULOMANDIBULOFACIAL SYNDROME see HALLERMANN–STREIFF SYNDROME

OCULO-OSTEOCUTANEOUS SYNDROME

Manifestations and Major Findings
short stature
prominent lower jaw
anodontia

OCULAR ABNORMALITIES
strabismus
downslanting palpebral fissures
myopia magna
nystagmus

SKELETAL ABNORMALITIES
malformed toes
short fingers and toes – especially third to fifth
short skull

Cutaneous Manifestations
congenital palmar hyperkeratosis
fine, blonde, sparse hair
absent pubic and axillary hair
thin eyelashes

> **References**
> Tuomaala P, Haapanen E: Three siblings with similar anomalies in the eyes, bones, and skin. Acta Ophthalmol 1968; 46:365-375.

OFD SYNDROME
see OROFACIODIGITAL SYNDROME

OFUJI SYNDROME, EOSINOPHILIC PUSTULAR FOLLICULITIS

Manifestations and Major Findings
characteristic sterile, eosinophilic, follicular pustules often in papules or plaques
seborrheic distribution on the face, upper arms, and trunk
eosinophilia
lymphadenopathy
condition responds to steroids
common in Japanese and AIDS patients
young males most commonly affected

> **References**
> Buchness MR, Lim HW, Hatcher VA, Sanchez M, Soter NA: Eosinophilic pustular folliculitis in the acquired immunodeficiency syndrome. N Engl J Med 1988; 318:1183–1186.
> Camacho-Martinez F: Eosinophilic pustular folliculitis. J Am Acad Dermatol 1987; 17:686–688.
> Colton AS, Schachner L, Kowalczyk AP: Eosinophilic pustular folliculitis. J Am Acad Dermatol 1986; 14:469–474.
> Isoda M, Doi F: Eosinophilic pustular folliculitis (Ofuji's disease) with response to indomethacin therapy. Cutis 1989; 44:407–409.
> Ofuji S, Ogino A, Horio T, Oheseko T, Uehara M: Eosinophilic pustular folliculitis. Acta Derm Venereol (Stockh) 1970; 50:195–203.

OGNA TYPE EPIDERMOLYSIS BULLOSA see EPIDERMOLYSIS BULLOSA; SIMPLEX

OID-OID DISEASE
see SULZBERGER–GARBE SYNDROME

OLLIER DYSCHONDROPLASIA,
ENCHONDROMATOSIS, OSTEOCHONDROMATOSIS, OLLIER SYNDROME

Manifestations and Major Findings
enchondromas causing firm, local, asymmetric, swellings of the fingers and/or toes
asymmetric growth of the extremities with shortening
hemihypertrophy
macrodactyly
bone fractures
malignant degeneration of enchondromas may occur in adulthood (5%)

> **References**
> Braddock GTF, Hadlow VD: Osteosarcoma in enchondromatosis (Ollier's disease): report of a case. J Bone Joint Surg 1966; 48B:145–149.

OLMSTED SYNDROME

Manifestations and Major Findings
severe, progressive, painful palmoplantar keratoderma
flexion deformities of the digits
digital constriction or spontaneous amputation
hyperkeratotic plaques around the mouth and other orifices
linear keratoses on the flexor forearms
retarded growth
alopecia universalis
delayed psychomotor development
nail abnormalities
dental anomalies

> **References**
> Atherton DJ, Sutton C, Jones BM: Mutilating palmoplantar keratoderma with periorificial keratotic plaques (Olmsted's Syndrome). Br J Dermatol 1990; 122:245–252.
> Poulin Y, Perry HO, Muller SA: Olmsted syndrome – congenital palmoplantar and periorificial keratoderma. J Am Acad Dermatol 1984; 10:600–610.

OMENN SYNDROME, FAMILIAL
RETICULOENDOTHELIOSIS WITH EOSINOPHILIA

Manifestations and Major Findings
severe combined immunodeficiency (variable)
severe, erythematous, scaly dermatitis
evolution into erythroderma
lymphadenopathy (massive)
prominent infiltraion of the lymph nodes with histiocyte-like cells
hepatosplenomegaly
peripheral eosinophilia with leukocytosis
onset early in life
failure to thrive
fatal at an early age

autosomal recessive

> **References**
> Businco L, DiFazio A, Ziruolo MG, Boner AL, Valletta EA, et al.: Clinical and immunological findings in four infants with Omenn's syndrome: a form of severe combined immunodeficiency with phenotypically normal T cells, elevated IgE, and eosinophilia. Clin Immunol Immunopathol 1987; 44:123–133.
> Junker AK, Chan KW, Massing BG: Clinical and immune recovery from Omenn syndrome after bone marrow transplantation. J Pediatr 1989; 114: 596–599.
> Omenn GS: Familial reticuloendotheliosis with eosinophilia. N Engl J Med 1965; 273:427–432.
> Pupo RA, Tyring SK, Raimer SS, Wirt DP, et al.: Omenn's syndrome and related combined immunodeficiency syndromes: diagnostic considerations in infants with persistent erythroderma and failure to thrive. J Am Acad Dermatol 1991; 25: 442–446.
> Schofer O, Blaha I, Mannhardt W, Zepp F, et al.: Omenn phenotype with short-limbed dwarfism. J Pediatr 1991; 118:86–88.

OROFACIODIGITAL SYNDROME,
OFD SYNDROME

Types of Orofaciodigital Syndrome and Features

type I, Papillon–Léage syndrome
oral abnormalities
– webbing between buccal mucosa and alveolar ridge (frenulum hypertrophy) ▷ ▷ ▷

▷ ▷ ▷
– clefting of lips, tongue, and gingiva
– dental abnormalities
– hamartomas of the tongue
facial dystrophies
– hypoplastic nasal alae
– dystopia canthorum
– broad nasal root
digital abnormalities
– asymmetric shortening (trident hand)
– clinodactyly
– syndactyly
– polydactyly
dry, rough, sparse hair and scalp
numerous milia on face, ears, and dorsum of hands
mental retardation
central nervous system anomalies
polycystic kidneys
lethal in males
X-linked dominant

type II, Mohr syndrome
oral abnormalities
– dental anomalies
– absent lower central incisors
– cleft lip and palate
– tongue hamartomas
facial dystrophies
– broad bifid tip of the nose
– broad nasal root
digital abnormalities
– polydactyly
– bilateral polysyndactyly
– hexadactyly
– syndactyly
hearing loss
mental retardation (rare)
normal skin and hair
autosomal recessive

References
Baraitser M: The orofaciodigital (OFD) syndromes. J Med Genet 1986; 23:116–119.
deLuna ML, Raspa ML, Ibargoyen J: Oral-facial-digital type I syndrome of Papillon-Léage and Psaume. Pediatr Dermatol 1992; 9:52–56.
Gustavson KH, Kreuger A, Petersson PO: Syndrome characterized by lingual malformation, polydactyly, tachypnea, and psychomotor retardation (Mohr syndrome). Clin Genet 1971; 2:261–266.
Shaw M, Gilkes JJH, Nally FF: Oral facial digital syndrome – case report and review of the literature. Br J Oral Surg 1981; 19:142–147.

OSLER–WEBER–RENDU SYNDROME, RENDU–OSLER–WEBER SYNDROME, HEREDITARY HEMORRHAGIC TELANGIECTASIA, OSLER DISEASE

Manifestations and Major Findings
recurrent epistaxis (usual presenting symptom)
telangiectasias
– mucous membranes
– gastrointestinal tract
– retina
• telangiectasias (Fig. 110)
– usually more prominent on the upper body
– conspicuous in the nailbeds
gastrointestinal/genitourinary hemorrhage from telangiectasias
central nervous system angiomas or aneurysms
focal neurologic signs

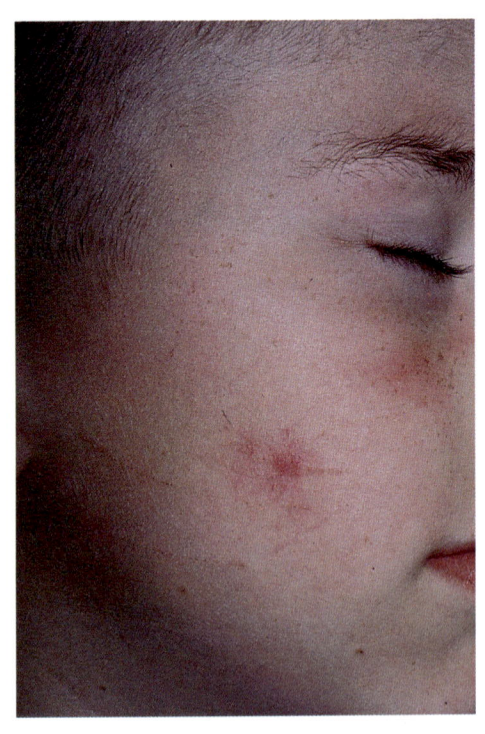

• *Figure 110* Cutaneous telangiectasias on the cheek in Osler–Weber–Rendu syndrome.

anemia (from bleeding)
pulmonary or hepatic arteriovenous fistulae
hepatic arteriovenous fistulae
hepatomegaly and cirrhosis

autosomal dominant

> **References**
> Gregory B, Ho VC: Cutaneous manifestations of gastrointestinal disorders. Part II. J Am Acad Dermatol 1992; 26:371–383.
> Peery WH: Clinical spectrum of hereditary hemorrhagic telangiectasia. Am J Med 1987; 82:989–997.
> Swanson DL, Dahl MV: Embolic abscesses in hereditary hemorrhagic telangiectasia. J Am Acad Dermatol 1991; 24:580–583.

OSTEOGENESIS IMPERFECTA

Ostegenesis imperfecta is a heterogenous group of heritable disorders characterized by fragile bones which are caused by a disorder of Type I collagen structure.

Types of Osteogenesis Imperfecta and Features

I mild form, Lobstein disease
osteoporosis
osseous fragility (minimal to moderately severe)
bone fractures
easy bruising
joint laxity
mitral valve prolapse
occasional aortic valve incompetence
near normal height
dentinogenesis imperfecta
blue sclerae
deafness caused by otosclerosis
decreased type I collagen proalpha 1 chains
autosomal dominant

II lethal perinatal form, Vrolik disease
extremely severe osseous fragility
multiple *in utero* fractures
marked tissue fragility
broad, crumpled long bones
skull calcification
broad ribs with beading
usually stillborn or early fatality
defective type I collagen proalpha 1 gene
autosomal recessive or dominant

III progressive deforming form
moderately severe to severe osseous fragility
fractures *in utero* or at birth
marked scoliosis or kyphoscoliosis
variable but severe deformities of the long bones
marked short stature
normal sclerae
normal hearing
defective type I collagen proalpha 2 gene
autosomal recessive or dominant

IV mild form with normal sclerae
osseous fragility
variable deformities of the long bones and spine
dentinogenesis imperfecta
kyphoscoliosis
short stature
normal sclerae
normal hearing
elastosis perforans serpiginosa
atrophic skin
wide scars
defective type I collagen proalpha 2 gene
autosomal dominant

> **References**
> Chines A, Petersen DJ, Schranck FW, et al.: Hypercalciuria in children severely affected with osteogenesis imperfecta. J Pediatr 1991; 119:51–57.
> Cole DE, Cohen MM: Osteogenesis imperfecta: an update. J Pediatr 1991; 119:73–74.
> Gahagan S, Rimsza ME: Child abuse or osteogenesis imperfecta: how can we tell? Pediatrics 1991; 88: 987–992.
> Tsipouras P 1993. Osteogenesis Imperfecta. In McKusick's Heritable Disorders of Connective Tissue, 5th edition, p.281–314. (St. Louis: Mosby-Year Book).

OUDSTHOORN DISEASE,
ERYTHROKERATOLYSIS HIEMALIS, WINTER ERYTHROKERATOLYSIS

Manifestations and Major Findings
palmoplantar erythema and hyperkeratosis
target-like lesions on the dorsum of the hands, feet, and buttocks
continuous peeling of lesions

characteristically seen in winter (cold weather), during fever, or after surgery

most often seen in white South Africans

autosomal dominant

References
Findlay GH, Morrison JGL: Erythrokeratolysis hiemalis–keratolytic winter erythema or 'Oudsthoorn skin' – a new epidermal genodermatosis with its histological features. Br J Dermatol 1978; 98:491–495.

P

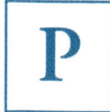

PACHYDERMOPERIOSTOSIS,
TOURAINE–SOLENTE-GOLÉ SYNDROME, PRIMARY HYPERTROPHIC OSTEOARTHROPATHY

Cutaneous Manifestations
hypertrophic skin changes
affects scalp, forehead, face, and other areas
cutis verticis gyrata (folded hyperplasia of scalp)
skin changes begin around puberty
sebaceous hyperplasia
hyperhidrosis of the hands and feet

OTHER FINDINGS
ptosis
periosteal lesions
hypertrophy of the long bones
clubbing of the fingers and toes
more severe in males
mental retardation
primary form of condition is autosomal dominant

Secondary form of condition (provoked by severe pulmonary disease, lung cancer, or other carcinomas) has relatively mild skin changes.

autosomal dominant

> **References**
> **Brenner S, Srebrnik A, Kisch ES:** Pachydermoperiostosis with new clinical and endocrinologic manifestations. Int J Dermatol 1992; 31:341–342.
> **Kucirka SJ, Scher RK:** Heritable Nail Disorders. Dermatol Clin 1987; 5:179–191.
> **Venencie PY, Boffa GA, Delmas PD, Verola O, et al.:** Pachydermoperiostosis with gastric hypertrophy, anemia, and increased serum bone Gla-protein levels. Arch Dermatol 1988; 124:1831–1834.

PACHYONYCHIA CONGENITA

Types of Pachyonychia Congenita and Features

type I, Jadassohn–Lewandowsky syndrome
- marked thickening of the nails (subungual hyperkeratosis) (Fig. 111)
recurrent nail shedding
palmoplantar keratoses
acral bullae
follicular keratoses on buttocks and extremities
palmoplantar hyperhidrosis
histology of leukoplakia resembles a white sponge nevus but no tendency toward malignant degeneration

type II
clinical findings of type I plus
– palmoplantar bullae
– no mucosal lesions
– steatocystoma multiplex
– epidermal cysts
– natal teeth

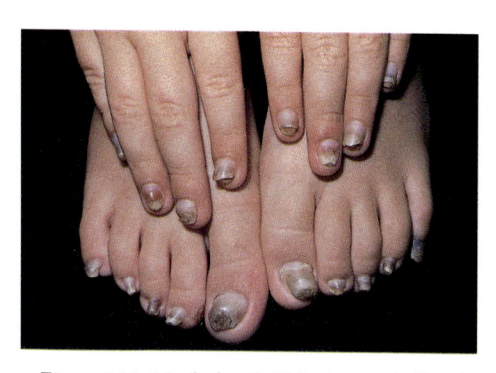

▷ ▷ ▷

• *Figure 111 Marked nail thickening is a hallmark of pachyonychia congenita.*

▷ ▷ ▷
type III
clinical findings of type II plus
- less severe nail thickening and keratoses
- ocular changes – cataracts, corneal dystrophy
- angular cheilosis

type IV
clinical findings of type III plus
- laryngeal lesions and hoarseness
- mental retardation
- hair anomalies
- alopecia
- macular pigmentation

autosomal dominant

References
Feinstein A, Friedman J, Schewach-Millet M: Pachyonychia congenita. J Am Acad Dermatol 1988; 19:705–711.
Su WPD, Chun SI, Hammond DE, Gordon H: Pachyonychia congenita: clinical study of 12 cases and review of the literature. Pediatr Dermatol 1990; 7:33–38.
Tidman MJ, Wells AS, MacDonald DM: Pachyonychia congenita with cutaneous amyloidosis and hyperpigmentation: a distinct variant. J Am Acad Dermatol 1987; 16:935–940.

PAGET DISEASE

Manifestations and Major Findings
progressive, marginated, scaly plaque on nipple and areola with underlying moist erythema
intraductal carcinoma of the breast
pruritus common
histology shows Paget cells with clear cytoplasm
extramammary Paget disease – most common in anogenital region and axillae

References
Anthony PP, Freeman K, Warin AP: Extramammary Paget's disease. Clin Exp Dermatol 1986; 11: 387–395.
Gregory B, Ho VC: Cutaneous manifestations of gastrointestinal disorders. Part I. J Am Acad Dermatol 1992; 26:153–166.
Guarner J, Cohen C, DeRose PB: Histogenesis of extramammary and mammary Paget cells: an immunohistochemical study. Am J Dermatopathol 1989; 11:313–319.
Ho TCN, St Jacques M, Schopflocher P: Pigmented Paget's disease of the male breast. J Am Acad Dermatol 1990; 23:338–341.

PAINFUL BRUISING SYNDROME
see AUTOERYTHROCYTE SENSITIZATION SYNDROME

PALMOPLANTAR KERATODERMA
see KERATODERMAS

PANGERIA see WERNER SYNDROME

PAPILLON–LÉAGE SYNDROME
see OROFACIODIGITAL SYNDROME; TYPE I

PAPILLON–LEFÈVRE SYNDROME,
KERATOSIS PALMOPLANTARIS WITH PERIODONTOSIS

Manifestations and Major Findings
palmoplantar hyperkeratosis with redness and thickening
childhood onset (1–5 years of age)
periodontosis with loss of teeth

OTHER FINDINGS
psoriasiform plaques on the elbows and knees
hyperhidrosis
calcification of dura (falx cerebri)
recurrent skin pyodermas
impaired immunity
mental retardation

autosomal recessive

References
Bergfeld WF, Derbes VJ, Elias PM, Frost P, et al.: The treatment of keratosis palmaris et plantaris with isotretinoin. J Am Acad Dermatol 1982; 6:727–731.
El Darouti MA, Al Raubaie SM, Eiada MA: Papillon–Lefèvre syndrome. Int J Dermatol 1988; 27:63–66.
Gelmetti C, Nazzaro V, Cerri D, Fracasso L: Long-term preservation of permanent teeth in a patient with Papillon–Lefèvre syndrome treated with etretinate. Pediatr Dermatol 1989; 6:222–225.
Nazzaro V, Blanchet-Bardon C, Mimoz C, et al.: Papillon–Lefèvre syndrome: ultrastructural study and successful treatment with acitretin. Arch Dermatol 1988; 533–539.   ▷ ▷ ▷

> > >
Nguyen TQ, Greer KE, Fisher GB, Cooper PH: Papillon–Lefèvre syndrome. J Am Acad Dermatol 1986; 15:46–49.
Trattner A, David M, Sandbank M: Papillon–Lefèvre syndrome with acroosteolysis. J Am Acad Dermatol 1991; 24:835–838.

References
Grob JJ, Collet-Villette AM, Horchowski N, et al.: Ofuji papuloerythroderma. J Am Acad Dermatol 1989; 20:927–931.
Nazzari G, Crovato F, Nigro A: Papuloerythroderma (Ofuji): two additional cases and review of the literature. J Am Acad Dermatol 1992; 26:499–501.

PAPULAR ACRODERMATITIS OF CHILDHOOD

see GIANOTTI–CROSTI SYNDROME

PAPULAR-PURPURIC 'GLOVES AND SOCKS' SYNDROME

Manifestations and Major Findings
pruritic edema and erythema of hands and feet
development of petechiae and purpura
oral lesions
fever
acute, self-limiting course
resolves within 1–2 weeks
associated with viral infections and drugs

References
Bagot M, Revuz J: Papular-purpuric 'gloves and socks' syndrome: primary infection with parvovirus B19. J Am Acad Dermatol 1991; 25:341–342.
Harms M, Feldmann R, Saurat J-H: Papular-purpuric 'gloves and socks' syndrome. J Am Acad Dermatol 1990; 23:850–854.

PAPULOERYTHRODERMA OF OFUJI

Manifestations and Major Findings
intensely pruritic papular eruption
widespread coalescing sheets of erythematous papules
sparing of body folds
blood eosinophilia
elevated serum immunoglobulin E
unknown etiology
associated with B cell or T cell lymphoma or visceral malignancy
affects older males

PAPULOVESICULAR ACROLOCATED SYNDROME see also GIANOTTI–CROSTI SYNDROME

Manifestations and Major Findings
symmetrical, erythematous, papular and/or vesicular lesions
acral distribution (may also be generalized)
pruritus
associated with viral infections
–adenovirus
–Epstein–Barr virus
–cytomegalovirus
self-limited course (20–50 days)
Papulovesicular acrolocated syndrome is a variant of Gianotti–Crosti syndrome and is vesicular, more pruritic, and may involve the trunk.

References
Patrizi A, DiLernia V, Ricci G, Masi M, et al.: Papular and papulovesicular acrolated eruptions and viral infections. Pediatr Dermatol 1990; 7:22–26.
Sagi EF, Linder N, Shouval D: Papular acrodermatitis of childhood associated with hepatitis A virus infection. Pediatr Dermatol 1985; 3:31–33.
Spear KL, Winkelmann RK: Gianotti–Crosti syndrome. Arch Dermatol 1984; 120:891–896.

PARACOCCIDIOIDAL GRANULOMA

see LUTZ–SPLENDORE–ALMEIDA DISEASE

PARANA HARD-SKIN SYNDROME

Manifestations and Major Findings
progressive rigidity of the skin
formation of an immovable body cast
all skin involved except eyelids, neck, and ears
onset in second month of life
growth retardation

OTHER FINDINGS
hirsutism
hyperpigmentation of the skin
enlargement of the parotid glands
pulmonary insufficiency leading to death

autosomal recessive

> **References**
> Cat I, Magdalena NIR, Marinoni LP, Wong MP: Parana hard-skin syndrome: study of seven families. Lancet 1974; 1:215–216.

PARINAUD OCULOGLANDULAR SYNDROME

Manifestations and Major Findings
unilateral granulomatous conjunctivitis
preauricular lymphadenopathy (ipsilateral)
Parinaud syndrome is caused by cat-scratch disease, tularemia, tuberculosis, sarcoidosis, leptospirosis, sporotrichosis, rhinosporidiosis, and other disorders.

> **References**
> Carithers HA: Oculoglandular disease of Parinaud. Am J Dis Child 1978; 132:1195–1200.

PARRY–ROMBERG SYNDROME,
PROGRESSIVE HEMIFACIAL ATROPHY, ROMBERG SYNDROME

Manifestations and Major Findings
progressive atrophy of the skin, fat, muscle and sometimes bone
usually affects half of the face (morphea-like)
early onset (before 20 years of age)
irregular hypo- or hyperpigmentation (initially in patches)
often results in sunken pigmentation
hair may be lost from involved skin
ipsilateral heterochromia iridis
associated with Horner syndrome

> **References**
> Abele DC, Bedingfield RB, Chandler FW, Given KS: Progressive facial hemiatrophy (Parry–Romberg syndrome) and borreliosis. J Am Acad Dermatol 1990; 22:531–533. ▷ ▷ ▷

> ▷ ▷ ▷
> Dintiman BJ, Shapiro RS, Hood AF, Guba AM: Parry–Romberg syndrome in association with contralateral Poland syndrome. J Am Acad Dermatol 1990; 22:371–373.

PASINI AND PIERINI ATROPHODERMA

Manifestations and Major Findings
- bluish-brown, sharply depressed plaques (Fig. 112)

single or multiple plaques
'cliff drop' border at the edge of each plaque
usually over 2cm in diameter
most common on the back, chest, and abdomen

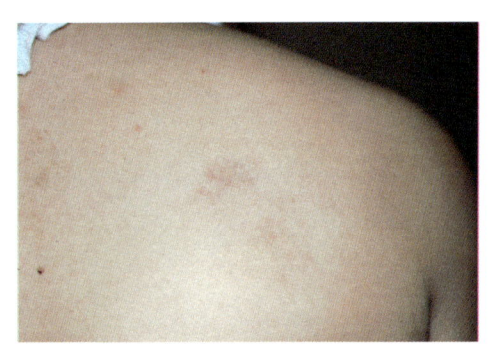

- *Figure 112 Pasini and Pierini atrophoderma presenting as depressed, bluish-brown plaques over the shoulder.*

> **References**
> Berman A, Berman GD, Winkelmann RK: Atrophoderma (Pasini–Pierini): findings on direct immunofluorescent, monoclonal antibody and ultrastructural studies. Int J Dermatol 1988; 27: 487–490.
> Buechner SA, Rufli T: Atrophoderma of Pasini and Pierini. J Am Acad Dermatol 1994; 30:441–446.

PASINI SYNDROME
see EPIDERMOLYSIS BULLOSA; DYSTROPHIC

PATTERSON–KELLY SYNDROME
see PLUMMER–VINSON SYNDROME

PEELING SKIN SYNDROME,
FAMILIAL CONTINUAL SKIN PEELING, DECIDUOUS SKIN
see also DISORDERS OF CORNIFICATION; DOC 21

Manifestations and Major Findings
continual generalized peeling of the skin
erythema
leaves polycyclic, denuded, red areas
no exudate
dry and dirty-looking skin
red, dry palms and soles – no true keratoderma
pruritus
childhood onset
no preceeding signs or symptoms
no oral or ocular involvement
histology shows cleavage below the stratum corneum

autosomal recessive

> **References**
> Abdel-Hafez K, Safer AM, Selim MM, Rehak A: Familial continual skin peeling. Dermatologica 1983; 166:22–31.
> Fine J-D, Johnson L, Wright T: Epidermolysis bullosa simplex superficialis. Arch Dermatol 1989; 125:633–638.
> Levy SB, Goldsmith LA: The peeling skin syndrome. J Am Acad Dermatol 1982; 7:606–613.
> Silverman AK, Ellis CN, Beals TF, Woo TY: Continual skin peeling syndrome. Arch Dermatol 1986; 122:71–75.

PELLEGRA *see* VITAMIN DEFICIENCIES

PEROXISOMOPATHIES

A group of disorders of peroxisomal biogenesis and peroxisomal enzyme deficiencies which include: Zellweger (cerebrohepatorenal) syndrome, Refsum disease, neonatal adrenoleukodystrophy, X-linked adrenoleukodystrophy, rhizomelic chondrodysplasia punctata, Conradi–Hünermann syndrome, hyperpipecolic acidemia, acatalasia, primary hyperoxaluria, and peroxisomal thiolase deficiency.

> **References**
> Kalter DC, Atherton DJ, Clayton PT: X-linked dominant Conradi–Hünermann syndrome presenting as congenital erythroderma. J Am Acad Dermatol 1989; 21:248–256.
> Pike MG, Applegarth DA, Dunn HG, Bamforth SJ, et al.: Congenital rubella syndrome associated with calcific epiphyseal stippling and peroxisomal dysfunction. J Pediatr 1990; 116:88–94.

PEUTZ–JEGHERS SYNDROME,
PERIORIFICIAL LENTIGINOSIS

Manifestations and Major Findings
• periorificial and digital lentigines (Fig. 113)
generalized intestinal polyposis (hamartomas)
polyposis most common in jejunum and ileum
abdominal pain with intussusception
malignant potential – mainly gastrointestinal tract and breast
ovarian tumors – sex cord tumors with annular tubules
clubbing of the digits

autosomal dominant

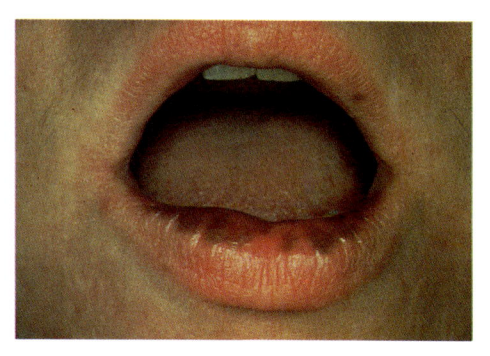

• *Figure 113 Perioral lentigines are found in Peutz–Jeghers syndrome.*

> **References**
> Giardiello FM, Welsh SB, Hamilton SR, Offerhaus GJA, et al.: Increased risk of cancer in the Peutz–Jeghers syndrome. N Engl J Med 1987; 316:1511–1514.
> Gregory B, Ho VC: Cutaneous manifestations of gastrointestinal disorders. J Am Acad Dermatol 1992; 26:153–166.

> > > Jeghers H, McKusick BA, Katz KH: Generalized intestinal polyposis and melanin spots of the oral mucosa, lips and digits. N Engl J Med 1949; 241: 1031–1036.
> Mallory SB, Stough DB: Genodermatoses with malignant potential. Dermatol Clin 1987; 5: 221–230.
> Spigelman AD, Murday V, Phillips RKS: Cancer and the Peutz–Jeghers syndrome. Gut 1989; 30: 1588–1590.

PEYRONIE DISEASE,
PENILE FIBROMATOSIS, INDURATIO PENIS PLASTICA

Manifestations and Major Findings
fibrosis of the dorsal penis
one or more irregular, hard, subcutaneous plaques
painful erection
curvature of the penis
affects middle-aged males
Peyronie disease is associated with Dupuytren contracture, keloids, and knuckle pads.

PHAKOMATOSIS PIGMENTOVASCULARIS

Manifestations and Major Findings
cutaneous vascular malformations
oculocutaneous melanosis
possible central nervous system malformation

Types of Phakomatosis Pigmentovascularis and Features

type I, Adamson–Best syndrome
vascular (capillary) malformations
linear epidermal nevus

type II, Takano–Krüger–Doi syndrome
vascular (capillary) malformations
aberrant mongolian spots
may also have nevus anemicus

type III, Kobori–Toda syndrome
vascular (capillary) malformations
nevus spilus
may also have nevus anemicus

type IV
vascular (capillary) malformations
aberrant mongolian spots
nevus spilus
may also have nevus anemicus
skeletal deformities

> **References**
> Hasegawa Y, Yasuhara M: Phakomatosis pigmentovascularis type IVa. Arch Dermatol 1985; 121:651–655.
> Ruiz-Maldonado R, Tamayo L, Laterza AM, et al.: Phakomatosis pigmentovascularis: a new syndrome? Report of four cases. Pediatr Dermatol 1987; 4: 189–196.
> Sigg C, Pelloni F: Oligosymptomatic form of Klippel–Trenaunay–Weber syndrome associated with giant nevus spilus. Arch Dermatol 1989; 125: 1284–1285.

PHENYLKETONURIA

Phenylketonuria arises from an accumulation of phenylalanine in the blood caused by hepatic phenylalanine hydroxylase deficiency or biopterin cofactor deficiency. In untreated cases, a number of clinical findings develop.

Manifestations and Major Findings
mental retardation
seizures
hyperreflexia
impaired growth

Cutaneous Manifestations
reduction of melanin in hair and skin (probably due to phenylalanine inhibition of tyrosine-tyrosinase reaction)
atopic dermatitis
acrocyanosis
scleroderma-like skin indurations
photosensitivity

autosomal recessive

> **References**
> Lee EB: Metabolic diseases and the skin. Pediatr Clin N Am 1983; 30:597–608. > > >

▷ ▷ ▷
Nova MP, Kaufman M, Halperin A: Scleroderma-like skin indurations in a child with phenylketonuria: a clinicopathologic correlation and review of the literature. J Am Acad Dermatol 1992; 26:329–333.
Okano Y, Eisensmith RC, Güttler F, Lichter-Konecki U, Konecki DS, et al.: Molecular basis of phenotypic heterogeneity in phenylketonuria. N Engl J Med 1991; 324:1232–1238

PHENYTOIN SYNDROME

see HYDANTOIN SYNDROME

PICKWICKIAN SYNDROME,
OBESITY-HYPOVENTILATION SYNDROME

Syndrome named after a character in Charles Dickens' The Pickwick Papers.

Manifestations and Major Findings
obesity (massive)
hypoventilation
daytime somnolence
noisy sleep

PIEBALDISM, PARTIAL ALBINISM

Manifestations and Major Findings
- congenital depigmentation (Fig. 114)
  – triangular shape on forehead
  – symmetrical on the anterior chest, mid-arms and legs
  – spares central spine, hands, feet, shoulders, and hips
  white forelock
  hyperpigmented thumbprint macules within the leukoderma

autosomal dominant; chromosome 4

References
Bolognia JL, Pawelek JM: Biology of hypopigmentation. J Am Acad Dermatol 1988; 19:217–255.
Mosher DB, Fitzpatrick TB: Piebaldism. Arch Dermatol 1988; 124:364–365.
Ortonne JP: Piebaldism, Waardenburg's syndrome, and related disorders. Dermatol Clin 1988; 6:205–216.

PIERRE ROBIN SYNDROME,
ROBIN SEQUENCE

Manifestations and Major Findings
micrognathia (mandibular hypoplasia)
glossoptosis
cleft palate

OTHER FINDINGS
fine, light-colored hair
ocular defects

References
Bull MJ, Givan DC, Sadove AM, Bixler D, et al.: Improved outcome in Pierre Robin sequence: effect of multidisciplinary evaluation and management. Pediatrics 1990; 86:294–301.
Mallory SB, Paradise JL: Glossoptosis revisited: on the development and resolution of airway obstruction in the Pierre Robin syndrome. Pediatrics 1979; 64:946–948.

PIGMENTED PURPURIC DERMATOSIS

see PURPURA PIGMENTOSA CHRONICA

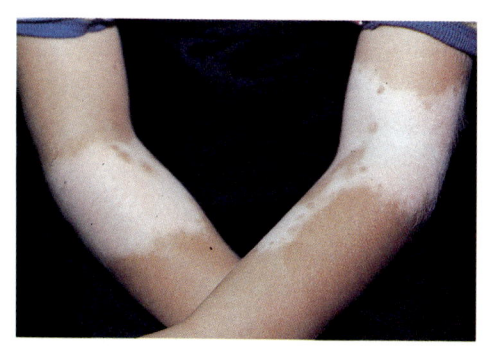

- *Figure 114* Congenital depigmentation affecting the arm, seen in piebaldism.

PILI TORTI SYNDROMES
see also HAIR SHAFT ANOMALIES

Pili Torti Syndromes and Features

1 classic type pili torti (Ronchese)
- irregular twisting of the hair shafts (Fig. 115)
  spangled or beaded appearance of the hair
  hairs may be brittle and easily broken
  eyebrows and eyelashes often involved
  widely-spaced teeth
  enamel hypoplasia
  nail dystrophy
  corneal opacities
  keratosis pilaris
  ichthyosis
  autosomal dominant

2 postpubertal pili torti (Beare)
  irregular twisting of the hair shafts
  scalp, beard, and body hair involvement
  mental retardation

3 Björnstad syndrome
  see Björnstad syndrome

4 Crandall syndrome
  see Crandall syndrome

5 Bazex syndrome
  see Bazex syndrome

6 trichothiodystrophy
  see trichothiodystrophy

7 Menkes kinky hair syndrome
  see Menkes syndrome

8 Salamon syndrome
  see Salamon syndrome

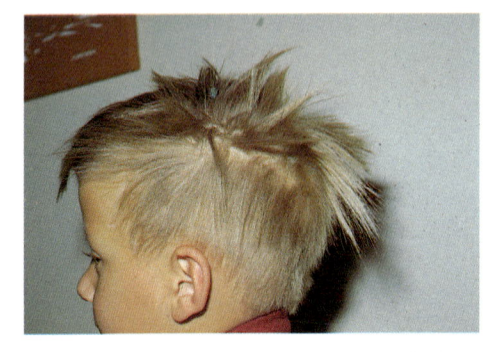

- *Figure 115* Irregular twisting of the hair shafts gives this untidy appearance in classic type pili torti.

References
Appel B, Messina SJ: Pili torti hereditaria. N Engl J Med 1942; 226:912–915.
Beare JM: Congenital pilar defect showing features of pili torti. Br J Dermatol 1952; 64:366–372.
Ronchese F: Twisted hairs (pili torti). Arch Dermatol Syphilol 1932; 26:98–109.
Whiting DA: Structural abnormalities of the hair shaft. J Am Acad Dermatol 1987; 16:1–25.

PILOMATRIXOMA OF MALHERBE,
MALHERBE CALCIFYING EPITHELIOMA, PILOMATRICOMA

Manifestations and Major Findings
solitary/multiple nodules with firm consistency composed of cells resembling hair matrix cells
commonly found on the scalp, face, neck, or arms
histology shows similarity to epidermal cysts with shadow cells and calcification
more common in children
rare association with myotonic dystrophy

References
Chiaramonte A, Gilgor RS: Pilomatricomas associated with myotonic dystrophy. Arch Dermatol 1978; 114:1363–1365.
Schlechter R, Hartsough NA, Guttman FM: Multiple pilomatricomas (calcifying epitheliomas of Malherbe. Pediatr Dermatol 1984; 2:23–25.
Taaffe A, Wyatt EH, Bury HPR: Pilomatricoma (Malherbe). A clinical and histopathologic survey of 78 cases. Int J Dermatol 1988; 27:477–480.

PINK DISEASE, ACRODYNIA, MERCURY POISONING

Manifestations and Major Findings
*p*ink tips of fingers, toes, and nose
*p*ainful hands and feet
*p*ruritus
*p*hotophobia
*p*aralysis or hypotonia
*p*rofuse salivation and sweating
elevated blood *p*ressure
disorder of infancy or childhood
fatal if untreated

> **References**
> Agocs MM, Etzel RA, Parrish RG, Paschal DC, et al.: Mercury exposure from interior latex paint. N Engl J Med 1990; 323:1096–1101.
> Clarkson TW: Mercury – an element of mystery. N Engl J Med 1990; 323:1137–1139.
> Dinehart SM, Dillard R, Raimer SS, Diven S, et al.: Cutaneous manifestations of acrodynia (Pink disease). Arch Dermatol 1988; 124:107–109.

PITYRIASIS LICHENOIDES ET VARIOLIFORMIS ACUTA (PLEVA)
see MUCHA–HABERMANN SYNDROME

PLUMMER–VINSON SYNDROME, SIDEROPENIC DYSPHAGIA, PATTERSON–KELLY SYNDROME

Manifestations and Major Findings
microcytic hypochromic anemia (iron deficiency)
atrophy of the mucosa – oral, lingual, pharyngeal, and esophageal
dysphagia
thinning of the lips
angular cheilitis
koilonychia
affects middle-aged women
predisposition to oral carcinoma

> **References**
> Gregory B, Ho VC: Cutaneous manifestations of gastrointestinal disorders. Part I. J Am Acad Dermatol 1992; 26:153–166.
> Marks J, Shuster S 1987. The Skin and Disorders of the Alimentary Tract. In Fitzpatrick TB, Eisen AZ, Wolff K et al. (eds.) Dermatology in General Medicine, 3rd edition, p.1965–1976. (New York: McGraw-Hill).

POEMS SYNDROME, CROW–FUKASE SYNDROME, TAKATSUKI SYNDROME, PEP SYNDROME

Manifestations and Major Findings
*p*olyneuropathy (peripheral sensory and motor neuropathy)
*o*rganomegaly (hepatosplenomegaly)
*e*ndocrinopathy
– diabetes mellitus
– primary gonadal failure
– hypothyroidism
– elevated prolactin levels
*m*onoclonal protein (plasma cell tumor)
*s*kin changes
– • sclerodermatous changes (Fig. 116)
– • diffuse hyperpigmentation (Fig. 116)
– edema of the legs
– clubbing of the fingers
– • hypertrichosis (Fig. 116)
– hyperhidrosis
– angiomas

> **References**
> Burton JL: Systemic plasmacytosis and the Crow–Fukase syndrome. Arch Dermatol 1987; 123: 425–426.
> Feddersen RM, Burgdorf W, Foucar K, Elias L, Smith SM: Plasma cell dyscrasia: a case of POEMS syndrome with a unique dermatologic presentation. J Am Acad Dermatol 1989; 21:1061–1068.
> Feingold KR, Elias PM: Endocrine–skin interactions. J Am Acad Dermatol 1988; 19:1–20
> Fishel B, Brenner S, Weiss S, Yaron M: POEMS syndrome assoicated with cryoglobulinemia, lymphoma, multiple seborrheic keratosis, and ichthyosis. J Am Acad Dermatol 1988; 19:979–982.
> Kanitakis J, Roger H, Soubrier M, Dubost J-J: Cutaneous angiomas in POEMS syndrome. Arch Dermatol 1988; 124:695–698.
> Miralles GD, O'Fallon JR, Talley NJ: Plasma-cell dyscrasia with polyneuropathy. N Engl J Med 1992; 327:1919–1923.
> Shelley WB, Shelley ED: The skin changes in the Crow–Fukase (POEMS) syndrome. Arch Dermatol 1987; 123:85–87.

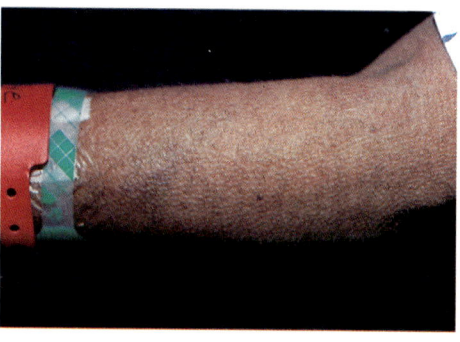

• *Figure 116 POEMS syndrome presents dermatologically as diffuse hyperpigmentation with sclerodermatous changes and hypertrichosis.*

POIKILODERMA CONGENITALE
see ROTHMUND–THOMSON SYNDROME

POIKILODERMA OF CIVATTE

Manifestations and Major Findings
hyper- and hypopigmentation on lateral neck
affects fair-skinned individuals
caused by excessive sun exposure
mild atrophy
telangiectasias
occurs in middle-aged and older Caucasians

> **References**
> Wheeland RG, Applebaum J: Flashlamp pumped pulse-dye laser therapy for poikiloderma of Civatte. J Dermatol Surg Oncol 1990; 16:12–16.

POLAND ANOMALY

Manifestations and Major Findings
hypoplasia/absence of pectoralis major muscle, nipple, and areola
rib defects (ipsilateral)
upper limb defects (ipsilateral)
–syndactyly
–brachydactyly
–limb reductions
–dermatoglyphic abnormalities

OTHER FINDINGS
axillary hair loss
renal anomalies
hemivertebrae
Sprengel anomaly

> **References**
> David TJ: Nature and etiology of the Poland anomaly. N Engl J Med 1972; 287:487–489.
> Dintiman BJ, Shapiro RS, Hood AF, Guba AM: Parry–Romberg syndrome in association with contralateral Poland syndrome. J Am Acad Dermatol 1990; 22:371–373.

POLYCYSTIC OVARY SYNDROME, STEIN–LEVENTHAL SYNDROME

Manifestations and Major Findings
nontumorous, dysfunctional condition of ovaries
enlarged cystic ovaries
luteinizing hormone-dependent hypersecretion of androgens from hyperplastic theca and stromal cells
obesity
menstrual irregularities/anovulation
infertility

Cutaneous Manifestations
hirsutism
acne
androgenic alopecia
acanthosis nigricans

> **References**
> Feingold KR, Elias PM: Endocrine–skin interactions. J Am Acad Dermatol 1988; 19:1–20.
> Sperling LC, Heimer WL: Androgen biology as a basis for the diagnosis and treatment of androgenic disorders in women. I. J Am Acad Dermatol 1993; 28: 669–683.

POLYGLANDULAR AUTOIMMUNE SYNDROME

Types of Polyglandular Autoimmune Syndrome and Features

type I
hypoparathyroidism
adrenal insufficiency (Addison disease)
gonadal failure
thyroid disorders
diabetes mellitus
cutaneous findings
– mucocutaneous candidiasis
– • vitiligo (Fig. 117)
– alopecia areata
– epidermolysis bullosa acquisita
pernicious anemia
chronic active hepatitis
nail dystrophy

type II
adrenal insufficiency (Addison disease)
gonadal abnormalities
thyroid disorders

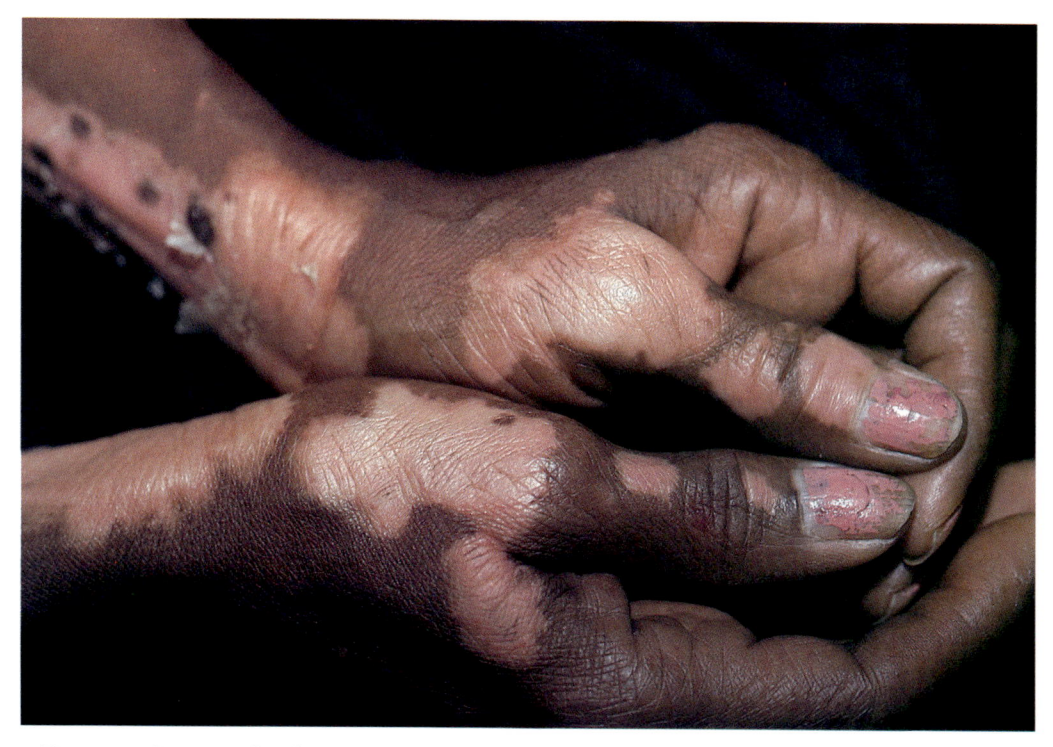

• *Figure 117* Symmetrical vitiligo seen in polyglandular autoimmune syndrome.

diabetes mellitus
cutaneous findings
– vitiligo
– alopecia
– Sjögren syndrome
pernicious anemia
myasthenia gravis
thrombocytopenic purpura
celiac disease
rheumatoid arthritis
nail dystrophy

type III
similar to type II without Addison disease

References
Ahonen P, Myllärniemi S, Sipilä I, Perheentupa J: Clinical variation of autoimmune polyendocrinopathy-candidiasis-ectodermal dystrophy (APECED) in a series of 68 patients. N Engl J Med 1990; 322: 1829–1836.
España A, Balsa J, Ledo A: Vitiligo and polyglandular autoimmune syndrome with selective IgA deficiency. Int J Dermatol 1992; 31:343–344.
Feingold KR, Elias PM: Endocrine–skin interactions. J Am Acad Dermatol 1988; 19:1–20. ▷ ▷ ▷

▷ ▷ ▷
Parker RI, O'Shea P, Forman EN: Acquired splenic atrophy in a sibship with the autoimmune polyendocrinopathy-candidiasis syndrome. J Pediatr 1990; 117:591–593.

POLYOSTOTIC FIBROUS DYSPLASIA
see McCUNE–ALBRIGHT SYNDROME

POPLITEAL PTERYGIUM SYNDROME, FACIOGENITOPOPLITEAL SYNDROME, POPLITEAL WEB SYNDROME

Manifestations and Major Findings
musculoskeletal abnormalities
– hypoplasia or agenesis of the digits
– valgus or varus deformities of the feet
– syndactyly
ankyloblepharon filiforme adnatum
oral frenula

genital abnormalities
- cryptorchidism
- absent or cleft scrotum or labia majora
- inguinal hernia

Cutaneous Manifestations
popliteal, facial, and genital webbing
cleft lip and/or palate
lip pits
nail anomalies
- reduction defects of the digits
- pterygium
dermal ridges over the toes
pili annulati (occasional)

autosomal dominant with variable expression

> **References**
> Bixler D, Poland C, Nance WE: Phenotypic variation in the popliteal pterygium syndrome. Clin Genet 1973; 4:220–228.
> Hall JG, Reed SD, Rosenbaum KN, Gershanik J, et al.: Limb pterygium syndromes: a review and report of eleven patients. Am J Med Genet 1982; 12:377–409.
> Oranje AP, Peereboom-Wynia JDR, Stolz E: Hair bands in facio-genito-popliteal syndrome. Pediatr Dermatol 1987; 4:346–347.
> Ramer JC, Ladda RL, Demuth WW: Multiple pterygium syndrome. Am J Dis Child 1988; 142:794–798.

POROKERATOSIS

Manifestations and Major Findings
raised, sharply marginated plaque(s) with a keratotic border
histology shows cornoid lamella at the edge of the lesion

Types of Porokeratosis and Features

1 porokeratosis of Mibelli
single or few discrete lesions
- • annular dry plaques (Fig. 118)
- surrounding fine keratotic wall
- atrophic center
centrifugal spread
appears in infancy or childhood
may be widely disseminated
autosomal dominant or sporadic

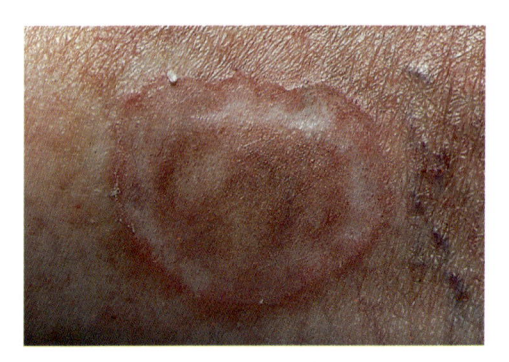

• *Figure 118* Porokeratosis of Mibelli; a dry, annular plaque with surrounding keratotic wall.

2 disseminated superficial actinic porokeratosis (DSAP)
multiple, small, flat lesions with cornoid lamellae
common on sun-exposed areas
commonly affects middle-aged Caucasian women
more numerous in third and fourth decades
autosomal dominant

3 palmoplantar porokeratosis
typical morphology of porokeratosis on the palms and soles
rare
autosomal dominant

4 linear porokeratosis
usually present at birth or in childhood
lesions in linear or zosteriform pattern
 (typical annular pattern with cornoid lamellae)
representative of aberrant keratinization
potential malignant degeneration of the lesion

5 disseminated superficial porokeratosis
widely disseminated, very flat lesions
asymptomatic
usually present at birth or in childhood
associated with renal or liver transplantation
autosomal dominant or sporadic

6 giant porokeratosis
large solitary lesion (10–20 cm diameter)
surrounding wall may be raised (1 cm)
most commonly found on foot
malignant degeneration of lesion

> **References**
> Chernosky ME: Porokeratosis. Arch Dermatol 1986; 122:869–870.
> Chernosky ME, Freeman RG: Disseminated superficial actinic porokeratosis (DSAP). Arch Dermatol 1967; 96:611–624. ▷ ▷ ▷

> Jurecka W, Neumann RA, Knobler RM: Porokeratoses: immunohistochemical, light and electron microscopic evaluation. J Am Acad Dermatol 1991; 24:96–101.
> Lestringant GG, Berge T: Porokeratosis punctata palmaris et plantaris: a new entity? Arch Dermatol 1989; 125:816–819.
> Rahbari H, Cordero AA, Mehregan AH: Linear porokeratosis: a distinctive clinical variant of porokeratosis of Mibelli. Arch Dermatol 1974; 109:526–528.
> Shumack SP, Commens CA: Disseminated superficial actinic porokeratosis: a clinical study. J Am Acad Dermatol 1989; 20:1015–1022.
> Spencer JM, Katz BE: Successful treatment of porokeratosis of Mibelli with diamond fraise dermabrasion. Arch Dermatol 1992; 128:1187–1188.

PORPHYRIA

Types of Porphyria with Clinical and Laboratory Findings

1. **erythropoietic porphyria (EP), Günther disease, congenital photosensitive porphyria, erythropoietic uroporphyria**
   onset in infancy
   dark urine
   marked photosensitivity to sunlight (with pain)
   vesicles and bullae
   hyperpigmentation
   hypertrichosis
   scleral ulcerations
   late-mutilating scars with acral deformities
   scarring alopecia
   sclerodermoid changes
   hemolytic anemia
   splenomegaly
   photophobia
   ectropion
   erythrodontia (fluorescent red teeth)
   laboratory findings
   – elevated urinary/fecal uroporphyrin I and coproporphyrin I
   – fluorescent urine
   – fluorescent red blood cells
   caused by uroporphyrinogen III cosynthetase deficiency
   autosomal recessive

2. **erythropoietic protoporphyria (EPP), erythrohepatic protoporphyria, protoporphyria**
   onset in first decade
   mild to severe photosensitivity

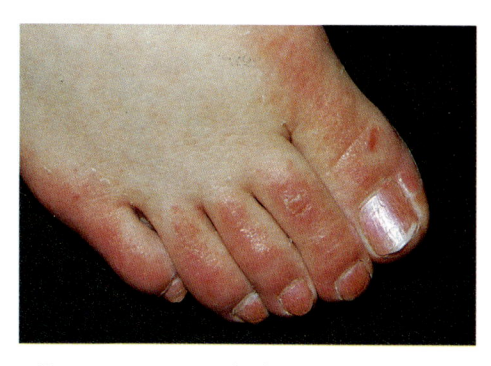

• *Figure 119* Urticarial, edematous, erythematous purpuric plaques on sun-exposed areas in erythropoietic protoporphyria.

   burning/stinging of the skin after sun exposure
   • edematous plaques with erythema, purpura, and urticaria in sun-exposed areas (Fig. 119)
   waxy/depressed scars on nose and dorsa of hands
   cholelithiasis
   terminal hepatic failure
   laboratory findings
   – elevated fecal protoporphyrin
   – fluorescent red blood cells
   – increased red blood cell and plasma protoporphyrin
   – normal urinary porphyrins
   caused by ferrochelatase deficiency
   autosomal dominant

3. **acute intermittent porphyria (AIP), Swedish porphyria**
   onset in second to fourth decade
   no photosensitivity
   no skin changes
   recurrent acute attacks
   – colicky abdominal pain lasting hours or days
   – muscle weakness
   – neuropathy
   – occasional paralysis (may be fatal)
   – bizarre, neurotic behavior or depression
   – limb, head, neck, or chest pain
   – hypertension
   – tachycardia
   – dark urine
   attacks often precipitated by drugs or environmental factors
   laboratory findings
   – elevated urinary δ-aminolevulinic acid
   – elevated urinary porphobilinogen
   caused by porphobilinogen deaminase deficiency or elevated δ-aminolevulinic acid synthetase activity
   autosomal dominant

▷ ▷ ▷

4 porphyria cutanea tarda (PCT), symptomatic porphyria, acquired hepatic porphyria, chemical porphyria
most common porphyria
onset in third to fourth decade
moderate to severe photosensitivity
vesicles
bullae
fragile skin
atrophic scars
hyperpigmentation
milia
facial hypertrichosis (particularly temples and cheeks)
alopecia
sclerodermoid plaques
diabetes mellitus (some cases)
liver iron overload
tumors of the liver (rare)
precipitated by environmental factors
– alcohol ingestion
– estrogens
– iron
– polyhalogenated cyclic hydrocarbons
laboratory findings
– urinary uroporphyrin I > uroporphyrin III
– increased coproporphyrin
– fecal isocoproporphyrin > protoporphyrin
caused by uroporphyrinogen decarboxylase deficiency
autosomal dominant (some cases) or sporadic

5 variegate porphyria (VP), porphyria variegata, mixed porphyria, South African porphyria, protocoproporphyria hereditaria
onset in second or third decade
mild to moderate photosensitivity
similar to PCT with vesicles on sun-exposed areas
vesicles evolve into hemorrhagic crusts
fragile skin
scars
milia
hypertrichosis
hypo- and hyperpigmentation
pseudoscleroderma
constipation
acute attacks (similar to AIP)
– bizarre behavior
– muscle weakness
– paralysis
– abdominal pain
most common in South Africa
laboratory findings
– increased urinary δ-aminolevulinic acid and porphobilinogen during attacks
– fecal protoporphyrin > coproporphyrin; both are elevated during and between attacks
caused by protoporphyrinogen oxidase deficiency, decreased erythrocyte ferrochelatase, and increased hepatic δ-aminolevulinic acid synthetase
autosomal dominant

6 hereditary coproporphyria (HCP), idiopathic coproporphyria
onset at any age
cutaneous lesions resemble PCT but are milder
blistering
photosensitivity (rare)
acute attacks (milder than AIP)
– mild neurologic symptoms (like AIP)
– abdominal pain
– vomiting
laboratory findings
– elevated fecal and urinary coproporphyrin III
caused by partial deficiency of coproporphyrinogen oxidase
autosomal dominant

7 hepatoerythropoietic porphyria (HEP)
onset before 2 years of age
dark urine from birth
marked photosensitivity
vesicles
bullae
hypertrichosis
sclerodermoid scarring (like PCT)
hyperpigmentation
hemolytic anemia
splenomegaly
laboratory findings
– elevated urinary uroporphyrins I and III
– elevated fecal uroporphyrin, coproporphyrin, and isocoproporphyrin
– elevated red blood cell protoporphyrin
– elevated plasma uroporphyrin
caused by deficiency of uroporphyrinogen decarboxylase (homozygous or compound heterozygous)
probably autosomal recessive

References
Logan GM, Weimer MK, Ellefson M, Pierach CA, Bloomer JR: Bile porphyrin analysis in the evaluation of variegate porphyria. N Engl J Med 1991; 324: 1408–1411.
Norris PG, Elder GH, Hawk JLM: Homozygous variegate porphyria: a case report. Br J Dermatol 1990; 122:253–257.
Poh-Fitzpatrick MB: Erythropoietic protoporphyria. Int J Dermatol 1978; 17:359–369.   ▷ ▷ ▷

> > >
Ross JB, Moss MA: Relief of photosensitivity of erythropoietic protoporphyria by pyridoxine. J Am Acad Dermatol 1990; 22:340–342.
Warner CA, Poh-Fitzpatrick MB, Zaider EF, Tsai S-F, et al.: Congenital erythropoietic porphyria. Arch Dermatol 1992; 128:1243–1248.

POTTER SYNDROME,
OLIGOHYDRAMNIOS SEQUENCE

Manifestations and Major Findings
renal agenesis
growth deficiency
fetal compression
pulmonary hypoplasia
limb position defects

PRADER–WILLI SYNDROME,
PRADER–LABHART–WILLI SYNDROME

Manifestations and Major Findings
hypotonia in infancy
feeding problems in infancy
poor weight gain
failure to thrive
obesity beginning after 12 months of age
behavioral problems especially with food/eating
hyperphagia/food foraging
small hands and feet
hypogonadism
hypopigmentation (fair skin and hair)
skin picking/ulcers
mental retardation (mild)
learning disabilities
chromosome 15 deletion in 60% of patients

Characteristic Facies (in Infancy)
dolichocephaly
narrow face
almond-shaped eyes
small mouth with thin upper lip
downward-slanting corners of the mouth

References
Fowler JF, Butler MG: Urticaria pigmentosa in a child with Prader–Labhart–Willi syndrome. J Am Acad Dermatol 1989; 21:147–148. > > >

> > >
Holm VA, Cassidy SB, Butler MG, Hanchett JM, et al.: Prader–Willi syndrome: consensus diagnostic criteria. Pediatrics 1993; 91:398–402.
Knoll JHM, Nicholls RD, Magenis RE, Graham JM, et al.: Angelman and Prader–Willi syndromes share a common chromosome 15 deletion but differ in parental origin of the deletion. Am J Med Genet 1989; 32:285–290.
Smeets DFCM, Hamel BCJ, Nelen MR, Smeets HJM, et al.: Prader–Willi syndrome and Angelman syndrome in cousins from a family with a translocation between chromosomes 6 and 15. N Engl J Med 1992; 326:807–811.

PROGERIA, HUTCHINSON-GILFORD SYNDROME

Manifestations and Major Findings
premature aging
short stature
profound growth failure after 6–12 months of age
'sculptured' nasal tip
pinched facies
micrognathia and thin lips
high-pitched voice
abnormal and delayed dentition
severe atherosclerosis
hypertension
myocardial infarction
bones show osteolysis, osteoporosis, and necrosis
joint dislocations
joint contractures
dystrophic, short clavicles
no sexual maturation
normal intelligence
life expectancy 10–15 years

Cutaneous Manifestations
alopecia of eyebrows, eyelashes, and scalp hair in first 2 years of life
midfacial cyanosis
prominent scalp veins
small, thin, dystrophic nails
atrophy of subcutaneous fat
scleroderma-like skin (thin, taut, shiny in some areas, but lax and wrinkled in others)
multiple keloids (rare)

autosomal recessive or sporadic

References

Badame AJ: Progeria. (Review). Arch Dermatol 1989; 125:540–544.
Beauregard S, Gilchrest BA: Syndromes of premature aging. Dermatol Clin 1987; 5:109–121.
DeBusk FL: The Hutchinson–Gilford progeria syndrome. J Pediatr 1972; 80:697–724.
Gillar PJ, Kaye CI, McCourt JW: Progressive early dermatologic changes in Hutchinson–Gilford progeria syndrome. Pediatr Dermatol 1991; 8:199–206.
Jimbow K, Kobayashi H, Ishii M, Oyanagi A, Ooshima A: Scar and keloidlike lesions in progeria. Arch Dermatol 1988; 124:1261–1266.

PROGRESSIVE HEMIFACIAL ATROPHY see PARRY–ROMBERG SYNDROME

PROGRESSIVE SYMMETRICAL ERYTHROKERATODERMIA
see GOTTRON SYNDROME

PROLIDASE DEFICIENCY

Manifestations and Major Findings
decreased prolidase enzyme (peptidase D)
causes abnormal collagen metabolism
mental retardation
dental abnormalities
hepatosplenomegaly
laxity of the joints
recurrent upper respiratory tract infections
iminodipeptiduria

Cutaneous Manifestations
skin fragility
chronic recurrent ulcers of the lower limbs
recurrent skin infections
eczematous dermatitis
diffuse telangiectasias
ecchymoses
purpura
photosensitivity
premature graying of hair (canities)
lymphedema

Characteristic Facies
flat facies
saddle nose
hypertelorism
hypoplasia of the jaw
ear abnormalities

autosomal recessive

References
Arata J, Umemura S, Yamamoto Y, Hagiyama M: Prolidase deficiency. Arch Dermatol 1979; 115:62–67.
Freij BJ, DerKaloustian VM: Prolidase deficiency. A metabolic disorder presenting with dermatologic signs. Int J Dermatol 1986; 25:431–433.
Ogata A, Tanaka S, Tomoda T, Murayama E, et al.: Autosomal recessive prolidase deficiency. Arch Dermatol 1981; 117:689–694.

POSTGASTRECTOMY SYNDROME
see DUMPING SYNDROME

PROTEIN C DEFICIENCY

Manifestations and Major Findings
homozygous state
– purpura fulminans (neonatal)
– vascular thrombosis
– disseminated intravascular coagulation
– severe bilateral vitreous hemorrhages
heterozygous state (*see* coumarin necrosis)

References
Dreyfus M, Magny JF, Bridey F, Schwarz HP, et al.: Treatment of homozygous protein C deficiency and neonatal purpura fulminans with a purified protein C concentrate. N Engl J Med 1991; 325:1565–1568.
Gladson CL, Groncy P, Griffin JH: Coumarin necrosis, neonatal purpura fulminans, and protein C deficiency. Arch Dermatol 1987; 123:1701a–1706a.
Peters C, Casella JF, Marlar RA, Montgomery RR, et al.: Homozygous protein C deficiency: observations on the nature of the molecular abnormality and effectiveness of warfarin therapy. Pediatrics 1988; 81:272–276.
Samlaska CP, James WD: Superficial thrombophlebitis I. Primary hypercoagulable states. J Am Acad Dermatol 1990; 22:975–989.

PROTEUS SYNDROME

Manifestations and Major Findings
an association of findings
- • asymmetrical overgrowth of body parts (Fig. 120)
- epidermal nevi
- vascular malformations
- lipomas

cerebriform hyperplasia of the skin – especially palms and soles

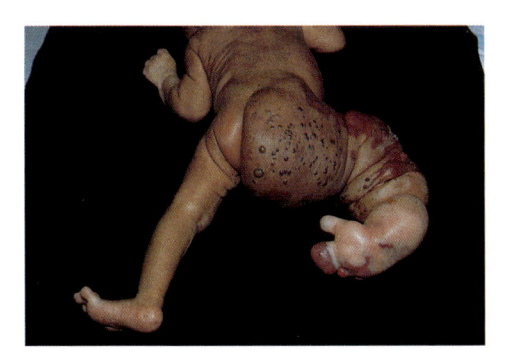

• *Figure 120* Asymmetric overgrowth of the leg, foot, and buttock in Proteus syndrome.

OCULAR ABNORMALITIES
epibulbar tumors
strabismus
enlargement of the globe
cataracts
ptosis

SKELETAL ABNORMALITIES
kyphosis
scoliosis
exostoses
skull abnormalities (enlarged or asymmetric)
osteoporosis

OTHER FINDINGS
subcutaneous tumors
hemihypertrophy or digital hypertrophy
partial gigantism of hands and/or feet
normal mentation
seizures
testicular tumors
accelerated growth in early life

Cutaneous Manifestations
epidermal nevi
nevocellular nevi
connective tissue nevi
café au lait macules
macular hyper- or hypopigmentation (linear or whorled)

References
Happle R: How many epidermal nevus syndromes exist? J Am Acad Dermatol 1991; 25:550–556.
Hornstein L, Bove KE, Towbin RB: Linear nevi, hemihypertrophy, connective tissue hamartomas, and unusual neoplasms in children. J Pediatr 1987; 110:404–408.
Nazzaro V, Cambiaghi S, Montagnani A, Brusasco A, et al.: Proteus syndrome. Ultrastructural study of linear verrucous and depigmented nevi. J Am Acad Dermatol 1991; 25:377–383.
Samlaska CP, Levin SW, James WD, Benson PM, Walker JC, et al.: Proteus syndrome. Arch Dermatol 1989; 125:1109–1114.
Viljoen DL, Saxe N, Temple-Camp C: Cutaneous manifestations of the Proteus syndrome. Pediatr Dermatol 1988; 5:14–21.

PRUNE BELLY SYNDROME,
APLASTIC ABDOMINAL MUSCULATURE SYNDROME

Manifestations and Major Findings
absence of abdominal muscles
protuberant lax abdomen with wrinkled skin
intestinal abnormalities
renal abnormalities
- megacystis
- megaureter
- hydronephrosis
- cystic dysplasia of the kidneys
bilateral cryptorchidism
hip dysplasia
talipes equinovarus
male predominence

References
Loder RT, Guiboux J-P, Bloom DA, Hensinger RN: Musculoskeletal aspects of prune-belly syndrome. Am J Dis Child 1992; 146:1224–1229.
Reinberg Y, Shapiro E, Manivel JC, Manley CB, et al.: Prune belly syndrome in females: a triad of abdominal musculature deficiency and anomalies of the urinary and genital systems. J Pediatr 1991; 118:395–398.

PSEUDOLYMPHOMA OF SPIEGLER–FENDT
see SPIEGLER–FENDT PSEUDOLYMPHOMA

PSEUDOLYMPHOMA SYNDROME
see HYDANTOIN SYNDROME

PSEUDOPELADE OF BROCQ

Manifestations and Major Findings
slowly progressive, cicatricial alopecia
no clinical evidence of folliculitis or marked inflammation
- follicular scarring of scalp – small, round or oval, bald patches (Fig. 121)

clinical syndrome ends in scarring
scarring may be due to lichen planus or other pathologic process
more common in females
long course (over 2 years)

> **References**
> Braun-Falco O, Imai S, Schmoeckel C, Steger O, et al.: Pseudopelade of Brocq. Dermatologica 1986; 172:18–23.
> Bulengo-Ransby SM, Headington JT: Pseudopelade of Brocq in a child. J Am Acad Dermatol 1990; 23: 944–945.

PSEUDOTHALIDOMIDE SYNDROME see ROBERTS SYNDROME

PSEUDOXANTHOMA ELASTICUM,
GRÖNBLAD–STRANDBERG SYNDROME

Manifestations and Major Findings
inherited disorder of connective (elastic) tissue
histology shows fragmented elastic tissue, clumped with calcium deposits

Types of Pseudoxathoma Elasticum and Features

type IA, classic type
- xanthoma-like papules ('plucked chicken') (Fig. 122)
  – found in flexural areas and neck
  – areas thicken with age
  small (1–3mm) yellowish papules
  – linear or reticular pattern
  – may form confluent plaques
  soft, lax, wrinkled skin hanging in folds
  perforating lesions with hyperkeratosis
  abnormal elastic tissue in arteries
  hypertension
  cerebrovascular accidents
  gastrointestinal hemorrhages
  severe vascular complications
  increased risk of miscarriage
  ocular abnormalities
  – angioid streaks in retina
  – 'punched-out' atrophic areas (breaks in Bruch's membrane)
  – speckled yellowish mottling of retina
  – pigmented dots on retina
  – loss of central vision due to hemorrhage of retinal vessels and choroiditis

autosomal dominant

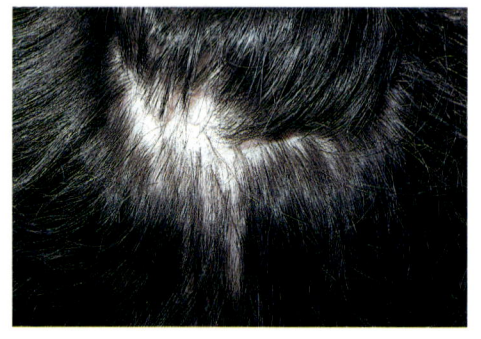

- *Figure 121* Oval patches of follicular scarring of the scalp in pseudopelade of Brocq.

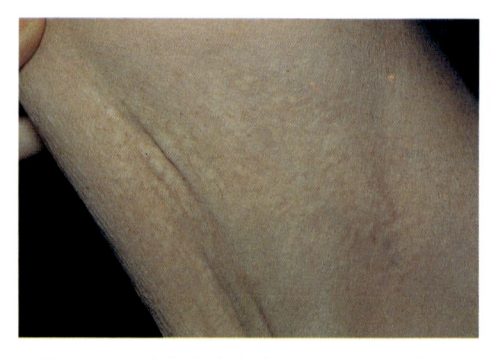

- *Figure 122* 'Plucked chicken' appearance of xanthoma-like papules in classic type pseudoxanthoma elasticum.

type IB
milder skin, vascular and retinal involvement than type IA
focal cutaneous involvement
hyperextensible skin
marfanoid features
– blue sclerae
– high-arched palate
– mitral valve prolapse
– loose joints
autosomal dominant

type IIA
cutaneous, vascular, and ocular manifestations similar to type IA
hematemesis common
autosomal recessive

type IIB
extensive cutaneous involvement
prominent cutaneous laxity
no vascular or ocular manifestations
autosomal recessive

type IIC
mild/moderate skin and cardiovascular changes until third decade
severe ocular changes after third decade
telangiectasias of the lips
bilateral cataracts
seen in Afrikaners
autosomal recessive

type III, localized acquired cutaneous pseudoxanthoma elasticum
periumbilical perforating lesions
most common in obese, middle-aged, multiparous black women

> **References**
> Eddy DD, Farber EM: Pseudoxanthoma elasticum. Internal manifestations: a report of cases and a statistical review of the literature. Arch Dermatol 1962; 86:729–740.
> Pruzan D, Rabbin PE, Heilman ER: Periumbilical perforating pseudoxanthoma elasticum. J Am Acad Dermatol 1992; 26:642–644.
> Rongioletti F, Rebora A: Pseudoxanthoma elasticum-like papillary dermal elastolysis. J Am Acad Dermatol 1992; 26:648–650.

PURPURA PIGMENTOSA CHRONICA, PIGMENTED PURPURIC DERMATOSIS

Manifestations and Major Findings
capillaritis of unknown etiology
petechiae and brown pigmentation
histology shows extravasation of red blood cells and hemosiderin in macrophages
chronic condition
not associated with hematologic disorders or venous insufficiency

Types of Purpura Pigmentosa Chronica and Features

1 **Schamberg purpura, progressive pigmentary disease**
   capillaritis of unknown cause
   • petechiae ('cayenne pepper') usually on lower legs (Fig. 123)
   usually asymptomatic
   more common in males ▷ ▷ ▷

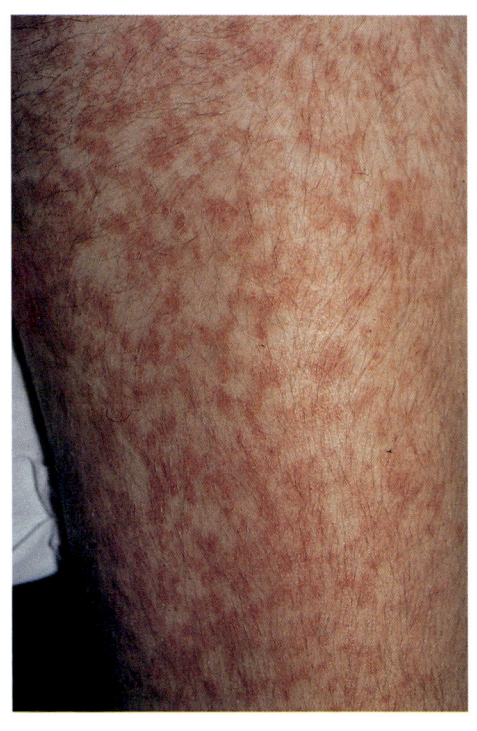

• *Figure 123* '*Cayenne pepper' macules on the lower leg in Shamberg purpura.*

▷ ▷ ▷

2 Majocchi disease, purpura annularis telangiectodes
macular, yellow/brown, annular plaques
1–3 cm diameter
lesions show hemosiderosis and telangiectasias
lesions may remain unchanged for months/years or slowly extend
slight atrophy may be found
most common in adolescents/young adults
lesions occur at any site
histology shows capillaritis with hemosiderin deposition

3 Gougerot–Blum disease, pigmented purpuric lichenoid dermatitis
lichenoid papules
petechial patches
usually seen on legs but also elsewhere
purpuric macules
similar to Schamberg purpura but with papules
affects males aged 40–60 years

4 lichen aureus, lichen purpuricus
localized, intensely purpuric eruption
- eruption is rust-colored or purple (sometimes with golden color) (Fig. 124)
resembles a bruise
zosteriform pattern

5 itching purpura
purpuric lesions
seen around ankles
often become widespread
spontaneous improvement within a few months
pruritus
histology shows spongiotic dermatitis with superficial mixed-cell perivascular infiltrate and extravasated red blood cells

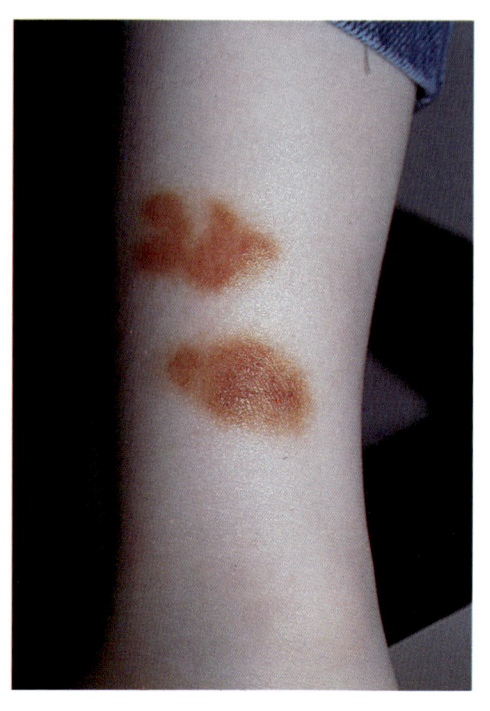

• *Figure 124* Rust-colored, localized, purpuric eruption of lichen aureus.

References
Aiba S, Tagami H: Immunohistologic studies in Schamberg's disease. Arch Dermatol 1988; 124: 1058–1062. ▷ ▷ ▷

▷ ▷ ▷
Gelmetti C, Cerri D, Grimalt R: Lichen aureus in childhood. Pediatr Dermatol 1991; 8:280–283.
Krizsa J, Hunyadi J, Dobozy A: PUVA treatment of pigmented purpuric lichenoid dermatitis (Gougerot–Blum). J Am Acad Dermatol 1992; 27:778–780.
Leal-Khouri SM, Sherman LD, Mallory SB: Segmental eruption in an 8-year-old girl. Pediatr Dermatol 1992; 9:154–156.
Ratnam KV, Su WPD, Peters MS: Purpura simplex (inflammatory purpura without vasculitis): a clinicopathologic study of 174 cases. J Am Acad Dermatol 1991; 25:642–647.

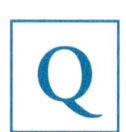

Q

QUEYRAT ERYTHROPLASIA
see ERYTHROPLASIA OF QUEYRAT

R

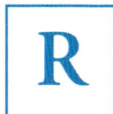

RAMSAY HUNT SYNDROME, HERPES ZOSTER OTICUS

Manifestations and Major Findings
herpes zoster of the external auditory canal
varicella-zoster virus infection causes
—edema and swelling of the auditory nerve (VIII)
—pressure on the facial nerve (V)
facial palsy (may be permanent)
tinnitus
vertigo
deafness
impaired taste sensation in the anterior two-thirds of the tongue
proximity of the geniculate ganglion of the facial nerve (VII) to the auditory nerve (VIII)

References
Feldman SR: Herpes zoster and facial palsy. Cutis 1988; 42:523–524.
Robillard RB, Hilsinger RL, Adour KK: Ramsey Hunt facial paralysis: clinical analyses of 185 patients. Otolaryngol Head Neck Surg 1986; 95:292–297.

RAPP–HODGKIN ECTODERMAL DYSPLASIA

Manifestations and Major Findings
hypohidrosis
hypotrichosis – sparse, coarse, wiry hair, pili torti
dystrophic, grooved, discolored nails
hypodontia (with conical teeth) or anodontia
cleft lip and/or palate

OCULAR ABNORMALITIES
atresia of the puncta
ectropion
corneal opacities
photophobia

OTHER FINDINGS
short stature
hypospadias

Characteristic Facies
high forehead
narrow nasal bridge with small nostrils
small mouth
maxillary hyperplasia

autosomal dominant with variable expression

References
Felding IB, Björklund LJ: Rapp–Hodgkin ectodermal dysplasia. Pediatr Dermatol 1990; 7:126–131.
O'Donnell BP, James WD: Rapp–Hodgkin ectodermal dysplasia. J Am Acad Dermatol 1992; 27:323–326.
Schroeder HW, Sybert VP: Rapp–Hodgkin ectodermal dysplasia. J Pediatr 1987; 110:72–75.

RAYNAUD DISEASE

Manifestations and Major Findings
Raynaud phenomenon
no associated disease or cause
more common in women
onset usually before 40 years of age

RAYNAUD PHENOMENON

Manifestations and Major Findings
paroxysmal sequential blanching, cyanosis, and redness of hands and feet (especially digits)
usually precipitated by cold or stress
typical attack lasts up to half an hour
pain and stiffness of the joints
superficial digital gangrene
variable course

Raynaud phenomenon is associated with trauma, neurovascular disease, occlusive disease, connective tissue disease, smoking, chemicals, and other disorders.

> **References**
> Dowd PA: The treatment of Raynaud's phenomenon. Br J Dermatol 1986; 114:527–533.
> **Duffy CM, Laxer RM, Lee P, Ramsay C, et al.:** Raynaud syndrome in childhood. J Pediatr 1989; 114:73–78.

RECRUDESCENT TYPHUS
see BRILL-ZINSSER DISEASE

RED MAN SYNDROME

Manifestations and Major Findings
Caused by rapid infusion/overdose of rifampin or vancomycin
histamine-induced flushing
maculopapular eruption
seen especially on the face and neck
red skin, urine, tears, feces, and sweat
pruritus
hypotension
tachycardia
respiratory distress
dizziness
agitation
mild hyperthermia

> **References**
> **Gross DJ, Dellinger RP:** Red/orange person syndrome. Cutis 1988; 42:175–177.
> **Levy M, Koren G, Dupuis L, Read SE:** Vancomycin-induced red man syndrome. Pediatrics 1990; 86:572–580.

REFSUM DISEASE, HEREDOPATHIA ATACTICA POLYNEURITIFORMIS see also DISORDERS OF CORNIFICATION; DOC 11

Manifestations and Major Findings
deficiency of phytanic acid α-hydroxylase
ichthyosis resembling ichthyosis vulgaris (DOC 1)
chronic polyneuritis
cerebellar ataxia
atypical retinitis pigmentosa (night blindness)
cataracts
progressive nerve deafness
presence of lipid vacuoles in the basal layer of the epidermis
symptoms appear insidiously
onset usually after 20 years of age

Dietary green vegetables are major source of phytanic acid.

autosomal recessive

> **References**
> **Reed WB, Stone VM, Boder E, Ziprkowski L:** Hereditary syndromes with auditory and dermatological manifestations. Arch Dermatol 1967; 95:456–461.
> **Williams ML, Elias PM:** Genetically transmitted, generalized disorders of cornification. The ichthyoses. Dermatol Clin 1987; 5:155–178.

REITER SYNDROME, URETHRO-OCULOSYNOVIAL SYNDROME, DYSENTERIC ARTHRITIS

Manifestations and Major Findings
predominantly occurs in young men
nonspecific urethritis and/or cervicitis (in women)
nonsuppurative polyarthritis
–seronegative for rheumatoid factor
–predominantly affects sacroiliac joints and lower extremities
ocular abnormalities with conjunctivitis, iritis, uveitis, corneal erosions – usually bilateral and may be transient

OTHER FINDINGS
ankylosing spondylitis
epididymitis
cardiac involvement uncommon
central nervous system involvement uncommon
episodes last longer than 1 month
Reiter syndrome is often associated with enteritis (Shigella, Yersinia, Klebsiella, Salmonella, Campylobacter) *or venereal disease* (Chlamydia, Ureaplasma).

Cutaneous Manifestations
- cutaneous lesions resembling psoriasis (Fig. 125)

circinate balanitis
keratoderma blenorrhagicum (palms, soles, glans penis) with limpet-like scales
oral ulcers
- nails show oil-drop lesions similar to psoriasis (Fig. 125)

HLA-B27

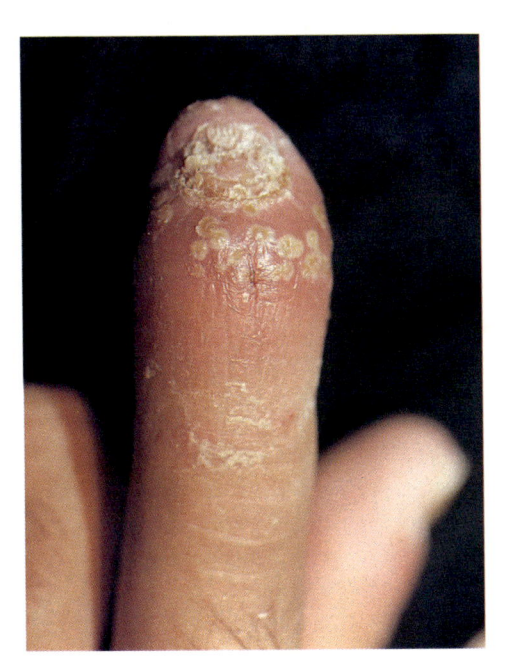

- *Figure 125* Lesions of the nail, resembling pustular psoriasis, in Reiter syndrome.

References
Edwards L, Hansen RC: Reiter's syndrome of the vulva. The psoriasis spectrum. Arch Dermatol 1992; 128:811–814.
O'Keefe E, Braverman IM, Cohen I: Annulus migrans. Arch Dermatol 1973; 107:240–244.

REM SYNDROME
see RETICULAR ERYTHEMATOUS MUCINOSIS

RENDU–OSLER–WEBER SYNDROME
see OSLER–WEBER–RENDU SYNDROME

RESTRICTIVE DERMOPATHY

Manifestations and Major Findings
abnormally tight skin from birth
generalized joint contractures
pulmonary hypoplasia
intrauterine growth retardation

Characteristic Facies
pinched nose
microstomia
micrognathia

References
Happle R, Stekhoven JHS, Hamel BCJ, Kollée LAA, et al.: Restrictive dermopathy in two brothers. Arch Dermatol 1992; 128:232–235.
Welsh KM, Smoller BR, Holbrook KA, Johnston K: Restrictive dermopathy. Arch Dermatol 1992; 128: 228–231.

RETICULAR ERYTHEMATOUS MUCINOSIS, REM SYNDROME, PLAQUE-LIKE CUTANEOUS MUCINOSIS

Manifestations and Major Findings
persistent, reticular, erythematous plaques found on upper chest and back – usually asymptomatic
most common in middle-aged females
histology shows dermal mucin with lymphocytic infiltrates
chronic course

Reticular erythematous mucinosis is associated with thyroid disease, diabetes, carcinoma, discoid lupus erythematosus, and thrombocytopenic purpura.

> **References**
> **Braddock SW, Davis CS, Davis RB:** Reticular erythematous mucinosis and thrombocytopenic purpura. J Am Acad Dermatol 1988; 19:859–868.
> **Cohen PR, Rabinowitz AD, Ruszkowski AM, DeLeo VA:** Reticular erythematous mucinosis syndrome: review of the world literature and report of the syndrome in a prepubertal child. Pediatr Dermatol 1990; 7:1–10.
> **Morison WL, Shea CR, Parrish JA:** Reticular erythematous mucinosis syndrome. Arch Dermatol 1979; 115:1340–1342.
> **Truhan AP, Roenigk HH:** The cutaneous mucinoses. J Am Acad Dermatol 1986; 14:1–18.

RETICULATE ACROPIGMENTATION OF KITAMURA see KITAMURA RETICULATE ACROPIGMENTATION

RETINOIC ACID EMBRYOPATHY,
ACCUTANE EMBRYOPATHY

Characteristic Facies
microcephaly or macrocephaly
bilateral microtia/anotia (may be asymmetric)
micrognathia
maldevelopment of the facial bones, calvarium
cleft palate
flat, depressed nasal bridge
ocular hypertelorism

NEUROLOGIC ABNORMALITIES
hydrocephalus
retinal or optic nerve abnormalities
structural abnormalities

CARDIOVASCULAR ABNORMALITIES
conotruncal heart defects
aortic arch abnormalities
ventricular septal defects
atrial septal defects

OTHER FINDINGS
thymic defects (ectopia, hypoplasia, aplasia)
limb anomalies

> **References**
> **Lammer EJ, Chen DT, Hoar RM, Agnish ND, et al.:** Retinoic acid embryopathy. N Engl J Med 1985; 313:837–841.

RETT SYNDROME

Manifestations and Major Findings
predominantly affects females
apparently normal development for 6–12 months
early behavioral, social, and psychomotor regression
deceleration of head growth between 6 months to 4 years
loss of purposeful hand skills (1–4 years)
stereotypic wringing/clapping/washing of hands
gait ataxia/apraxia
cutis marmorata
hyperventilation

OTHER FINDINGS
seizures
respiratory dysfunction
apneic spells during wakefulness
dysphagia
scoliosis
progressive rigidity

> **References**
> **Moeschler JB, Charman CE, Berg SZ, Graham JM:** Rett syndrome: natural history and management. Pediatrics 1988; 82:1–10.
> **Trevathan E:** Rett syndrome. Pediatrics Suppl 1989; 83:636–637.

RICHNER–HANHART SYNDROME,
TYROSINEMIA TYPE II, OCULOCUTANEOUS TYROSINEMIA

Manifestations and Major Findings
hepatic tyrosine aminotransferase deficiency
growth failure
progressive mental retardation (mild to moderate)
fine motor coordination defects
self-mutilation

OCULAR ABNORMALITIES
corneal erosions with scarring
glaucoma
photophobia
corneal neovascularization

Cutaneous Manifestations
painful, punctate palmoplantar keratoses, blisters, and erosions
commonly found on the distal phalanges, thenar and hypothenar eminences
hyperhidrosis
prepatellar keratoses
hyperkeratosis of the tongue

autosomal recessive

> **References**
> **Goldsmith LA:** Tyrosinemia II: lessons in molecular pathophysiology. Pediatr Dermatol 1983; 1:25–34.
> **Lestringant GG:** Tyrosinemia type II with incomplete Richner–Hanhart's syndrome. Int J Dermatol 1988; 27:43–44.
> **Ney D, Bay C, Schneider JA, Kelts D, Nyhan WL:** Dietary management of oculocutaneous tyrosinemia in an 11 year old child. Am J Dis Child 1983; 137: 995–1000.
> **Shimizu N, Ito M, Ito K, Nakamura A, et al.:** Richner–Hanhart's syndrome, electron microscopic study of the skin lesion. Arch Dermatol 1990; 126: 1342–1346.

RIEHL MELANOSIS, FEMALE FACIAL MELANOSIS

Manifestations and Major Findings
brown/grey reticular pigmentation
lesions on the face – may extend to the chest, neck, and scalp
possibly caused by tar derivatives or cosmetics
most frequent in middle-aged females

> **References**
> **Nakayama H, Harada R, Toda M:** Pigmented cosmetic dermatitis. Int J Dermatol 1976; 15: 673–675.
> **Serrano G, Pujol C, Cuadra J, Gallo S, et al.:** Riehl's melanosis: pigmented contact dermatitis caused by fragrances. J Am Acad Dermatol 1989; 21:1057–1060.

RILEY–DAY SYNDROME, FAMILIAL AUTONOMIC DYSFUNCTION SYNDROME, FAMILIAL DYSAUTONOMIA

Manifestations and Major Findings
impaired pharyngeal and esophageal motility
feeding difficulties
recurrent fevers
drooling continues beyond infancy
failure to produce tears when crying
absent corneal reflexes
absence of deep tendon reflexes
delayed growth
episodes of hypertension or postural hypotension
pulmonary infections
most common in Ashkenazi Jews

Cutaneous Manifestations
intermittent blotchy erythema during eating or excitement
acrocyanosis of the hands and feet
excessive sweating
complete absence of fungiform and vallate papillae of the tongue
abnormal intradermal histamine test (no flare produced)

autosomal recessive

> **References**
> **Brunt PW, McKusick VA:** Familial dysautonomia: a report of genetic and clinical studies with a review of the literature. Medicine 1970; 49:343–374.
> **Fellner MJ:** Manifestations of familial autonomic dysautonomia: report of a case with an analysis of 125 cases in the literature. Arch Dermatol 1964; 89:190–195.

RILEY–SMITH SYNDROME, MACROCEPHALY WITH PSEUDOPAPILLEDEMA AND HEMANGIOMAS

Manifestations and Major Findings
macrocephaly without hydrocephalus
pseudopapilledema
vascular malformations (may be progressive)
gastrointestinal polyposis

OTHER FINDINGS
absence of lipomas
lymphatic anomalies
macrodactyly
frequent respiratory infections

autosomal dominant

> **References**
> Dvir M, Beer S, Aladjem M: Heredofamilial syndrome of mesodermal hamartomas, macrocephaly, and pseudopapilledema. Pediatrics 1988; 81: 287–290.
> Riley HD, Smith RW: Macrocephaly, pseudopapilledema, and multiple hemangiomata. A previously undescribed heredofamilial syndrome. Pediatrics 1960; 26:293–300.

RITTER DISEASE see STAPHYLOCOCCAL SCALDED SKIN SYNDROME

ROBERTS SYNDROME,
PSEUDOTHALIDOMIDE SYNDROME, ROBERTS-SC PHOCOMELIA SYNDROME, HYPOMELIA-HYPOTRICHOSIS-FACIAL HEMANGIOMA SYNDROME

Manifestations and Major Findings
cleft lip and/or palate
midface capillary malformation (port-wine stain)
sparse, silvery-blond hair
limb-reduction malformations
–hypomelia (more severe in upper limbs)
–phocomelia
–oligodactyly
–syndactly
–flexion positioning of the joints
marked growth retardation

OTHER FINDINGS
mental retardation
genital abnormalities
–large genitalia
–cryptorchidism
cystic kidneys
congenital heart disease

Characteristic Facies
hypertelorism
malformed ears
blue sclerae
clouded corneae
hypoplastic nasal alae and tip
anteverted nostrils

autosomal recessive

> **References**
> Freeman MVR, Williams DW, Schimke RN, et al.: The Roberts syndrome. Clin Genet 1974; 5:1–16.
> Hall BD, Greenberg MH: Hypomelia-hypotrichosis-facial hemangioma syndrome (pseudothalidomide, SC syndrome, SC phocomelia syndrome). Am J Dis Child 1972; 123:602–604.
> Romke C, Froster-Iskenius U, Heyne K, et al.: Roberts syndrome and SC phocomelia: a single genetic entity. Clin Genet 1987; 31:170–177.

ROBIN SYNDROME
see PIERRE ROBIN SYNDROME

ROCKY MOUNTAIN SPOTTED FEVER

Manifestations and Major Findings
acute infectious disease caused by *Rickettsia rickettsii*
transmitted by tick bite *(Dermacentor)*
occurs in North and South America
malaise/myalgia
headache
fever
• maculopapular rash (Fig. 126)
–typically begins on the wrists and ankles
–centripetal spread (limbs, trunk, face)
–rash becomes hemorrhagic and purpuric
periorbital edema
conjunctivitis

> **References**
> Nichols MM, Walker DH, Frates RC, Davis A: Three-month-old infant with diarrhea, fever, and rash. J Pediatr 1989; 114:154–160. ▷ ▷ ▷

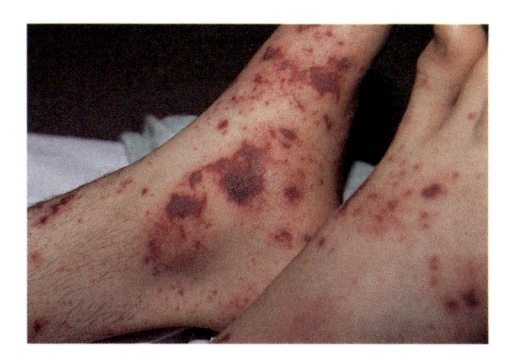

Figure 126 Purpuric lesions on the ankles in Rocky Mountain spotted fever.

▷ ▷ ▷
Prose NS, Resnick SD: Cutaneous manifestations of systemic infection in children. Curr Probl Dermatol 1993; 94–95.
Walker DH, Gay RM, Valdes-Dapena M: The occurrence of eschars in Rocky Mountain spotted fever. J Am Acad Dermatol 1981; 4:571–576.

ROMBERG–PARRY SYNDROME

see PARRY–ROMBERG SYNDROME

ROMBO SYNDROME

Manifestations and Major Findings

atrophoderma vermiculatum (grainy appearance of the skin)
milia
multiple trichoepitheliomas
multiple basal cell carcinomas
peripheral vasodilation/cyanosis of the hands, feet, and lips
hypotrichosis
eyelashes and eyebrows progressively disappear
facial lesions begin in late childhood

autosomal dominant

References
Ashinoff R, Jacobson M, Belsito DV: Rombo syndrome: a second case report and review. J Am Acad Dermatol 1993; 28:1011–1014.
Frosch PJ, Brumage MR, Schuster-Pavlovic C, Bersch A: Atrophoderma vermiculatum. J Am Acad Dermatol 1988; 18:538–542. ▷ ▷ ▷

▷ ▷ ▷
Michaëlsson G, Olsson E, Westermark P: The Rombo syndrome: a familial disorder with vermiculate atrophoderma, milia, hypotrichosis, trichoepitheliomas, basal cell carcinomas and peripheral vasodilation with cyanosis. Acta Derm Venereol (Stockh) 1981; 61:497–503.

ROSAI–DORFMAN DISEASE, SINUS HISTIOCYTOSIS WITH MASSIVE LYMPHADENOPATHY

Manifestations and Major Findings

reactive proliferation of lymphoid and histiocytic cell lines
painless marked adenopathy (especially cervical)
extranodal involvement – nasal cavity, bones, salivary glands, thyroid, central nervous system, gastrointestinal, genitourinary, heart
skin lesions – yellow, violaceous or purple papules, nodules, or plaques
night-time sweats
fever
weight loss
leukocytosis
usually self-limited but protracted course
most often seen in young adults

References
Foucar E, Rosai J, Dorfman RF: Sinus histiocytosis with masive lymphadenopathy (Rosai–Dorfman disease): review of the entity. Semin Diagn Pathol 1990; 7:19–73.
Foucar E, Rosai J, Dorfman RF: Sinus histiocytosis with massive lymphadenopathy. Arch Dermatol 1988; 124:1211–1214.
Suster S, Cartagena N, Cabello-Inchausti B, Robinson MJ: Histiocytic lymphophagocytic panniculitis. Arch Dermatol 1988; 124:1246–1249.

ROSENTHAL–KLOEPFER SYNDROME

Manifestations and Major Findings

corneal leukomata (opaque)
acromegalic facial features
large hands and feet
prognathism
cutis verticis gyrata – onset in the fourth to fifth decade

autosomal dominant

> **References**
> Rosenthal JW, Kloepfer HW: An acromegaloid, cutis verticis gyrata, corneal leukoma syndrome. A new medical entity. Arch Ophthalmol 1962; 68:722–726.

ROTHMANN–MAKAI SYNDROME, MAKAI SUBCUTANEOUS LIPOGRANULOMATOSIS

Manifestations and Major Findings
spontaneous circumscribed panniculitis (spontaneously involuting)
usually found on the trunk and extremities
afebrile
no systemic symptoms
most common in children

> **References**
> Laymon CW, Peterson WC: Lipogranulomatosis subcutanea (Rothmann and Makai). Arch Dermatol 1964; 90:288–292.
> Matukas T, Reisner RM: Panniculitis, possibly Rothmann–Makai type. Arch Dermatol 1972; 105:287.

ROTHMUND–THOMSON SYNDROME, POIKILODERMA CONGENITALE

Manifestations and Major Findings
photosensitivity
generalized poikiloderma
– reticulated erythema
– telangiectasias
– hyper- and hypopigmentation
lesions begin as red, edematous plaques
lesions may be accompanied by blistering
onset in infancy
progressive until 3–5 years of age
hyperkeratosis of the palms, soles, hands, wrists, ankles, and other areas (squamous cell carcinoma may develop)
calcinosis cutis (rare)
sparse, fine scalp hair – may progress to partial/total alopecia
nail dystrophy
microdontia/hypoplastic or conical teeth
osteosarcoma (rare)
hypogonadism
microcephaly
mental retardation (rare)
normal life expectancy

OCULAR ABNORMALITIES
juvenile cataracts (bilateral)
exophthalmos
corneal atrophy
glaucoma
blue sclerae

SKELETAL ABNORMALITIES
absence/shortening of the long bones (especially radii)
joint contractures
short stature (under 1.2 m)
frontal bossing
osteosclerosis or cystic changes of the long bones
small hands and feet

autosomal recessive (female predominance)

> **References**
> Beauregard S, Gilchrest BA: Syndromes of premature aging. Dermatol Clin 1987; 5:109–121.
> Collins P, Barnes L, McCabe M: Poikiloderma congenitale: case report and review of the literature. Pediatr Dermatol 1991; 8:58–60.
> Hall JG, Pagon RA, Wilson KM: Rothmund–Thomson syndrome with severe dwarfism. Am J Dis Child 1980; 134:165–169.
> Moss C: Rothmund–Thomson syndrome: a report of two patients and a review of the literature. Br J Dermatol 1990; 122:821–829.
> Nanda A, Kanwar AJ, Kapoor MM, Thappa DM, et al.: Rothmund–Thomson syndrome in two siblings Pediatr Dermatol 1989; 6:325–328.
> Potozkin JR, Geronemus RG: Treatment of the poikilodermatous component of the Rothmund–Thomson Syndrome with the flashlamp-pumped pulsed dye laser: a case report. Pediatr Dermatol 1991; 8:162–165.
> Roth DE, Campisano LC, Callen JP, Hersh JH, et al.: Rothmund–Thomson syndrome: a case report. Pediatr Dermatol 1989; 6:321–324.
> Shuttleworth D, Marks R: Epidermal dysplasia and skeletal deformity in congenital poikiloderma (Rothmund–Thomson syndrome). Br J Dermatol 1987; 117:377–384. ▷ ▷ ▷

> > >
Vennos EM, Collins M, James WD: Rothmund–Thomson syndrome: review of the world literature. J Am Acad Dermatol 1992; 27:750–762.

ROWELL SYNDROME

Manifestations and Major Findings
lupus erythematosus (discoid or systemic)
annular lesions resembling erythema multiforme
chilblains

References
Parodi A, Drago EF, Varaldo G, Rebora A: Rowell's syndrome. J Am Acad Dermatol 1989; 21:374–377.
Rowell NR, Beck JS, Anderson JR: Lupus erythematosus and erythema multiforme-like lesions. Arch Dermatol 1963; 88:176–180.

RUBELLA SYNDROME,
CONGENITAL RUBELLA SYNDROME

Manifestations and Major Findings
deafness
cataracts
cardiovascular defects
intrauterine growth retardation
growth failure
mental retardation
caused by fetus contracting rubella before 20th week of gestation

OTHER FINDINGS
microcephaly
microphthalmia
thrombocytopenia

Cutaneous Manifestations
discrete, erythematous or purplish, infiltrated macules (3–8 mm diameter) – dermal erythropoiesis or 'blueberry muffin' lesions
lesions present in first two days of life
cutis marmorata
seborrhea
hyperpigmentation

References
Naeye RL, Blanc W: Pathogenesis of congenital rubella. J Am Med Assoc 1965; 194:1277–1283.
Orenstein WA, Bart KJ, Hinman AR, et al.: The opportunity and obligation to eliminate rubella from the United States. J Am Med Assoc 1984; 251: 1988–1994.

RUBINSTEIN–TAYBI SYNDROME

Manifestations and Major Findings
mental retardation (mild to severe)
microcephaly
broad thumbs and great toes (with or without angulation)
growth retardation

OTHER FINDINGS
capillary malformation (port-wine stain) on the forehead or nape of the neck
hypertrichosis – especially over the back
cardiac defects
genitourinary anomalies
hypospadias
cryptorchidism
renal malformations

Characteristic Facies
hypoplastic maxillae
downward-slanting palpebral fissures
high-arched palate
crowded irregular teeth
strabismus
low-set or malformed auricles
beak-shaped nose
heavy eyebrows
long eyelashes

References
Filippi G: The Rubinstein–Taybi syndrome, report of 7 cases. Clin Genet 1972; 3:303–318.
Rubinstein JH, Taybi H: Broad thumbs and toes and facial abnormalities. Am J Dis Child 1963; 105: 588–608.

RUSSELL–SILVER SYNDROME,
SILVER SYNDROME

Manifestations and Major Findings
short stature of prenatal onset
skeletal asymmetry
premature sexual development

OTHER FINDINGS
clinodactyly
syndactyly
normal intelligence
ivory epiphyses
genitourinary anomalies including ambiguous genitalia

Cutaneous Manifestations
café au lait macules
diffuse brown pigmentation
–with few small achromic spots
–covering most of trunk and limbs
–sparing of the face
excess sweating

Characteristic Facies
large calvarium with triangular facies
frontal bossing
micrognathia
downward curvature of the mouth

usually sporadic inheritance

> **References**
> **Duncan PA, Hall JG, Shapiro LR, Vibert BK:** Three generation dominant transmission of the Silver–Russell syndrome. Am J Med Genet 1990; 35:245–250.
> **Herman TE, Crawford JD, Cleveland RH, Kushner DC:** Hand radiographs in Russell–Silver syndrome. Pediatrics 1987; 79:743–744.
> **Hansen KK, Latson LA, Buehler BA:** Silver–Russell syndrome with unusual findings. Pediatrics 1987; 79: 125–128.
> **Partington MW:** X-linked short stature with skin pigmentation: evidence for heterogeneity of the Russell–Silver syndrome. Clin Genet 1986; 29: 151–156.

RUVALCABA–MYHRE–SMITH SYNDROME

Manifestations and Major Findings
macrocephaly (present at birth)
large for gestational age
hypotonia or developmental delay
hamartomatous intestinal polyps
lobulated tongue
ocular abnormalities
–prominent Schwalbe lines
–corneal nerves
mental retardation or normal intelligence
lipid storage myopathy
Some findings are similar to Riley–Smith syndrome, Bannayan syndrome and Sotos syndrome.

Cutaneous Manifestations
pigmented penile macules
acanthosis nigricans
angiolipomas/lipomas

possible autosomal dominant

> **References**
> **Dvir M, Beer S, Aladjem M:** Heredofamilial syndrome of mesodermal hamartomas, macrocephaly, and pseudopapilledema. Pediatrics 1988; 81: 287–290.
> **Gregory B, Ho VC:** Cutaneous manifestations of gastrointestinal disorders. J Am Acad Dermatol 1992; 26:153–166.
> **Gretzula JC, Hevia O, Schachner LS, DiLiberti JH, Ruvalcaba RHA, et al.:** Ruvalcaba–Myhre–Smith syndrome. Pediatr Dermatol 1988; 5:28–32.
> **Ruvalcaba RH, Myhre S, Smith DW:** Sotos syndrome with intestinal polyposis and pigmentary changes of the genitalia. Clin Genet 1980; 18: 413–416.

S

SAMMAN SYNDROME
see YELLOW NAIL SYNDROME

SANFILIPPO SYNDROME
see MUCOPOLYSACCHARIDOSES; TYPE III

SARCOIDOSIS, SCHAUMANN SYNDROME, BESNIER–BOECK–SCHAUMANN SYNDROME

Manifestations and Major Findings
pulmonary bilateral hilar lymphadenopathy
histology shows naked granulomas of epithelioid cells with multinucleated cells

Cutaneous Manifestations
erythema nodosum
lesions arising in scars
papular/nodular lesions
lupus pernio
subcutaneous, psoriasiform, annular, ulcerated lesions
erythroderma

OCULAR ABNORMALITIES
uveitis
conjunctivitis
lacrimal gland involvement (see Mikulicz disease)
iris nodules
Löfgren syndrome – acute iridocyclitis with erythema nodosum and hilar adenopathy
Heerfordt syndrome – uveitis, parotid gland enlargement, fever, cranial nerve palsies (usually facial nerve (VII))

OTHER FINDINGS
hypercalcemia/hypercalciuria
lymphadenopathy
central nervous system involvement
– meningoencephalitis
– peripheral neuropathy
– psychiatric changes
– multiple sclerosis-like changes
bone and joint changes
polyarthralgias/arthritis
muscular involvement
– polymyositis
– myopathy
– weakness
– tenderness
cardiac involvement
heart block
arrhythmias
sudden death
renal involvement with renal failure

References
Clark SK: Sarcoidosis in children. Pediatr Dermatol 1987; 4:291–299.
Kerdel FA, Moschella SL: Sarcoidosis. An updated review. J Am Acad Dermatol 1984; 11:1–19.

SCALDED SKIN SYNDROME
see STAPHYLOCOCCAL SCALDED SKIN SYNDROME

SCHAMBERG PURPURA
see PURPURA PIGMENTOSA CHRONICA

SCHAUMANN SYNDROME
see SARCOIDOSIS

SCHEIE SYNDROME
see MUCOPOLYSACCHARIDOSES; TYPE I-S

SCHNITZLER SYNDROME

Manifestations and Major Findings
chronic urticarial vasculitis
histology shows leukocytoclastic vasculitis
macroglobulinemia (IgM)
bone pain
hyperostosis
intermittent fever
hepatosplenomegaly
lymphadenopathy

> **References**
> Janier M, Bonvalet D, Blanc MF, Lemarchand F, et al.: Chronic urticaria and macroglobulinemia (Schnitzler's syndrome): report of two cases. J Am Acad Dermatol 1989; 20:206–211.
> Machet L, Vaillant L, Machet MC, Esteve E, et al.: Schnitzler's syndrome (urticaria and macroglobulinemia) associated with pseudoxanthoma elasticum. Acta Derm Verereol (Stockh) 1992; 72:22–24.
> Pujol RM, Barnadas MA, Brunet S, de Moragas JM: Urticarial dermatosis associated with Waldenström's macroglobulinemia. J Am Acad Dermatol 1989; 30: 855–857.

SCHWENINGER–BUZZI ANETODERMA

Manifestations and Major Findings
idiopathic, noninflammatory, localized depressions or outpouchings of the skin
numerous, small, round, slightly protuberant lesions with herniation of subcutaneous tissues
histology shows loss of elastic fibers
mainly found on the trunk

> **References**
> Hodak E, Shamai-Lubovitz O, David M, Hazaz B, et al.: Immunologic abnormalities associated with primary anetoderma. Arch Dermatol 1992; 128: 799–803.
> Venencie PY, Winkelmann RK: Histopathologic findings in anetoderma. Arch Dermatol 1984; 120: 1040–1044.
> Venencie PY, Winkelmann RK, Moore BA: Anetoderma: clinical findings, associations, and long-term follow-up evaluations. Arch Dermatol 1984; 120:1032–1039.

SCLEROMYXEDEMA, LICHEN MYXEDEMATOSUS, GOTTRON–ARNDT SYNDROME, PAPULAR MUCINOSIS

Manifestations and Major Findings
diffuse thickening of the skin with lichenoid papules
lack of skin mobility simulating scleroderma
affects middle-aged men and women
abnormal circulating immunoglobulin (usually IgG with λ light chains)

OTHER FINDINGS
neurologic abnormalities
muscle weakness
myopathy
psychosis
depression
paralysis
cardiovascular abnormalities (uncommon)
leonine facies
amyloidosis

> **References**
> Harris AO, Altman AR, Tschen JA, Wolf JE: Scleromyxedema. Int J Dermatol 1989; 28:661–667.
> Milam CP, Cohen LE, Fenske NA, Ling NS: Scleromyxedema: therapeutic response to isotretinoin in the three patients. J Am Acad Dermatol 1988; 19: 469–477.
> Schmidt KT, Gattuso P, Messmore H, Shrit MA, et al.: Scleredema and smoldering myeloma. J Am Acad Dermatol 1992; 26:319–321.
> Westheim AI, Lookingbill DP: Plasmapheresis in a patient with scleromyxedema. Arch Dermatol 1987; 123:786–789.
> Wright RC, Franco RS, Denton MD, Blaney DJ: Scleromyxedema. Arch Dermatol 1976; 112:63–66.

SCURVY
see VITAMIN DEFICIENCIES; ASCORBIC ACID

SEABRIGHT BANTAM SYNDROME
see ALBRIGHT HEREDITARY OSTEODYSTROPHY

SEBACEOUS NEVUS SYNDROME
see NEVUS SEBACEUS SYNDROME

SECKEL SYNDROME, BIRD-HEADED DWARFISM

Manifestations and Major Findings
short stature of prenatal onset
severe microcephaly
mental retardation
clinodactyly

OTHER FINDINGS
canities (premature graying of hair)
sparse hair
missing ribs
eczema
wrinkled and redundant skin of the palms
ptosis
cryptorchidism

Characteristic Facies
small face
large nose
small ears
hypoplastic mandible

autosomal recessive

> **References**
> Fitch N, Pinsky L, Lachance RL: A form of bird-headed dwarfism with features of premature senility. Am J Dis Child 1970; 120:260–264.
> McKusick VA, Mahloudji M, Abbott MH, et al.: Seckel's bird-headed dwarfism. N Engl J Med 1967; 277:279–286.

SENEAR–USHER SYNDROME, PEMPHIGUS ERYTHEMATOSUS

Manifestations and Major Findings
clinical features of lupus erythematosus
– facial lesions
– erythema and scaling

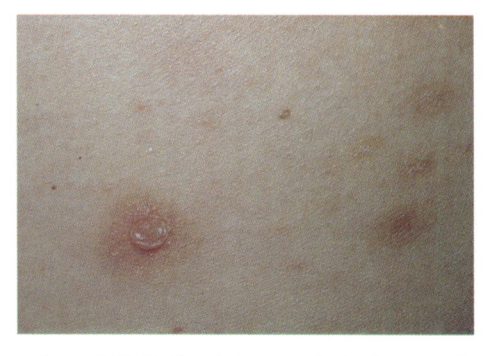

• *Figure 127* Bullous lesions are classic dermatologic findings in Senear–Usher syndrome.

• crusted bullous lesions (Fig. 127)
– face (butterfly distribution)
– chest and extremities
– may become generalized
positive Nikolsky sign
oral involvement (rare)
aggravated by sunlight or penicillamine-induced
histology shows acantholysis in the upper epidermis
direct immunofluorescence shows IgG and/or complement in intercellular spaces

Senear–Usher syndrome is associated with thymoma and myasthenia gravis.

> **References**
> Amerian ML, Ahmed RA: Pemphigus erythematosus. Presentation of four cases and review of the literature. J Am Acad Dermatol 1984; 10:215–222.
> Lever WF: Pemphigus and pemphigoid: a review of advances since 1964. J Am Acad Dermatol 1979; 1:2–31.

SENTER SYNDROME
see KID SYNDROME

SEPTIC SYNDROME, SEPTIC SHOCK

Manifestations and Major Findings
focus of marked infection or inflammation triggering circulatory shock
fever or hypothermia
tachypnea

tachycardia
impaired organ system function or perfusion
–altered mentation
–hypoxemia
–elevated plasma lactate
–oliguria

Cutaneous Manifestations
poor perfusion
cutis marmorata
necrosis
gangrene

OTHER FINDINGS
coagulation abnormalities
disseminated intravascular coagulation

> **References**
> **Balk RA, Bone RC:** The septic syndrome: definition and clinical implications. Crit Care Clin 1989; 5:1–8.
> **Boyd JL, Stanford GG, Chernow B:** The pharmacotherapy of septic shock. Crit Care Clin 1989; 5:133–151.
> **Pavillo JE:** Pathogenetic mechanisms of septic shock. New Engl J Med 1993; 328:1471–1477.

SEVERE COMBINED IMMUNODEFICIENCY

Manifestations and Major Findings
marked T and B lymphocyte deficiencies
failure to thrive
recurrent infections
chronic diarrhea
pneumonia
This phenotype may be caused by enzyme deficiencies (adenosine deaminase, purine nucleoside phosphorylase), defective interleukin-2 production, or bare lymphocyte syndrome.

Cutaneous Manifestations
candidiasis
seborrheic dermatitis or eczema
cutaneous infections – *Staphylococcus aureus*, group A streptococci, herpes simplex
morbilliform eruptions
graft versus host disease
erythroderma
alopecia
absence of eyelashes and eyebrows
skin ulcerations

> **References**
> **DeRaeve L, Song M, Levy J, Mascart-Lemone F:** Cutaneous lesions as a clue to severe combined immunodeficiency. Pediatr Dermatol 1992; 9:49–51.
> **Llorente CP, Amorós JI, deFrutos FJO, Regueiro JR, et al.:** Cutaneous lesions in severe combined immunodeficiency: two case reports and a review of the literature. Pediatr Dermatol 1991; 8:314–321.

SÉZARY SYNDROME

Manifestations and Major Findings
cutaneous T-cell lymphoma with atypical circulating cells
triad of findings
–generalized exfoliative erythroderma
–lymphadenopathy
–10% or more Sézary cells (circulating atypical cells with cerebriform nuclei) in the peripheral blood (T-helper cells, CD4-positive lymphocytes)

OTHER FINDINGS
affects elderly males
intense pruritus
edema
hepatomegaly
onychodystrophy
palmoplantar keratoderma
alopecia
histology shows epidermotropism, Pautrier microabscesses, and atypical lymphocytes in the dermis

> **References**
> **Wieselthier JS, Koh HK:** Sézary syndrome: diagnosis, prognosis, and critical review of treatment options. J Am Acad Dermatol 1990; 22:381–401.

SHEEHAN SYNDROME,
POSTPARTUM PITUITARY NECROSIS

Manifestations and Major Findings
thrombosis of the pituitary circulation during delivery
increasing lethargy
loss of appetite
skin pallor with a yellow tinge
dry, wrinkled skin
wasting and asthenia
loss of axillary and pubic hair
onycholysis
ridging and brownish discoloration of nail plate
discoid lupus erythematous (possibly associated)

> **References**
> Trattner A, Weingarten MW: Discoid lupus erythematosus coexistent with Sheehan's Syndrome. Int J Dermatol 1992; 31:182–183.

SHPRINTZEN SYNDROME
see VELOCARDIOFACIAL SYNDROME

SHULMAN SYNDROME
see EOSINOPHILIC FASCIITIS

SHWACHMAN SYNDROME

Manifestations and Major Findings
exocrine pancreatic insufficiency
malabsorption
steatorrhea
failure to thrive
growth retardation
neutropenia

OTHER FINDINGS
recurrent skin and lung infections
skeletal abnormalities
–short ribs
–coxa vara
–metaphyseal dysplasia
bone marrow hypoplasia with anemia
thrombocytopenia with petechiae or bleeding
predisposition to hematologic malignancies

autosomal recessive

> **References**
> Goeteyn M, Oranje AP, Vuzevski VD, de Groot R, et al.: Ichthyosis, exocrine pancreatic insufficiency, impaired neutrophil chemotaxis, growth retardation and metaphyseal dysplasia (Shwachman syndrome). Arch Dermatol 1991; 127:225-230.
> Mortwreux P, Taüb A, Bazeille J-ES, Hehunstre JP, Maleville J: Shwachman Syndrome: a case report. Pediatr Dermatol 1992; 9:57–61.
> Shwachman H, Diamond LK, Oski FA, Khaw K-T: Pancreatic insufficiency and bone marrow dysfunction: a new clinical entity. J Pediatr 1963; 63:835–837.
> Woods WG, Roloff JS, Lukens JN, et al.: The occurrence of leukemia in patients with the Shwachman syndrome. J Pediatr 1981; 99:425–428.

SICCA SYNDROME see SJÖGREN SYNDROME

SICKLE CELL DISEASE

Manifestations and Major Findings
chronic hemolytic anemia
intermittent 'pain crises' with pallor, fever, and swelling of the extremities
red blood cells are sickle-shaped when deoxygenated
hemoglobin (Hb) electrophoresis shows
–sickle cell Hb
–absent Hb A (or other Hb)
–variable quantities of Hb F
aplastic crisis
occurs predominantly in African and Mediterranean races

OTHER FINDINGS
oral manifestations
–jaw deformities
–osteomyelitis or pain
chronic pallor
jaundice
Howell–Jolly bodies in peripheral red blood cells
hyposthenuria (inability to concentrate urine)
Associated complications include ischemia of bones and organs, splenic enlargement, osteomyelitis (most commonly due to Salmonella), gallstones, acute splenic sequestration crises, and priapism.

Cutaneous Manifestations

hand-foot syndrome (dactylitis) with swelling of hands and feet during a crisis
hyperpigmentation of the lower legs
chronic unhealing leg ulcers (often indolent and unhealing)

autosomal recessive

> **References**
> **Platt OS, Thorington BD, Brambilla DJ, Milner PF:** Pain in sickle cell disease. N Engl J Med 1991; 325: 11–16.
> **Stevens MCG, Padwick M, Serjeant GR:** Observations on the natural history of dactylitis in homozygous sickle cell disease. Clin Pediatr 1981; 20:311–317.

SIEMENS SYNDROME, KERATOSIS PALMOPLANTARIS AREATA/STRIATA

Manifestations and Major Findings

hyperkeratotic lesions (islands or linear) found on the palms and soles but may be diffuse
may be associated with deafness

autosomal dominant

> **References**
> **Roth W, Penneys NS, Fawcett N:** Hereditary painful callosities. Arch Dermatol 1978; 114:591–592.
> **Tezuka T:** Circumscribed palmo-plantar keratoderma. Unusual histological findings. Dermatologica 1982; 165:30–38.

SILVER SYNDROME

see RUSSELL–SILVER SYNDROME

SINUS HISTIOCYTOSIS WITH MASSIVE LYMPHADENOPATHY

see ROSAI–DORFMAN SYNDROME

SIPPLE SYNDROME see MULTIPLE ENDOCRINE NEOPLASIA SYNDROMES; TYPE 2A

SISTER MARY JOSEPH NODULE

Manifestations and Major Findings

nodule in the umbilicus which is a sign of metastases
common primary malignancies
– adenocarcinomas from the gastrointestinal tract (stomach)
– tumors from the reproductive or urinary tract

> **References**
> **Edoute Y, Ben-Haim SA, Malberger E:** Umbilical metastasis from urinary bladder carcinoma. J Am Acad Dermatol 1992; 26:656–657.
> **Gregory B, Ho VC:** Cutaneous manifestations of gastrointestinal disorders. Part I. J Am Acad Dermatol 1992; 26:153–166.
> **Powell FC, Cooper AJ, Massa MC, Goellner JR, et al.:** Sister Mary Joseph's nodule: a clinical and histologic study. J Am Acad Dermatol 1984; 10: 610–615.

SJÖGREN–LARSSON SYNDROME

see also DISORDERS OF CORNIFICATION; DOC 10

Manifestations and Major Findings

triad of findings
– • ichthyosis (Fig. 128) – three types of scaling: dandruff-like, lamellar type, and nonscaly, thickly adherent type (onset in first months of life or as a collodion baby)
– mental retardation
– spasticity (more pronounced in the lower extremities)

OTHER FINDINGS

seizures
degenerative retinitis – 'glistening dots' on retinoscopy
palmoplantar hyperkeratosis
collodion membrane-like scaling at birth
dermatoglyphic abnormalities
dry hair
short stature
skeletal abnormalities
kyphosis
dental abnormalities
speech disturbances

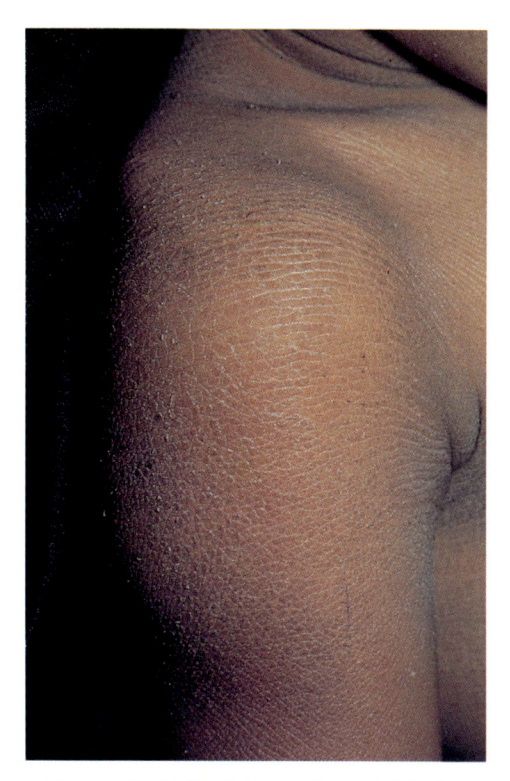

Figure 128 Ichthyosis is one of a triad of findings in Sjögren–Larsson syndrome.

fatty alcohol: NAD oxidoreductase (FAO) deficiency
fatty alcohol accumulation in cells

autosomal recessive

References
Fivenson DP, Lucky AW, Iannoccone S: Sjögren–Larsson syndrome associated with the Dandy–Walker malformation: report of a case. Pediatr Dermatol 1989; 6:312–315.
Hofer P-A, Jagell S: Sjögren–Larsson syndrome: a dermato-histopathologic study. J Cutan Pathol 1982; 9:360–376.
Hooft C, Kriekemans J, van Acker K, Devos E, et al.: Sjögren–Larsson syndrome with exudative enteropathy. Influence of medium-chain triglycerides on the symptomatology. Helv Paediatr Acta 1967; 22: 447–458.
Jagell S, Liden S: Ichthyosis in the Sjögren–Larsson syndrome. Clin Genet 1982; 21:243–252.
Koone MD, Rizzo WB, Elias PM, Williams ML, et al.: Ichthyosis, mental retardation, and asymptomatic spasticity. Arch Dermatol 1990; 126:1485–1490.
▷ ▷ ▷

Levisohn D, Dintiman B, Rizzo WB: Sjögren–Larsson syndrome: case reports. Pediatr Dermatol 1991; 8:217–220.
Liden S, Jagell S: The Sjögren–Larsson syndrome. Int J Dermatol 1984; 23:247–253.
Rizzo WB, Dammann AL, Craft DL, et al.: Sjögren–Larsson syndrome: Inherited defect in the fatty alcohol cycle. J Pediatr 1989; 115:228–234.

SJÖGREN SYNDROME, SICCA SYNDROME (PRIMARY SJÖGREN SYNDROME), GOUGEROT–HOUWER–SJÖGREN SYNDROME

Manifestations and Major Findings
dryness and atrophy of the conjunctivae and cornea (keratoconjunctivitis sicca)
positive Schirmer test indicating few tears
dry mouth (xerostomia)
decreased salivary flow rate
lymphocytic infiltrate in salivary gland biopsy

OTHER FINDINGS
dryness of all mucous membranes and skin
scleroderma-like cutaneous changes
alopecia
telangiectasias
swelling of lacrimal and salivary glands
anti-Ro (SSA) and/or anti-La (SSB) antibody-positive
Sjögren syndrome is associated with rheumatoid arthritis, lupus erythematosus, and scleroderma (secondary Sjögren syndrome).

References
Atkinson JC, Travis WD, Pillemer SR, Bermudez D, et al.: Major salivary gland function in primary Sjögren's syndrome and its relationship to clinical features. J Rheumatol 1990; 17:318–322.
Deprettere AJ, Van Acker KJ, De Clerck LS, Docx MK, et al.: Diagnosis of Sjögren's syndrome in children. Am J Dis Child 1988; 142:1185–1187.
Kawamura H, Taniguchi N, Itoh K, Kano S: Salivary gland echography in patients with Sjögren syndrome. Arthritis Rheum 1990; 33:505–510.
Provost TT, Talal N, Harley JB, Reichlin M, Alexander E: The relationship between anti-Ro (SSA) antibody-positive Sjögren's syndrome and Anti-Ro (SS-A) antibody-positive lupus erythematosus. Arch Dermatol 1988; 124:63–71.

SLY SYNDROME

see MUCOPOLYSACCHARIDOSES; TYPE VII

SNEDDON SYNDROME

Manifestations and Major Findings
livedo reticularis (usually extensive)
occlusive vascular disease – may involve cerebral, ocular, coronary, renal, and peripheral arteries
occasional Raynaud phenomenon
hypertension (may be transient)
common involvement of fundi, peripheral nerves, heart, and kidneys – usually asymptomatic
slowly progressive course

CEREBROVASCULAR FINDINGS
headaches/dizziness (early stages)
hemiplegia
aphasia
hemianopia
strokes
transient ischemic attacks
seizures
progressive cognitive impairment

> **References**
> **Alegre VA, Winkelmann RK, Gastineau DA:** Cutaneous thrombosis, cerebrovascular thrombosis, and lupus anticoagulant – the Sneddon syndrome. Int J Dermatol 1990; 29:45–49.
> **Deffer TA, Berger TG, Gelinas-Sorell D:** Sneddon's syndrome. J Am Acad Dermatol 1987; 16:1084–1087.
> **Fine RM:** Sneddon syndrome: a diagnosis you do not want to miss. Int J Dermatol 1990; 29:479–480.
> **Manganelli P, Lisi R, Saginario A, Benoldi D:** Sneddon's syndrome and primary antiphospholipid syndrome: a case report. J Am Acad Dermatol 1992; 26:309–311.
> **Zelger B, Sepp N, Stockhammer G, Dosch E, et al.:** Sneddon's syndrome. A long-term follow-up of 21 patients. Arch Dermatol 1993; 129:437–447.

SNEDDON–WILKINSON SYNDROME,
SUBCORNEAL PUSTULAR DERMATOSIS

Manifestations and Major Findings
discrete sterile pustules
subcorneal neutrophilic abscesses
pustules form annular or gyrate groups
predominantly seen in the axillae, groin, and abdomen
lesions dry within a few days
remaining crust or postinflammatory hyperpigmentation
most common in women aged 40–50 years

> **References**
> **Kalaher KM, Scott DW:** Subcorneal pustular dermatosis in dogs and in human beings: comparative aspects. J Am Acad Dermatol 1990; 22:1023–1028.
> **Kasha EE, Epinette WW:** Subcorneal pustular dermatosis (Sneddon–Wilkinson disease) in association with a monoclonal IgA gammopathy: a report and review of the literature. J Am Acad Dermatol 1988; 19:854–858.

SOTOS SYNDROME, CEREBRAL GIGANTISM

Manifestations and Major Findings
congenital macrosomia (large body size)
poor coordination
developmental delay
macrocephaly/dolichocephaly
large hands and feet
unusual dermatoglyphics
malignant tumors
prominent palatine ridges
congenital nonprogressive cerebral impairment
scoliosis common
congenital heart defects

Characteristic Facies
prominent forehead
hypertelorism
downward-slanting palpebral fissures
pointed chin

References
Bale AE, Drum MA, Parry DM, Mulvihill JJ: Familial Sotos syndrome. Am J Med Genet 1985; 20:613–624.
Sotos JF, Cutler EA, Dodge P: Cerebral gigantism. Am J Dis Child 1977; 131:625–627.

SPIEGLER–FENDT PSEUDOLYMPHOMA, LYMPHOCYTOMA CUTIS, SPIEGLER–FENDT SARCOID, LYMPHADENOSIS BENIGNA CUTIS

Manifestations and Major Findings
benign, reactive hyperplasia or pre-existing lymphoid elements in the skin
red/brown asymptomatic nodules
predilection for the head and neck (especially the ear lobes)
usually solitary or grouped – rarely disseminated
histology shows
–grenz zone
–heavy infiltrate of histiocytes and lymphocytes (predominantly B cells)
–occasional germinal centers
benign process
most common in adult females

SPITZ NEVUS, BENIGN JUVENILE MELANOMA, SPINDLE AND EPITHELIOID CELL NEVUS, EPITHELIOID CELL–SPINDLE CELL NEVOMELANOCYTIC NEVUS, SPITZ TUMOR

Manifestations and Major Findings
firm papule or (rarely) aggregated papules
• papule may be light (tan/pink) or dark (Fig. 129)
benign
reports of malignant transformation (rare)
histology can be confused with melanoma with epithelioid and spindle cells
seen mainly in children

References
Kaye VN, Dehner LP: Spindle and epithelioid cell nevus (Spitz nevus). Arch Dermatol 1990; 126: 1581–1583. ▷ ▷ ▷

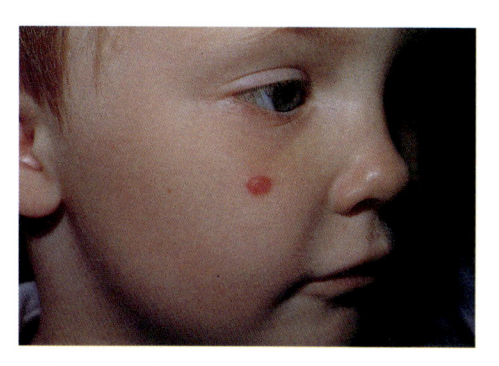

• *Figure 129* Spitz nevus presenting as a firm, pink papule on the cheek.

▷ ▷ ▷
Omura EF, Kheir SM: Recurrent Spitz's nevus. Am J Dermatopathol 1984; 6:207–212.
Smith KJ, Barrett TL, Skelton HG, Lupton GP, Graham JH: Spindle cell and epithelioid cell nevi with atypia and metastasis (malignant Spitz nevus). Am J Surg Pathol 1989; 13:931–939.
Weedon D, Little JH: Spindle and epithelioid cell nevi in children and adults: a review of 211 cases of the Spitz nevus. Cancer 1977; 40:217–225.

SPUN GLASS HAIR SYNDROME
see UNCOMBABLE HAIR SYNDROME and HAIR SHAFT ANOMALIES

STAPHYLOCOCCAL SCALDED SKIN SYNDROME, RITTER DISEASE

Manifestations and Major Findings
Staphylococcus aureus infection (phage group II usually)
usually affects skin, pharynx, conjunctiva, or circumcision site
initial widespread erythema, pain, and skin edema
extensive loosening of the skin (with or without bulla)
• denudation with raw, red, oozing surfaces or dry peeling (Fig. 130)
sometimes involves the entire body
toxicity (fever, painful skin)
symptoms caused by exfoliative toxin
increased neonatal mortality rate

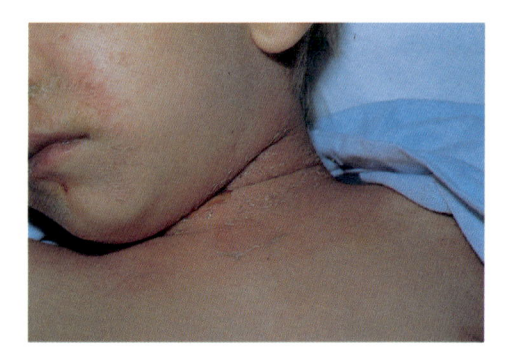

• *Figure 130* Erythema and skin peeling on the neck in staphylococcal scalded skin syndrome.

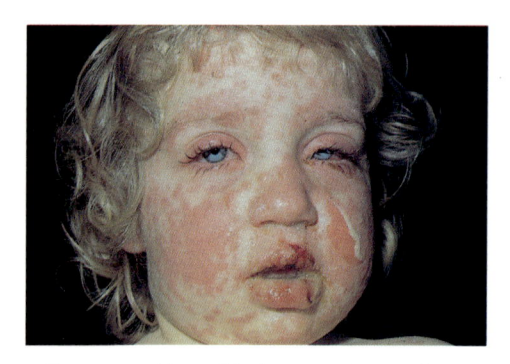

• *Figure 131* Target-like lesions and mucosal ulcerations in Stevens–Johnson syndrome due to an antibiotic.

> **References**
> Elias PM, Fritsch P, Epstein EH: Staphylococcal scalded skin syndrome. Arch Dermatol 1977; 113: 207–219.
> Reid LH, Weston WL, Humbert JR: Staphylococcal scalded skin syndrome. Adult onset in a patient with deficient cell-mediated immunity. Arch Dermatol 1974; 109:239–241.
> Snyder RA, Elias PM: Toxic epidermal necrolysis and staphylococcal scalded skin syndrome. Dermatol Clin 1983; 1:235–248.

STEINERT SYNDROME
see MYOTONIC DYSTROPHY

STEIN–LEVENTHAL SYNDROME
see POLYCYSTIC OVARY SYNDROME

STEVENS–JOHNSON SYNDROME,
ERYTHEMA MULTIFORME EXUDATIVUM MAJOR

Manifestations and Major Findings
- target-like skin lesions (Fig. 131)
lesions become bullous and hemorrhagic
- mucosal involvement (Fig. 131) – ulceration of mouth, eyes, urethra, anal mucosa, bronchi, and alveoli
severe constitutional symptoms
purulent conjunctivitis, keratitis, uveitis, and even panophthalmitis
corneal scarring
corneal opacities
residual synechiae
blindness
can involve all mucosal and cutaneous surfaces
caused by herpes simplex, drugs, infections, or other unknown etiologies

OTHER FINDINGS
diarrhea
paronychia
nail shedding
polyarthritis
renal involvement

> **References**
> Prendiville JS, Hebert AA, Greenwalt MJ, Esterly NB: Management of Stevens–Johnson syndrome and toxic epidermal necrolysis in children. J Pediatr 1989; 115:881–887.

STEWART–TREVES SYNDROME,
POSTMASTECTOMY LYMPHANGIOSARCOMA

Manifestations and Major Findings
lymphangiosarcoma of an extremity arising in an extremity with chronic lymphedema
edematous upper extremity – usually after a radical mastectomy
sarcoma begins as a bluish discoloration
blue or red nodules develop
nodules may ulcerate or form blisters
dissemination of tumor occurs early

> **References**
> MacKenzie DH: Lymphangiosarcoma arising in chronic congenital and idiopathic lymphedema. J Clin Pathol 1971; 24:524–529.

STIFF SKIN SYNDROME,
CONGENITAL FASCIAL DYSTROPHY

Manifestations and Major Findings
localized areas of stony, hard skin and subcutaneous tissue
onset at birth or in infancy
mild hypertrichosis
restricted joint mobility – particularly lower limbs
functional impairment of the lungs

autosomal dominant

> **References**
> Jablonska S, Groniowski J, Krieg T, Nerlich A, et al.: Congenital fascial dystrophy – a noninflammatory disease of fascia: the stiff skin syndrome. Pediatr Dermatol 1984; 2:87–97.
> Jablonska S, Schubert H, Kikuchi I: Congenital fascial dystrophy: stiff skin syndrome – a human counterpart of the tight-skin mouse. J Am Acad Dermatol 1989; 21:943–950.
> Kikuchi I, Inoue S, Hamada K, Ando H: Stiff skin syndrome. Pediatr Dermatol 1985; 3:48–53.

STILL DISEASE,
JUVENILE RHEUMATOID ARTHRITIS

Manifestations and Major Findings
acute onset in childhood
monoarticular, pauciarticular, or polyarticular arthritis
high fever
chronic iridocyclitis – may lead to band keratitis or cataracts

OTHER FINDINGS
lymphadenopathy
splenomegaly
myocarditis/pericarditis
pneumonitis

Cutaneous Manifestations
small, erythematous, evanescent macules and papules with irregular margins and central pallor
occur on the trunk and extremities
rash characteristically appears at midday or during high fever
subcutaneous nodules

> **References**
> Calabro JJ, Marchesano JM: Juvenile rheumatoid arthritis. N Engl J Med 1967; 277:696–699.

STREETER ANOMALY
see AMNIOTIC BAND SYNDROME

STURGE–WEBER SYNDROME,
ENCEPHALOTRIGEMINAL ANGIOMATOSIS,
ENCEPHALOFACIAL ANGIOMATOSIS

Manifestations and Major Findings
vascular malformation of the leptomeninges overlying the cerebral cortex (usually posterior parietal and occipital lobes)
- ipsilateral port-wine stain (capillary malformation) of face along first branch of trigeminal nerve (Fig. 132) – may be bilateral
vascular malformations of various internal organs
gradual calcification of cerebrovascular malformations

NEUROLOGIC ABNORMALITIES
seizures
paralysis
mental retardation

OCULAR ABNORMALITIES
glaucoma
buphthalmos (congenital glaucoma)

> **References**
> Bebin EM, Gomez MR: Prognosis in Sturge–Weber disease: comparison of unihemispheric and bihemispheric involvement. J Child Neurol 1988; 3:181–184. ▷ ▷ ▷

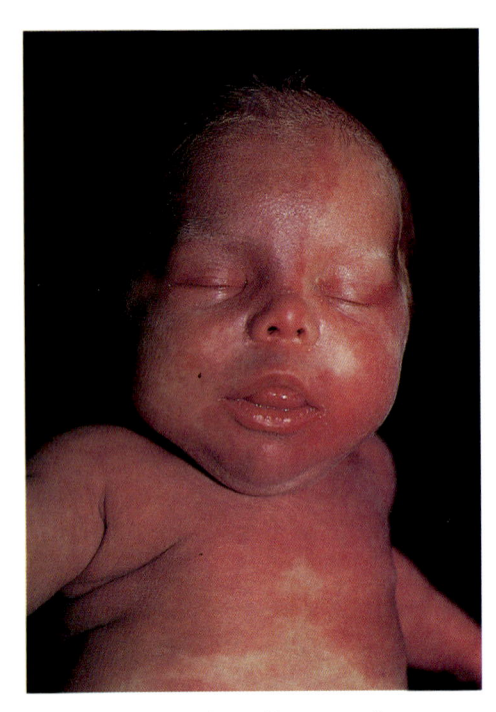

Figure 132 Vascular malformation of leptomeninges and ipsilateral port-wine stain are classic findings in Sturge–Weber syndrome.

▷ ▷ ▷
Enjolras O, Riche MC, Merland JJ: Facial port-wine stains and Sturge–Weber syndrome. Pediatrics 1985; 76:48–51.
Paller AS: The Sturge–Weber syndrome. Pediatr Dermatol 1987; 4:300–304.

SUBCORNEAL PUSTULAR DERMATOSIS see SNEDDON–WILKINSON SYNDROME

SUBCUTANEOUS LIPOGRANULOMATOSIS
see ROTHMANN–MAKAI SYNDROME

SULZBERGER–GARBE SYNDROME, OID-OID DISEASE, EXUDATIVE DISCOID AND LICHENOID DERMATITIS, POLYMORPHIC PRURIGO

Manifestations and Major Findings
several polymorphous forms of atopic dermatitis
 – exudative, weeping, discoid or oval plaques (scattered but sparing scalp, palms, and soles)
 – lichenified plaques and papules (may be follicular)
 – urticarial lesions
progressive cases may develop exfoliative dermatitis
marked pruritus – especially at night
aggravated by stress
resistant to treatment

References
Rongioletti F, Corbella L, Rebora A: Exudative discoid and lichenoid chronic dermatosis (Sulzberger–Garbe) – a fictional disease? Int J Dermatol 1989; 28: 40–43.

SUPERIOR VENA CAVA SYNDROME

Manifestations and Major Findings
obstruction of superior vena cava or its main tributaries
usually caused by a neoplasm or goiter
marked facial and eyelid edema
dilated blood vessels around lower chest wall
gynecomastia

SUTTON NEVUS, HALO NEVUS, LEUKODERMA ACQUISITUM CENTRIFUGUM

Manifestations and Major Findings
pigmented cutaneous tumor, usually a nevus but may be a neurofibroma or melanoma
surrounding hypomelanosis (halo)
nevus gradually disappears leaving hypopigmented macule
mostly found in children or young adults

References
Frank SB, Cohen HJ: The halo nevus. Arch Dermatol 1964; 89:367–373.
Kopf AW, Morrill SD, Silberberg I: Broad spectrum of leukoderma acquisitum centrifugum. Arch Dermatol 1965; 92:14–35.

SWEET SYNDROME,
ACUTE FEBRILE NEUTROPHILIC DERMATOSIS

Manifestations and Major Findings
- raised, painful, red plaques or nodules (Fig. 133)

found on the limbs, face, and neck

no mucosal involvement

sterile pustules may later develop in plaques

neutrophilic polymorphonuclear leukocytosis

high, persistent fever

variable degrees of malaise, arthralgia, headache, vomiting, abdominal pain, prostration, and episcleritis

middle-aged women most commonly affected

skin biopsy shows numerous neutrophils but no true vasculitis

responds to steroids

Sweet syndrome may be associated with lymphoma, leukemia, ulcerative colitis, carcinomas, cellulitus, and upper respiratory tract infections.

References
Cohen PR, Kurzrock R: Sweet's syndrome and malignancy. Am J Med 1987; 82:1220–1226.

▷ ▷ ▷

Cohen PR, Talpaz M, Kurzrock R: Malignancy-associated Sweet's syndrome: review of the world literature. J Clin Oncol 1988; 6:1887–1897.
Delaporte E, Gaveau DJ, Piette FA, Bergoënd HA: Acute febrile neutrophilic dermatosis (Sweet's syndrome). Arch Dermatol 1989; 125:1101–1104.
Jorizzo JL, Solomon AR, Zanolli MD, Leshin B: Neutrophilic vascular reactions. J Am Acad Dermatol 1988; 19:983–1005.
Kemmett D, Harrison DJ, Hunter JAA: Antibodies to neutrophil cytoplasmic antigens: a serologic marker for Sweet's syndrome. J Am Acad Dermatol 1991; 24:967–969.
Kemmett D, Hunter JAA: Sweet's syndrome: a clinicopathologic review of twenty-nine cases. J Am Acad Dermatol 1990; 23:503–507.
Kibbi AG, Zaynoun ST, Kurban AK, Najjar SS: Acute febrile neutrophilic dermatosis (Sweet's syndrome): case report and review of the literature. Pediatr Dermatol 1985; 3:40–44.

SYPHILIS (CONGENITAL)

Features of Congenital (Prenatal) Syphilis at Early and Late Stages

1 presentation at birth
spontaneous abortion during pregnancy or stillbirth
presentation of live births
  – analagous to secondary syphilis
  – marasmus
  – hepatosplenomegaly with jaundice
  – blistered, oozing, erosions on ears or extremities
  – pallor
  – split papules at angles of mouth or lateral nares
  – snuffles
  – bone lesions (osteochondritis, periostitis)
  – anemia
  – thrombocytopenia

2 early presentation at 2–6 weeks
snuffles
mucous patches
condylomata lata
copper-colored macules and papules on palms, soles, and diaper area
rhagades
saddle nose
osteochondritis and periostitis
pseudoparalysis of Parrot (local tenderness or pain immobilizing limb) caused by osteochondritis
meningitis
seizures

▷ ▷ ▷

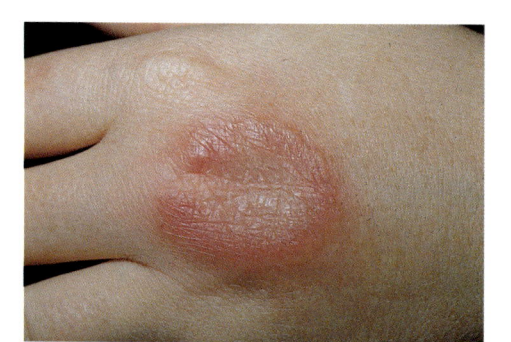

- *Figure 133 Sweet syndrome presents as raised, painful, red plaques or nodules – commonly on the limbs.*

▷ ▷ ▷
lymphadenopathy
hepatosplenomegaly
jaundice
renal disease

3 late presentation at 2–30 years
similar to acquired late syphilis
interstitial keratitis leading to blindness
neurosyphilis
eighth cranial nerve deafness
tinnitus
gummata
Clutton joints (bilateral painless hydroarthrosis of knees)
von Gies joints with ankylosis
saber shins (periostitis of tibiae)
Higoumenakis sign (sternoclavicular joint) – periostitis of inner ends of clavicles
cardiovascular syphilis (very rare)

4 late stigmata of congenital syphilis
Hutchinson teeth (barrel or peg-shaped upper central incisors with notching)
Mulberry/Moon/Fournier molars (first lower molars with numerous, poorly developed cusps)
Hutchinson triad
– Hutchinson teeth
– interstitial keratitis
– eighth cranial nerve deafness
saddle nose
frontal bossae of Parrot
scarred choroiditis ('salt and pepper' fundus)
short maxillae
protuberance of mandible
high-arched palate
Higoumenakis sign
rhagades
saber shins
scaphoid scapulae

References
Brion LP, Manuli M, Rai B, Kresch MJ, et al.: Long-bone radiographic abnormalities as a sign of active congenital syphilis in asymptomatic newborns. Pediatrics 1991; 88:1037–1040.
Dorfman DH, Glaser JH: Congenital syphilis presenting in infants after the newborn period. N Engl J Med 1990; 323:1299–1302.
Felman YM: Syphilis (editorial). Arch Dermatol 1989; 125:1698–1700.
Ikeda MK, Jenson HB: Evaluation and treatment of congenital syphilis. J Pediatr 1990; 117:843–851.

SYSTEMIC LUPUS ERYTHEMATOSUS
see LUPUS ERYTHEMATOSUS

T

TAKAHARA SYNDROME, ACATALASEMIA, ACATALASIA

Manifestations and Major Findings
defect of blood and tissue catalase activity
recurrent painful ulcers of the gingiva and dental alveoli
tooth loss
possible destruction of bone and tissue
oral organisms produce H_2O_2 which accumulates and injures exposed tissues by oxidation
blood turns dark brown upon contact with H_2O_2 (no foaming)

autosomal recessive

TAKAYASU DISEASE, PULSELESS DISEASE

Manifestations and Major Findings
focal inflammatory granulomatous vasculitis of the aorta and its branches
most common in Southeast Asia
Takayasu disease is associated with tuberculosis, syphilis, systemic lupus erythematosus, and rheumatoid arthritis.

Cutaneous Manifestations
skin necrosis over the scalp
malar flush
erythema nodosum
erythema induratum
Raynaud phenomenon

References
Hall S, Barr W, Lie JT, et al.: Takayasu arteritis. A study of 32 North American patients. Medicine 1985; 64:89–99.

TANGIER DISEASE, ANALPHALIPOPROTEINEMIA, FAMILIAL HIGH DENSITY LIPOPROTEIN DEFICIENCY, α-LIPOPROTEIN DEFICIENCY DISEASE

Manifestations and Major Findings
red/orange enlarged tonsils/adenoids
low apolipoproteins A-I and A-II
low plasma cholesterol
elevated plasma triglyceride
hepatosplenomegaly
peripheral neuropathy
dermal deposition of cholesterol esters in the generalized papular eruption

autosomal recessive

References
Assmann G, Herbert PN, Fredrickson DS, Forte T: Isolation and characterization of an abnormal high density lipoprotein in Tangier disease. J Clin Invest 1977; 60:242–252.
Waldorf DS, Levy RI, Fredrickson DS: Cutaneous cholesterol ester deposition in Tangier disease. Arch Dermatol 1967; 95:161–165.

TAR SYNDROME
see THROMBOCYTOPENIA-ABSENT RADII SYNDROME

TAY SYNDROME
see TRICHOTHIODYSTROPHY

TESTICULAR FEMINIZATION,
ANDROGEN INSENSITIVITY SYNDROME

Manifestations and Major Findings
end organ insensitivity to androgens
normal male karyotype
female external genitalia or ambiguous genitalia
lack of pubic and axillary hair
sterility

> **References**
> Feldman SR: Androgen insensitivity syndrome (testicular feminization): a model for understanding steroid hormone receptors. J Am Acad Dermatol 1992; 27:615–619.

THOST–UNNA SYNDROME
see UNNA–THOST SYNDROME

THROMBOANGIITIS OBLITERANS
see BUERGER DISEASE

THROMBOCYTOPENIA–ABSENT RADII SYNDROME, TAR SYNDROME

Manifestations and Major Findings
foreshortened forearms
bilateral absence or hypoplasia of the radii
radially-deviated hands
profound thrombocytopenia (present at birth)
abnormal megakaryocytes in the bone marrow

OTHER FINDINGS
vascular malformations (port-wine stains) of the head and neck
musculoskeletal malformations
cardiac anomalies
anemia
neutropenia
allergies

autosomal recessive

> **References**
> Ashinoff R, Geronemus RG: Thrombocytopenia-absent radii syndrome and lack of response to the pulsed dye laser. Arch Dermatol 1990; 126:1520–1521.
> Brochstein JA, Shank B, Kernan NA, Terwilliger JW, et al.: Marrow transplantation thrombocytopenia-absent radii syndrome. J Pediatr 1992; 121:587–589.

TIETZ SYNDROME

Manifestations and Major Findings
hypopigmentation of the skin and hair
eyebrow hypoplasia
deafness
blue eyes
no ocular abnormalities

autosomal dominant

> **References**
> Tietz W: A syndrome of deaf-mutism associated with albinism showing dominant autosomal inheritance. Am J Hum Genet 1963; 15:259–264.

TORCH SYNDROME

Manifestations and Major Findings
intrauterine infection with the following organisms
– *T*oxoplasma
– *o*ther (*Treponema pallidum*, etc.)
– *r*ubella virus
– *c*ytomegalovirus
– *h*erpes simplex virus
infections show similar clinical and laboratory neonatal findings
small for gestational age
hepatosplenomegaly
pneumonitis/respiratory distress
hypo- or hyperthermia
heart defects/myocarditis

NEUROLOGIC ABNORMALITIES
microcephaly
seizures
calcifications

hyper- or hypotonia
encephalitis
cerebrospinal fluid pleocytosis

OCULAR ABNORMALITIES
chorioretinitis
cataracts
glaucoma
microphthalmia
keratitis

Cutaneous Manifestations
icterus
petechiae
purpura
vesicles

References
Leland D, French MLV, Kleiman MB, Schreiner RL: The use of TORCH titers. Pediatrics 1983; 72:41–43.

TORRE–MUIR SYNDROME,
TORRE SYNDROME, MUIR–TORRE SYNDROME

Manifestations and Major Findings
sebaceous gland neoplasms (adenoma, carcinoma, or hyperplasia)
visceral malignancies
–lungs
–gastrointestinal tract
–genitourinary system
keratoacanthomas (multiple)

OTHER FINDINGS
thyroid disease (adenoma, thyroiditis)
uterine fibroids
renal cysts
adenofibromatous hyperplasia of the prostate
Peyronie disease
carpal tunnel syndrome

autosomal dominant

References
Banse-Kupin L, Morales A, Barlow M: Torre's syndrome: report of two cases and review of the literature. J Am Acad Dermatol 1984; 10:803–817.

▷ ▷ ▷

Finan MC, Connolly SM: Sebaceous gland tumors and systemic disease: a clinicopathologic analysis. Medicine 1984; 63:232–242.
Gregory B, Ho VC: Cutaneous manifestations of gastrointestinal disorders. Part I. J Am Acad Dermatol 1992; 26:153–166.
Guitart J, McGillis ST, Bergfeld WF, et al.: Muir–Torre syndrome associated with alpha-1-antitrypsin deficiency and cutaneous vasculitis. J Am Acad Dermatol 1991; 24:875–877.
Rothenberg J, Lambert WC, Vail JT, Nemlick AS, et al.: The Muir–Torre (Torre's) syndrome: the significance of a solitary sebaceous tumor. J Am Acad Dermatol 1990; 23:638–640.
Torre D: Multiple sebaceous tumors. Arch Dermatol 1968; 98:549–551.
Umbert I, López-Gil F, Torné R, Umbert P: 'Sebaceoma' associated with centroblastic-centrocytic lymphoma. J Am Acad Dermatol 1990; 22:533–534.

TOURAINE–SOLENTE–GOLÉ SYNDROME see PACHYDERMOPERIOSTOSIS

TOURAINE SYNDROME
see NEUROCUTANEOUS MELANOSIS

TOURETTE SYNDROME,
GILLES DE LA TOURETTE SYNDROME

Manifestations and Major Findings
multiple involuntary tics
–eye twitching
–sounds or words
–facial grimacing
–head jerks
–echolalia
–coprolalia
involuntary vocalizations
spontaneous remission with minimal coordination problems
never completely resolves
onset at 2–15 years of age (mean 7 years)
normal mentation – may have attention deficits or learning disabilities
sleep disturbances
somnabulism (sleep walking)
feelings of imminence
more common in males

References
Golden GS: Tourette syndrome: Recent advances. Neurol Clin 1990; 8:705–714.
Pauls DL, Leckman JF: The inheritance of Gilles de la Tourette's syndrome and associated behavior. N Engl J Med 1986; 315:993–937.

TOURNIQUET SYNDROME

Manifestations and Major Findings
threads, hairs, or other strands encircling digit, nipple, or penis
distal soft tissue swelling caused by the ligating band

References
Barton DJ, Sloan GM, Nichter LS, Reinisch JF: Hair-thread tourniquet syndrome. Pediatrics 1988; 82:925–928.

TOXIC EPIDERMAL NECROLYSIS, LYELL SYNDROME

Manifestations and Major Findings
whole epidermis becomes necrotic
damage primarily to basal cells
begins as inflammation of the eyelids, conjunctivae, mouth, and genitalia
erythema and tenderness of the skin
fever, malaise, and anorexia
sheet-like loss of epidermis involving over 10% of body surface
positive Nikolsky sign
mucous membrane involvement
multisystem involvement
usually caused by drugs, graft versus host disease, or idiopathic
may result in scarring with loss of nails and hair
high mortality rate

References
Avakian R, Flowers FP, Araujo OE, Ramos-Caro FA: Toxic epidermal necrolysis: a review. J Am Acad Dermatol 1991; 25:69–79.
Roujeau J-C, Chosidow O, Saiag P, Guillaume J-C: Toxic epidermal necrolysis (Lyell syndrome). J Am Acad Dermatol 1990; 23:1039–1058.

TOXIC SHOCK SYNDROME (TSS)

Manifestations and Major Findings
usual cause is *Staphylococcus aureus* infection (producing TSS toxin I)
other cause is *Streptococcus* pyogenes
fever (over 38.9°C) for up to 14 days
hypotension or shock

OTHER FINDINGS
muscular involvement with myalgia
gastrointestinal involvement
vomiting and diarrhea
cardiopulmonary involvement
renal involvement
elevated creatinine
hematologic involvement
 —thrombocytopenia
 —disseminated intravascular coagulation
hepatic involvement
 —elevated enzymes
neurologic involvement with disorientation

Cutaneous Manifestations
diffuse macular erythroderma
no discrete lesions or Nikolsky sign
rash usually clears within 3 days
convalescent desquamation 10–21 days after onset
edema of hands and feet
mucous membrane hyperemia (conjunctival, pharyngeal, strawberry tongue)
telogen effluvium/Beau lines (later)

References
Bach MC: Dermatologic signs in toxic shock syndrome – clues to diagnosis. J Am Acad Dermatol 1983; 8:343–347.
Elbaum DJ, Wood C, Abuabara F, Morhenn VB: Bullae in a patient with toxic shock syndrome. J Am Acad Dermatol 1984; 10:267–272.
Huntley AC, Tanabe JL: Toxic shock syndrome as a complication of dermatologic surgery. J Am Acad Dermatol 1987; 16:227–229.
Wiesenthal AM, Ressman M, Caston SA, Todd JK: Toxic shock syndrome. Am J Epidemiol 1985; 122:847–856.
Working Group on Severe Streptococcal Infections. Defining the Group A streptococcal toxic shock syndrome. J Am Med Assoc 1993; 269:390–391.

TRANSIENT ACANTHOLYTIC DERMATOSIS *see also* GROVER DISEASE

TREACHER COLLINS SYNDROME, MANDIBULOFACIAL DYSOSTOSIS, FRANCESCHETTI–ZWAHLEN–KLEIN SYNDROME

Manifestations and Major Findings
probably caused by arrested development of the structures of the first branchial arch at 5–9 weeks gestation
circumscribed scarring alopecia (occasional)
hearing loss

Characteristic Facies
downward-slanting palpebral fissures
coloboma of the lower eyelids
partial/total absence of lower eyelashes
malar hypoplasia (especially zygomatic area)
mandibular hypoplasia
microtia
extension of scalp hair onto the cheeks
skin tags between the ear and the angle of mouth
cleft palate

autosomal dominant or sporadic

> **References**
> Fazen LE, Elmore J, Nadler HL: Mandibulo-facial dysostosis (Treacher Collins syndrome). Am J Dis Child 1967; 113:405–410.
> Sulik KK, Johnston MC, Smiley SJ, et al.: Mandibulo-facial dysostosis (Treacher Collins syndrome): a new proposal for its pathogenesis. Am J Med Genet 1987; 27:359–372.

TRICHODENTOOSSEOUS SYNDROME, TDO SYNDROME, AMELOGENESIS IMPERFECTA-TAURODONTISM-SCLEROTIC BONES

Manifestations and Major Findings
thick, curly hair at birth – may straighten with age
teeth are pitted, small, and widely spaced with poor enamel, taurodontism (asymptomatic increase in pulp chamber size), and impaction
increased bone density
frontal bossing
dolichocephaly (elongated head)
square jaw

OTHER FINDINGS
normal physical and mental development
nails peel and break easily
children have white bands on nails
hypohidrosis

autosomal dominant

> **References**
> Kucirka SJ, Scher RK: Heritable nail disorders. Dermatol Clin 1987; 5:179–191.
> Lichtenstein J, Warson R, Jorgenson R, et al: The tricho-dento-osseous syndrome. Am J Hum Genet 1972; 24:569–582.
> Shapiro SD, Quattromani FL, Jorgenson RJ, et al.: Tricho-dento-osseous syndrome: heterogeneity or clinical variability. Am J Med Genet 1983; 16:225–236.

TRICHORHINOPHALANGEAL SYNDROME

Types of Trichorhinophalangeal Syndrome and Features

type I
sparse, brittle hair
pili torti and/or trichorrhexis nodosa
prominent nose (pear-shaped)
broad, high nasal bridge
long philtrum
multiple cone-shaped digital epiphyses
crooked fingers/toes or brachydactyly
thin, brittle nails
short stature
winged scapulae
deep voice
degenerative hip disease in early adulthood

type II Langer–Giedion syndrome, trichorhinophalangeal syndrome with exostoses
sparse hair
pear-shaped nose (bulbous)
cone-shaped phalangeal epiphyses
multiple exostoses
prominent ears (protruding)
microcephaly ▷ ▷ ▷

▷ ▷ ▷
short stature
hyperextensible joints
loose, redundant skin in infancy
increased number of nevi
mental retardation

> **References**
> Bühler UK, Beutler C, et al.: A final word on the tricho-rhino-phalangeal syndrome. Clin Genet 1987; 31:273–275.
> Cope R, Beals RK, Bennett RM: The trichorhinophalangeal dysplasia syndrome: report of eight kindreds with emphasis on hip complications, late presentations, and premature osteoarthrosis. J Pediatr Orthop 1986; 6:133–138.
> McCloud DJ, Solomon LM: The tricho-rhino-phalangeal syndrome. Br J Dermatol 1977; 96: 403–407.
> Wilson WG, Herrington RT, Sylsworth AS: The Langer–Giedion syndrome: report of a 22-year-old woman. Pediatrics 1979; 64:542–545.
> Yáñez S, Hernández-Vicente I, Armijo M: Trichorhinophalangeal syndrome. Int J Dermatol 1992; 31:706–709.

TRICHOTHIODYSTROPHY,

SULFUR-DEFICIENT BRITTLE HAIR, BIDS/IBIDS/PIBIDS SYNDROME, TAY SYNDROME *see also* DISORDERS OF CORNIFICATION; DOC 14

Manifestations and Major Findings
*i*chthyosiform erythroderma
- *b*rittle hair – short and sulfur-deficient (Fig. 134)

*i*ntellectual impairment (variable mental retardation)
*d*ecreased fertility
*s*hort stature (growth retardation)
under polarizing microscope hairs show
– alternating bands of light
– pili torti
– trichoschisis (clean breaks)
– trichorrhexis nodosa

OTHER FINDINGS
*p*hotosensitivity – association with xeroderma pigmentosum and decreased DNA repair (ultraviolet light) in some cases
dystrophic nails
dental caries

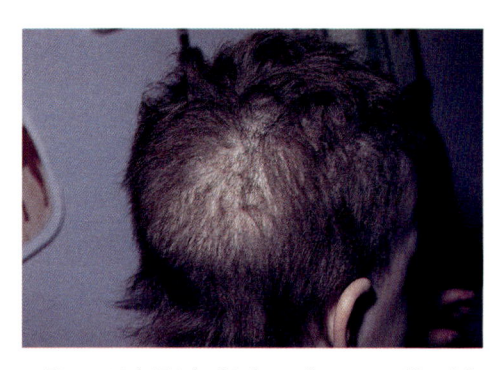

• *Figure 134* Trichothiodystrophy causes sulfur-deficient hair to break easily, leaving patches of short hair.

congenital cataracts
dysmorphic facies
spasticity
ataxia
microcephaly
deafness
hypogonadism

autosomal recessive

> **References**
> Itin PH, Pittelkow MR: Trichothiodystrophy: review of sulfur-deficient brittle hair syndromes and association with the ectodermal dysplasias. J Am Acad Dermatol 1990; 22:705–717.
> Kousseff BC: Collodion baby, sign of Tay syndrome. Pediatrics 1991; 87:571–574.
> Lucky PA, Kirsch N, Lucky AW, Carter DM: Low-sulfur hair syndrome associated with UVB photosensitivity and testicular failure. J Am Acad Dermatol 1984; 11:340–346.
> Motley RJ, Finlay AY: A patient with Tay's syndrome. Pediatr Dermatol 1989; 6:202–205.
> Price VH, Odom RB, Ward WH, Jones FT: Trichothiodystrophy. Arch Dermatol 1980; 116:1375–1384.
> Rebora A, Crovato F: PIBI(D)S syndrome – trichothiodystrophy with xeroderma pigmentosum (group D) mutation. J Am Acad Dermatol 1987; 16:940–947.

TRIGEMINAL TROPHIC SYNDROME

Manifestations and Major Findings
neurotrophic ulceration following minor trauma to anesthetic skin within the trigeminal area

pronounced paresthesias causes patient to repeatedly touch or pick the skin
usually begins at the ala nasi
tip of the nose spared
anesthesia may be result of infarction, degeneration, or tumor growth
psychologic problems common

> **References**
> **Finlay AY:** Trigeminal trophic syndrome. Arch Dermatol 1979; 115:1118.
> **Walton S, Keczkes K:** Trigeminal neurotrophic ulceration – a report of four patients. Clin Exp Dermatol 1985; 10:485–490.
> **Westerhof W, Bos JD:** Trigeminal trophic syndrome: a successful treatment with transcutaneous electrical stimulation. Br J Dermatol 1983; 108:601–604.

TRISOMY 13, PATAU SYNDROME, BARTHOLIN–PATAU SYNDROME

Manifestations and Major Findings
mental retardation (severe)
malformed brain (holoprosencephaly)
deafness
cryptorchidism
rocker-bottom feet (prominent heels)
polydactyly
cardiac anomalies (ventricular septal defects)

Characteristic Facies
microcephaly
microphthalmia/anophthalmia
abnormal helices of the ears
micrognathia
cleft lip and palate
bulbous nose
sloping forehead

Cutaneous Manifestations
aplasia cutis of the scalp
hemangiomas/vascular malformations
narrow hyperconvex fingernails
cutis laxa of the neck

> **References**
> **Hodes ME, Cole J, Palmer CG, Reed T:** Clinical experience with trisomies 18 and 13. J Med Genet 1978; 15:48–60.

TRISOMY 18 SYNDROME, EDWARDS SYNDROME

Manifestations and Major Findings
clenched hand with overlapping of index over third fingers and fifth over fourth fingers
rocker-bottom feet (prominent heels)
short sternum
prematurity or postmaturity
single umbilical artery
inguinal or umbilical hernia
cryptorchidism (male)
cardiac anomalies
hypertonia
severe mental retardation
reduced life expectancy

Characteristic Facies
small chin
prominent occiput
low-set, malformed ears
epicanthal folds
cleft lip and/or palate

Cutaneous Manifestations
webbing of the neck
little subcutaneous fat
cutis marmorata
hemangiomas/vascular malformations
hypoplasia of the nails
hypertrichosis of the forehead and back
small nipples
dermatoglyphic abnormalities with low-arch dermal ridge patterning on the fingertips

> **References**
> **Hodes ME, Cole J, Palmer CG, et al.:** Clinical experience with trisomies 18 and 13. J Med Genet 1978; 15:48–60.
> **Van Dyke DC, Allen M:** Clinical management considerations in long-term survivors with trisomy 18. Pediatrics 1990; 85:753–759.

TRISOMY 21 SYNDROME
see DOWN SYNDROME

TROUSSEAU SYNDROME

Manifestations and Major Findings
recurrent migratory thrombophlebitis
involves numerous sites – especially the upper extremities and the trunk
crops of tender, linear or oval lesions
Trousseau syndrome is often associated with malignancy (pancreatic, gastric, lung, prostate, colon, ovary, and gallbladder neoplasms) and is believed to be secondary to a low-grade, intravascular hypercoagulable state.

> **References**
> **Samlaska CP, James WD:** Superficial thrombophlebitis. J Am Acad Dermatol 1990; 23:1–18.

TUBEROUS SCLEROSIS,
BOURNEVILLE DISEASE

Manifestations and Major Findings
classic triad of findings
– angiofibromas of face (adenoma sebaceum)
– seizures or infantile spasms
– mental retardation

OCULAR ABNORMALITIES
retinal gliomas
papilledema
optic atrophy

OTHER FINDINGS
multiple hamartomas of skin, brain, eyes, kidneys, heart, adrenal glands, liver, pancreas, testes, and thyroid
neurologic abnormalities
– calcifications
– hamartomas
cardiac rhabdomyomas
renal cysts or tumors (angiomyolipomas)
lung cysts
spontaneous pneumothorax
lymphangiomyomatosis of the lung
phalangeal bone cysts
periosteal thickening
gastrointestinal polyps

Cutaneous Manifestations
shagreen patch (collagenoma in the lumbosacral area)
• hypopigmented macules (Fig. 135)
– ash-leaf
– confetti
– dermatomal
– polygonal
poliosis
• periungual fibromas (Koenen tumors) (Fig. 136)
gingival fibromas
diffuse bronzing
café au lait macules

autosomal dominant or sporadic

> **References**
> **Bolognia JL, Pawelek JM:** Biology of hypopigmentation. J Am Acad Dermatol 1988; 19:217–255.
> **Hanno R, Beck R:** Tuberous sclerosis. Neurol Clin 1987; 5:351–359. ▷ ▷ ▷

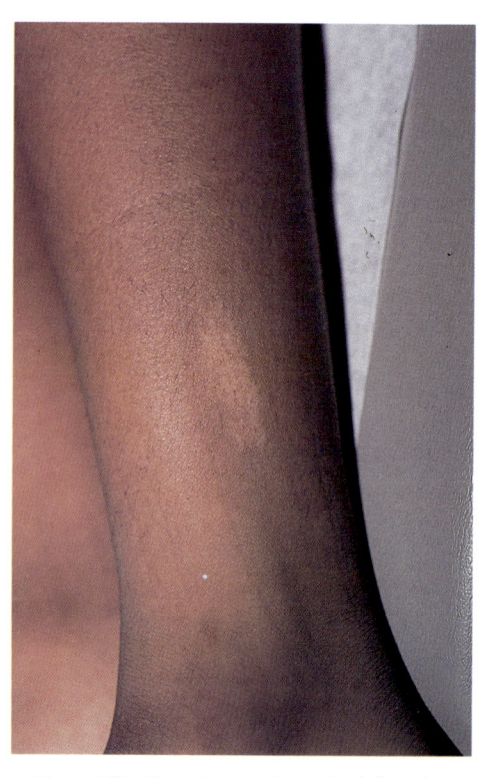

• *Figure 135* Hypopigmented macules (of varying shapes) on the skin are seen in tuberous sclerosis.

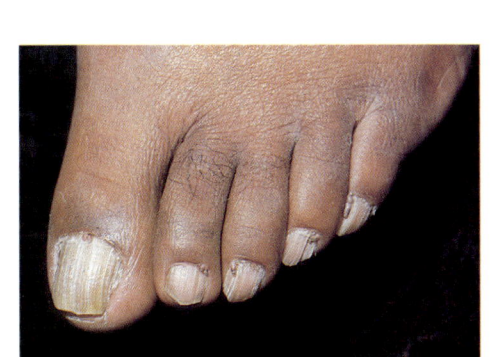

• *Figure 136* Periungual fibromas seen in tuberous sclerosis, usually more prominent on the feet.

▷ ▷ ▷
Kegel MF: Dominant disorders with multiple organ involvement. Dermatol Clin 1987; 5:205–219.
Osborne JP: Diagnosis of tuberous sclerosis. Arch Dis Child 1988; 63:1423–1425.
Park Y-K, Hann SK: Cluster growths in adenoma sebaceum associated with tuberous sclerosis. J Am Acad Dermatol 1989; 20:918–920.
Weinblatt ME, Kahn E, Kochen J: Renal cell carcinoma in patients with tuberous sclerosis. Pediatrics 1987; 80:898–903.

TURNER SYNDROME, ULLRICH–TURNER SYNDROME, BONNEVIE–ULLRICH SYNDROME

Manifestations and Major Findings
single X (XO) 45 chromosome pattern or mosaic forms

OTHER FINDINGS
short stature from birth
cystic hygroma
primary amenorrhea
shield chest (broad chest)
cubitus valgus of the elbow
narrow palate
small mandible
bicuspid aortic valve
coarctation of the aorta
anomalous auricles
impaired hearing
ptosis
kidney anomalies

Cutaneous Manifestations
lymphedema of the hands and feet at birth
residual puffiness of the hands and feet
low posterior hairline
pterygium colli (webbed neck)
widely spaced nipples
increased number of nevi
tendency toward keloid formation
narrow, hyperconvex nails

References
Moore JW, Kirby WC, Rogers WM, Poth MA: Partial anomalous pulmonary venous drainage associated with 45, X Turner's Syndrome. Pediatrics 1990; 86:273–276.
Van Dyke DL, Wiktor A, Roberson JR, Weiss L: Mental retardation in Turner syndrome. J Pediatr 1991; 118:415–417.

TYROSINEMIA

Tyrosinemias and Features

type I
acute and chronic liver failure
failure to thrive
vomiting
renal tubular dysfunction
hepatocellular carcinoma
neurologic crises
– severe peripheral neuropathy
– muscle weakness
– paralysis
abdominal crises
deficiency of fumarylacetoacetate hydrolase
elevated levels of plasma tyrosine as well as other amino acids

type II
see Richner–Hanhart syndrome

References
Mitchell G, Larochelle J, Lambert M, Michaud J, et al.: Neurologic crises in hereditary tyrosinemia. N Engl J Med 1990; 322:432–437.
Rank JM, Pascual-Leone A, Payne W, Glock M, et al.: Hematin therapy for the neurologic crisis of tyrosinemia. J Pediatr 1991; 118:136–139.

U

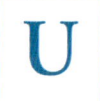

ULERYTHEMA OPHRYOGENES,
KERATOSIS PILARIS ATROPHICANS

Manifestations and Major Findings
- inflammatory, keratotic, facial papules (Fig. 137)

keratosis pilaris
onset at birth or in infancy
may result in scarring alopecia and atrophy
Ulerythema ophryogenes is sometimes associated with Noonan syndrome, developmental retardation, woolly hair, and atopy.

possible autosomal dominant

> **References**
> **Burnett JW, Schwartz MF, Berberian BJ:** Ulerythema ophyrogenes with multiple congenital anomalies. J Am Acad Dermatol 1988; 18:437–440.
> **Snell JA, Mallory SB:** Ulerythema ophryogenes in Noonan syndrome. Pediatr Dermatol 1990; 7:77–78.

UNCOMBABLE HAIR SYNDROME,
SPUN GLASS HAIR SYNDROME *see also* HAIR SHAFT ANOMALIES

Manifestations and Major Findings
- unmanageable, silvery-blonde scalp hair in childhood (Fig. 138)

slow hair growth
pili trianguli et canaliculi
– longitudinal grooves in the hair shafts
– triangular cross-section of shafts
possibly familial

autosomal dominant

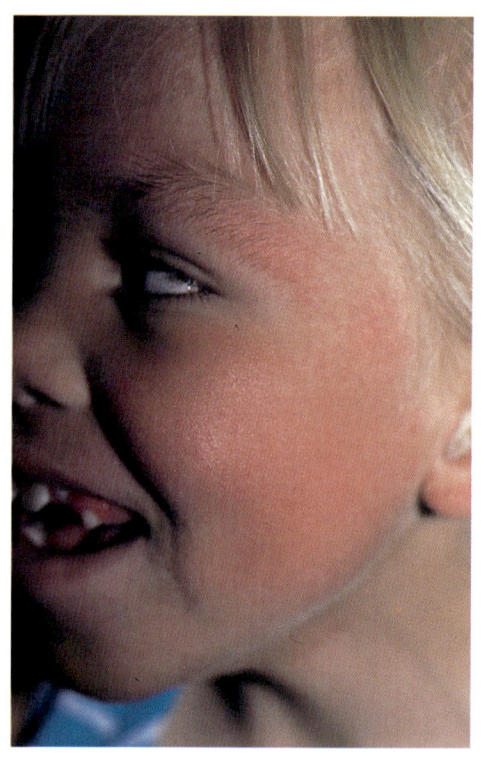

• *Figure 137 Inflammatory, keratotic, facial papules are a feature of ulerythema ophryogenes.*

> **References**
> **Matis WL, Baden H, Green R, Boiko S, Lucky AW, et al.:** Uncombable-hair syndrome. Pediatr Dermatol 1987; 4:215–219.
> **Rest EB, Fretzin DF:** Quantitative assessment of scanning electron microscope defects in uncombable-hair syndrome. Pediatr Dermatol 1990; 7:93–96.
> **Whiting DA:** Structural abnormalities of the hair shaft. J Am Acad Dermatol 1987; 16:1–25.

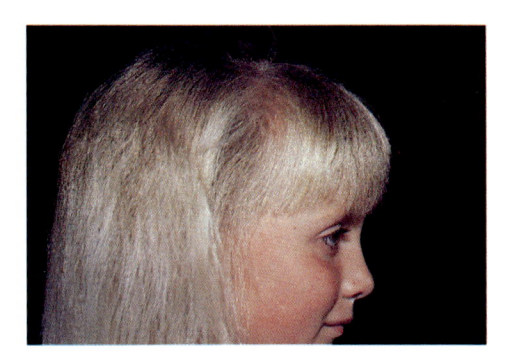

• *Figure 138* Unmanageable, silvery-blonde hair (spun glass hair) in uncombable hair syndrome.

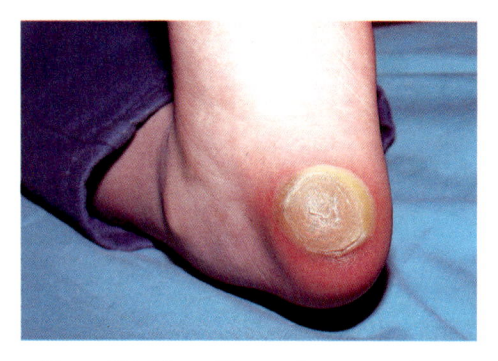

• *Figure 139* Unna–Thost syndrome presenting as keratosis of the heel causing pain when walking.

UNNA–THOST SYNDROME, TYLOSIS, DIFFUSE PALMOPLANTAR KERATODERMA

Manifestations and Major Findings
- diffuse, waxy, palmoplantar keratoderma (Fig. 139)
  painful fissuring frequent
  sharp 'cut-off' at the wrist
  no spread to the extensor surfaces
  childhood onset
  keratosis of the knees and elbows
  hyperhidrosis of the palms and soles
  dermatophyte infections common
  normal hair and teeth
  oral leukoplakia (not premalignant)

autosomal dominant

References
Küster W, Becker A: Indication for the identity of palmoplantar keratoderma type Unna–Thost with type Vörner. Acta Derm Venereol (Stockh) 1992; 72:120–122.
Sybert VP, Dale BA, Holbrook KA: Palmar-plantar keratoderma. J Am Acad Dermatol 1987; 18:75–86.

URBACH–WIETHE DISEASE
see LIPOID PROTEINOSIS

UVEOPAROTID FEVER
see HEERFORDT SYNDROME

V

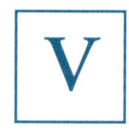

VACTERL ASSOCIATION,
VATER ASSOCIATION

Manifestations and Major Findings
*v*ertebral anomalies
*a*nal atresia – with or without fistula
*c*ardiac defects (ventricular septal)
*t*racheo-*e*sophageal fistula
*r*adial anomalies
*l*imb anomalies (radial and lower extremity defects)

> **References**
> Levine F, Muenke M: VACTERL association with high prenatal lead exposure: similarities to animal models of lead teratogenicity. Pediatrics 1991; 87: 390–392.

VANISHING BONE SYNDROME
see GORHAM SYNDROME

VELOCARDIOFACIAL SYNDROME,
SHPRINTZEN SYNDROME

Manifestations and Major Findings
cleft palate
cardiac abnormalities
 – ventricular septal defect
 – right aortic arch defect
 – aberrant subclavian arteries
 – tetralogy of Fallot
ear anomalies
hearing loss
long, thin fingers
learning disabilities

Characteristic Facies
long, prominent nose
wide or high, square nasal bridge
narrow alar base
long face
malar hypoplasia

autosomal dominant

> **References**
> Jedele KB, Michels VV, Puga FJ, Feldt RH: Velo-cardio-facial syndrome associated with ventricular septal defect, pulmonary atresia, and hypoplastic pulmonary arteries. Pediatrics 1992; 89:915–919.
> Stevens CA, Carey JC, Shigeoka AO: DiGeorge anomaly and velocardiofacial syndrome. Pediatrics 1990; 85:526–530.

VINCENT INFECTION, ACUTE
NECROTIZING ULCERATIVE GINGIVITIS, TRENCH MOUTH

Manifestations and Major Findings
acute, painful, ulcerative infection of the gingiva
soreness and bleeding upon minor oral trauma
severe fetid breath
punched-out papillae
affects young adults
probably caused by a complex of microorganisms (fusiform bacilli and spirochetes) plus host factors

VITAMIN DEFICIENCIES

Causes and Symptoms of Vitamin Deficiencies

1 vitamin A (retinol) deficiency, phrynoderma
Retinol reacts with fatty acids to form esters to be incorporated into chylomicrons and transported with retinol-binding protein. Dietary retinol is found in liver, fish, milk, eggs, and vegetables (especially dark green leafy ones).
poor night vision
scaliness
atrophy of sebaceous and sweat glands
follicular plugging
dull scalp hair
conjunctival xerosis
Bitot spots in the eyes
impaired bone growth
cranial nerve lesions
causative drugs/factors:
– fat malabsorption
– liver disease

2 vitamin B$_1$ (thiamine) deficiency, beriberi
Unable to decarboxylate pyruvate, making pyruvate unavailable to the citric acid cycle and causing build-up of pyruvate and lactate. Dietary thiamine is found in milk, yeast, and the germ and husk of grain.
wet (cardiac) beriberi
– myocarditis with congestive heart disease
– edema
dry (neurologic) beriberi
– peripheral neuropathy with wrist and/or foot drop
– motor disturbances
– digestive disturbances
Wernicke–Korsakoff syndrome (encephalopathy with psychosis)
orogenital dermatitis
causative drugs/factors:
– rice-dependent diets
– chronic alcoholism

3 vitamin B$_2$ (riboflavin) deficiency
Glutathione reductase is activated by riboflavin and acts as a coenzyme in oxidation-reduction reactions. Dietary riboflavin is found in meat, fish, milk, and eggs.
oculo-orogenital syndrome
angular cheilitis
black tongue
seborrheic dermatitis/dyssebacia
anemia
scrotal dermatitis
mental retardation
causative drugs/factors:
– borate poisoning
– neonatal phototherapy for hyperbilirubinemia
– protein deficiency
– hypothyroidism

4 vitamin B$_3$ (niacin) deficiency, pellagra
One-third of niacin is absorbed, two-thirds is synthesized from tryptophan. Cereals contain niacin (lime juice releases niacin).
the four D's
– diarrhea
– dementia
– dermatitis
– death
Casal necklace
dermatitis on sun-exposed areas
angular stomatitis
glossitis
weakness
oral and perirectal sores
causative drugs/factors:
– isoniazid
– sulfonamides
– anticonvulsants and antidepressants
– 6-mercaptopurine
– 5-fluorouracil
– chloramphenicol
– plain corn diet (niacin not bioavailable)
– alcoholic disease
– gastrointestinal disease (malabsorption)
– carcinoid syndrome
Hartnup disease is associated with niacin deficiency.

5 vitamin B$_6$ (pyridoxine) deficiency
Among other metabolic roles, a pyridoxine metabolite is a coenzyme in tryptophan conversion to niacin. Most classes of foodstuffs provide pyridoxine.
periorificial dermatitis
pellagra-like rash
seborrhea
polyneuritis
gastrointestinal symptoms
cheilosis
glossitis
anorexia
confusion
lymphopenia
causative drugs/factors:
– isoniazid
– hydralazine
– penicillamine
– uremia
– cirrhosis ▷ ▷ ▷

▷ ▷ ▷
6 vitamin B₁₂ (cobalamin) deficiency
Cobalamin lowers glutathione levels (sulfhydryl balance). Reduced glutathione results in increased tyrosinase activity which increases melanogenesis. Animal foodstuffs are the main dietary source.
hyperpigmentation (finger pulps, neck, axillae)
hyperpigmented macules
glossitis
poliosis
megaloblastic anemia
paresthesias
ataxia
mental status changes
causative drugs/factors:
– decreased gastric synthesis of intrinsic factor
– pernicious anemia
– tropical sprue
– strict vegetarianism
– ileal destruction or bypass
– chronic alcoholism

7 vitamin C (ascorbic acid) deficiency, scurvy
Ascorbic acid is a cofactor for enzymes (e.g. proline hydroxylase) essential in collagen formation and is contained in citrus fruit.
follicular hyperkeratosis
perifollicular petechiae
poor wound healing
'corkscrew' hairs
koilonychia
gingival hemorrhage
sclerodermatous changes
weakness
fatigue
depression

8 vitamin D deficiency, rickets
Vitamin D is synthesized from 7-dehydrocholesterol in the skin by the body on exposure to sunlight. Deficiency can be due to malabsorption, liver disease, vitamin D resistance, and renal disease.
rickets
muscle weakness

9 vitamin H (biotin) deficiency
(See also *biotin deficiency and biotin-responsive disorders* for the three forms of biotin deficiency)
Biotin acts as a coenzyme in a diverse series of metabolic processes. Biotin is found in animal and vegetable foodstuffs and deficient diets are rare.
looks similar to zinc deficiency
acrodermatitis enteropathica
intertriginous and periorificial dermatitis
conjunctivitis
glossitis
cheilitis

xerosis
alopecia
neuropsychiatric symptoms
causative drugs/factors:
– anticonvulsants
– raw egg-white (avidin) – binds biotin in gut preventing absorption
– total parenteral nutrition (without biotin)
– chronic gastrointestinal disease
– short bowel

10 vitamin K deficiency
Vitamin K is necessary for the production of blood coagulation factors II (prothrombin), VII, IX, and X by the liver. About half of the requirement is synthesized by normal intestinal flora. Dietary vitamin K is found in green, leafy vegetables, meat, and dairy products.
intracutaneous hemorrhage
gastrointestinal, nasal, subgaleal, and intracranial bleeding
causative drugs/factors:
– coumarin
– antibiotics
– liver disease
– neonates
– fat malabsorption

11 folic acid deficiency
The folic acid coenzyme form assists in early purine and pyrimidine synthesis, generation and use of formate, and amino acid conversions. Dietary folic acid is found in liver, green vegetables, and yeast.
similar to vitamin B₁₂ deficiency
hyperpigmentation of tongue and genitals
glossitis
angular cheilitis
megaloblastic anemia
causative drugs/factors:
– phenytoin
– barbiturates
– methotrexate
– celiac disease
– diet of goat's milk only
– pregnancy

References
Barthelemy H, Chouvet B, Cambazard F: Skin and mucosal manifestations in vitamin deficiency. J Am Acad Dermatol 1986; 15:1263–1274.
Ellis CN, Vanderveen EE, Rasmussen JE: Scurvy: a case caused by peculiar dietary habits. Arch Dermatol 1984; 120:1212–1214.
Grob JJ, Collet-Villette AM, Aillaud MF, Capo C, et al.: Spontaneous adult scurvy in a developed country: new insight in an ancient disease. Arch Dermatol 1990; 126:249–251. ▷ ▷ ▷

> **Lifshitz AY, Stern F, Kaplan B, Sofer E, et al.:** Pellagra complicating Crohn's disease. J Am Acad Dermatol 1992; 27:620.
> **Miller SJ:** Nutritional deficiency and the skin. J Am Acad Dermatol 1989; 21:1–30.
> **Pinnell SR, Murad S, Darr D:** Induction of collagen synthesis by ascorbic acid. Arch Dermatol 1987; 123: 1684–1686.
> **Sanders MN, Winkelmann RK:** Cutaneous reactions to vitamin K. J Am Acad Dermatol 1988; 19:699–704.

VOGT–KOYANAGI–HARADA SYNDROME, UVEOMENINGITIS SYNDROME

Manifestations and Major Findings
prodromal febrile episode
meningeal irritation with pleocytosis (aseptic) or encephalitis
bilateral uveitis
iritis (1–2 weeks later) may lead to blindness
deafness (usually temporary)
tinnitus or dysacusis

Cutaneous Manifestations
alopecia – circumscribed (alopecia areata) or diffuse
symmetrical vitiligo
poliosis of the eyelashes, eyebrows, scalp, and body hair
halo nevi

> **References**
> **Bologna JL, Pawelek JM:** Biology of hypopigmentation. J Am Acad Dermatol 1988; 19:217–255.

VOHWINKEL SYNDROME, KERATOMA HEREDITARIA MUTILANS, MUTILATING KERATODERMA

Manifestations and Major Findings
onset in infancy
diffuse palmoplantar keratoderma honeycombed by small depressions
starfish-shaped keratoses on the dorsa of the hands and feet
constricting, fibrous bands on fingers and toes causing autoamputation (ainhum)
irregular, linear keratoses of knees and elbows

OTHER FINDINGS
cicatricial alopecia
deafness
spastic paraplegia
myopathy
transient plantar bullae

autosomal dominant or recessive

> **References**
> **Gibbs RC, Frank SB:** Keratoma hereditaria mutilans (Vohwinkel). Arch Dermatol 1966; 94:619–624.
> **Goldfarb MT, Woo TY, Rasmussen JE:** Keratoderma hereditaria mutilans (Vohwinkel's syndrome): a trial of isotretinoin. Pediatr Dermatol 1984; 2:216–218.

VOIGT LINES

Manifestations and Major Findings
sharply demarcated, bilateral lines of hyperpigmentation seen at the anterolateral junctions (extensor and flexor surface junctions)
usually affects the upper arms
lines show patterned configurations
– cape-like on the upper chest
– open hourglass on anterior trunk
– lateral vertical lines on posterior trunk

VON HIPPEL–LINDAU SYNDROME, ANGIOMATOSIS RETINAE ET CEREBELLI SYNDROME, LINDAU DISEASE

Manifestations and Major Findings
angiomatosis of the retina and central nervous system (especially cerebellum)
may lead to blindness if untreated
tumors, angiomas, and cysts (kidney, pancreas, liver, epididymis)
renal cell carcinoma (often bilateral)
pheochromocytoma
vascular malformations of the face (rare)
symptoms usually begin in third decade

autosomal dominant

References
Greenwald MJ, Weiss A: Ocular manifestations of the neurocutaneous syndromes. Pediatr Dermatol 1984; 2:98–117
Neumann HPH: Prognosis of von Hippel–Lindau syndrome. Vasa 1987; 16:309–311.
Neumann HPH, Eggert HR, Weigel K, Friedburg H, et al.: Hemangioblastomas of the central nervous system: a ten year study with special reference to von Hippel–Lindau syndrome. J Neurosurg 1989; 70: 24–30.
Seizinger BR, Rouleau GA, Ozelius LJ, Lane AH, et al.: Von Hippel–Lindau disease maps to the region of chromosome 3 associated with renal cell carcinoma. Nature 1988; 332:268–269.

VON RECKLINGHAUSEN DISEASE
see NEUROFIBROMATOSIS; CLASSIC TYPE

VON WILLEBRAND DISEASE

Manifestations and Major Findings
prolonged bleeding time
decreased factor VIII activity
normal platelet count
epistaxis
menorrhagia
easily bruised

autosomal dominant and recessive types

References
Ruggeri ZM, Zimmerman TS: Von Willebrand factor and von Willebrand disease. Blood 1987; 70:895–904.

VON ZUMBUSCH SYNDROME,
ACUTE GENERALIZED PUSTULAR PSORIASIS

Cutaneous Manifestations
• sheets of erythema and pustules (Fig. 140)
usually involves the flexural areas
thickened nails with pus underneath
oral mucosa involvement
telogen effluvium

OTHER FINDINGS
high fever
severe malaise
hypoalbuminemia
hypocalcemia
liver dysfunction
polyarthritis
malabsorption

References
Aronsson A, Nilsson A: Pustular psoriasis of v. Zumbusch type associated with recurring cholestatic jaundice. Acta Derm Venereol (Stockh) 1986; 66:164–167.
Fradin MS, Ellis CN, Voorhees JJ: Rapid response of von Zumbusch psoriasis to cyclosporine. J Am Acad Dermatol 1990; 23:925–926.
Hubler WR: Lingual lesions of generalized pustular psoriasis. J Am Acad Dermatol 1984; 11:1069–1076.

VÖRNER DISEASE
see also EPIDERMOLYTIC HYPERKERATOSIS

Manifestations and Major Findings
epidermolytic palmoplantar hyperkeratosis
presents as diffuse keratoderma
mild hyperhidrosis
no spreading to the extensor surfaces
onset in the first decade

Vörner disease is associated with breast and ovarian cancer.

autosomal dominant

References
Blanchet-Bardon C, Nazzaro V, Chevrant-Breton J, et al.: Hereditary epidermolytic palmoplantar keratoderma associated with breast and ovarian cancer in a large kindred. Br J Dermatol 1987; 117: 363–370.
Kanitakis J, Tsoitis G, Kanitakis C: Hereditary epidermolytic palmoplantar keratoderma (Vörner type). J Am Acad Dermatol 1987; 17:414–422.

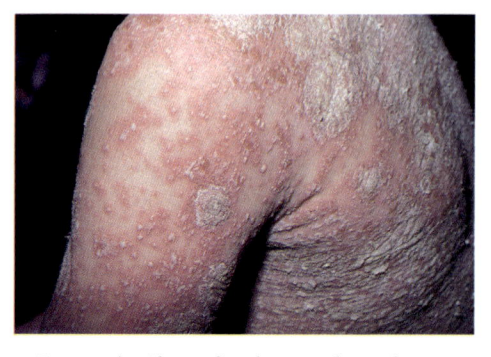

• *Figure 140* Sheets of erythema and pustules in von Zumbusch syndrome.

W

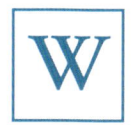

WAARDENBURG SYNDROME,
WAARDENBURG–KLEIN SYNDROME,
KLEIN–WAARDENBURG SYNDROME

Manifestations and Major Findings
congenital sensorineural deafness
- depigmentation of hair and skin (Fig. 141)
white (occasionally black) forelock
premature graying of hair
congenital megacolon (Hirschsprung disease)

Characteristic Facies
confluent, thick eyebrows (synophrys)
broad nasal root
upturned nasal tip
square or asymmetric face
massive jaw

OCULAR ABNORMALITIES
heterochromic irides
- hypopigmentation of iris (isohypochromia) (Fig. 141)
laterally displaced inner canthi (dystopia canthorum)

Waardenburg syndrome type I features dystopia canthorum, in type II this finding is not a feature.

autosomal dominant

> **References**
> **Bolognia JL, Pawelek JM:** Biology of hypopigmentation. J Am Acad Dermatol 1988; 19:217–255.
> **Mallory SB, Wiener E, Nordlund JJ:** Waardenburg's syndrome with Hirschsprung's disease: a neural crest defect. Pediatr Dermatol 1986; 3:119–124.

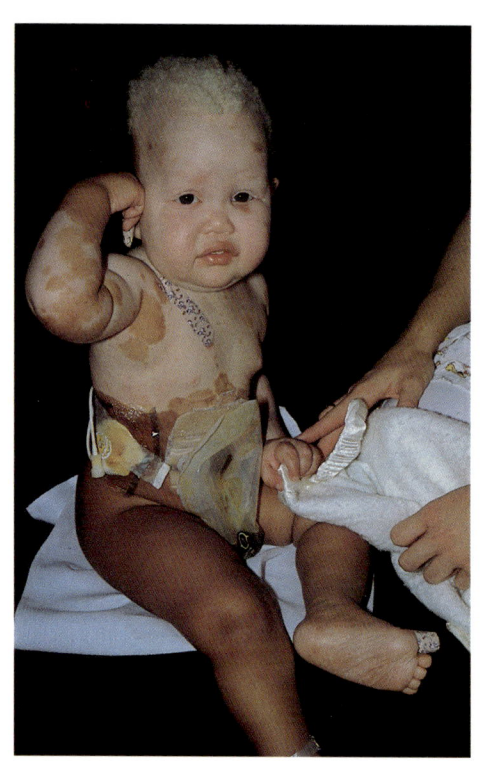

• *Figure 141* Depigmentation of the hair and skin seen in Waardenburg syndrome. This child also had Hirschsprung disease.

WALDENSTRÖM MACROGLOBULINEMIA,
HYPERGAMMAGLOBULINEMIC PURPURA OF WALDENSTRÖM

Manifestations and Major Findings
chronic lymphoreticular disorder
marked increase in serum IgM
hepatosplenomegaly

lymphadenopathy
high erythrocyte sedimentation rate
blood hyperviscosity
cryoglobulinemia
xerostomia
xerophthalmia
weakness
weight loss
anemia
epistaxis
neurologic symptoms

Cutaneous Manifestations
relapsing nonthrombocytopenic purpura
papules with IgM paraprotein deposits
lymphocytoma cutis
brown macular lesions
vasculitis
livedo reticularis
Raynaud phenomenon
diffuse infiltration of the ears
Waldenström macroglobulinemia is associated with autoimmune diseases – Sjögren syndrome and systemic lupus erythematosus.

> **References**
> Cobb MW, Domloge-Hultsch N, Frame JN, Yancey KB: Waldenström macroglobulinemia with an IgM-kappa antiepidermal basement membrane zone antibody. Arch Dermatol 1992; 128:372–376.
> Finder KA, McCollough ML, Dixon SL, Majka AJ, et al.: Hypergammaglobulinemic purpura of Waldenström. J Am Acad Dermatol 1990; 23: 669–676.
> Lowe L, Fitzpatrick JE, Huff JC, Shanley PF, Golitz LE: Cutaneous macroglobulinosis. Arch Dermatol 1992; 128:377–380.

WATERHOUSE–FRIDERICHSEN SYNDROME

Manifestations and Major Findings
fulminating meningococcemia or
  other septicemia
hemorrhage into the adrenal glands
fever
purpura
shock

WATSON–ALAGILLE SYNDROME
see ALAGILLE SYNDROME

WEARY–KINDLER SYNDROME
see HEREDITARY ACROKERATOTIC POIKILODERMA

WEAVER SYNDROME

Manifestations and Major Findings
accelerated skeletal maturation of prenatal onset
macrosomia (large organs)
camptodactyly (relative shortness of the flexor
  tendons causing flexion contractures) –
  usually the third, fourth, and fifth digits
broad thumbs
limited elbow and knee extension
progressive spasticity

Characteristic Facies
large ears
long philtrum
large bifrontal diameter of the skull
ocular hypertelorism
micrognathia

Cutaneous Manifestations
relatively loose skin
inverted nipples
thin hair
thin, deeply set nails
prominent fingertip pads

> **References**
> Ramos-Arroyo MA, Weaver DD, Banks ER: Weaver Syndrome: a case without early overgrowth and review of the literature. Pediatrics 1991; 88:1106–1111.

WEBER–CHRISTIAN DISEASE,
RELAPSING FEBRILE NODULAR NONSUPPURATIVE PANNICULITIS

Manifestations and Major Findings
recurrent, localized, inflammatory,
  nonsuppurative subcutaneous nodules
  (panniculitis) – may show atrophy

recurrent attacks of malaise, fever, abdominal pain, and arthritis
subcutaneous atrophy at the nodule sites
may present as severe systemic illness with inflammation of heart, lungs, liver, or kidney
self-limiting course

> **References**
> Hendrick SJ, Silverman AK, Solomon AR, Headington JT: Alpha-1-antitrypsin deficiency associated with panniculitis. J Am Acad Dermatol 1988; 18:684–692.
> Patterson JW: Panniculitis (editorial). Arch Dermatol 1987; 123:1615–1618.
> Sharma BK, Talukdar B, Mathur RP: Weber–Christian disease, an unusual occurrence in a 12-year-old child. Int J Dermatol 1990; 29:358–359.
> Sorenson RU, Abramowsky C, Stern RC: Corticosteroid-sparing effect of hydroxychloroquine in a patient with early onset Weber–Christian syndrome. J Am Acad Dermatol 1990; 23: 1172–1174.

WEBER–COCKAYNE SYNDROME
see EPIDERMOLYSIS BULLOSA; SIMPLEX

WEGENER GRANULOMATOSIS

Manifestations and Major Findings
generalized necrotizing angiitis of the upper respiratory tract and lungs
severe sinopulmonary inflammation
persistent, crusty, hemorrhagic granulomas of the nostrils, nasal septum, or pharynx

OTHER FINDINGS
glomerulonephritis causing renal insufficiency
arthritis
asthma
parotid gland involvement with granulomas
ocular involvement
antineutrophilic cytoplasmic antibodies (ANCA)

Cutaneous Manifestations
symmetric, papulonecrotic lesions of the extremities
widespread vesicular, urticarial, or vasculitic lesions
pyoderma gangrenosum
erythema elevatum diutinum
gingivitis and oral ulcerations

> **References**
> Cohen Tervaert JW, van der Woude FJ, Fauci AS, et al.: Association between active Wegener's granulomatosis and anticytoplasmic antibodies. Arch Intern Med 1989; 149:2461–2465.
> Fauci AS, Haynes BF, Katz P, Wolff SM: Wegener's granulomatosis: prospective clinical and therapeutic experience with 85 patients for 21 years. Ann Intern Med 1983; 98:76–85.
> Mangold MC, Callen JP: Cutaneous leukocytoclastic vasculitis associated with active Wegener's granulomatosis. J Am Acad Dermatol 1992; 26:579–584.
> Patten SF, Tomecki KF: Wegener's granulomatosis: cutaneous and oral mucosal disease. J Am Acad Dermatol 1993; 28:710–718.
> Valeriano-Marcet J, Spiera H: Treatment of Wegener's granulomatosis with sulfamethoxazole-trimethoprim. Arch Intern Med 1991; 151: 1649–1652.
> Wegener F: Wegener's granulomatosis: thoughts and observations of a pathologist. Eur Arch Otorhinolaryngol 1990; 247:133–142.

WELLS SYNDROME,
EOSINOPHILIC CELLULITIS

Manifestations and Major Findings
- recurrent dermatitis (Fig. 142) resembling cellulitis or persistent urticaria

lesions may be pruritic or painful
eosinophilia (peripheral and bone marrow)
may resolve spontaneously (or with steroids)
histology shows 'flame figures' and tissue eosinophilia

> **References**
> Aberer W, Konrad K, Wolff K: Wells' syndrome is a distinctive disease entity and not a histologic diagnosis. J Am Acad Dermatol 1988; 18:105–114.
> Wells GC, Smith NP: Eosinophilic cellulitis. Br J Dermatol 1979; 100:101–109.
> Wolf C, Pehamberger H, Breyer S, Leiferman KM, et al.: Episodic angioedema with eosinophilia. J Am Acad Dermatol 1989; 20:21–27.

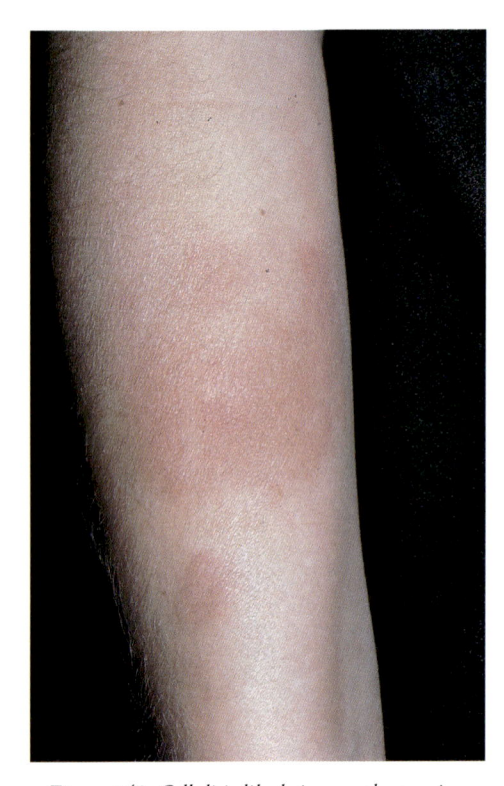

Figure 142 Cellulitis-like lesions on the arm in Wells syndrome.

WERMER SYNDROME see MULTIPLE ENDOCRINE NEOPLASIA SYNDROMES; TYPE 1

WERNER SYNDROME, ADULT PROGERIA SYNDROME, ADULT PREMATURE AGING SYNDROME, PANGERIA

Manifestations and Major Findings
acceleration of many aging-associated processes
onset at 14–18 years of age
short stature – growth cessation at 12 years
severe atherosclerotic vascular disease
increased risk of malignancy
  (sarcoma, meningioma)
high-pitched, hoarse voice
flat feet
small hands and feet
thin extremities
hyperreflexia
endocrine abnormalities
–diabetes mellitus
–hypogonadism
–early menopause
life expectancy of 40–60 years

Characteristic Facies
bird-like facies with beaked nose
dystrophic teeth
juvenile cataracts and glaucoma
premature graying and baldness

Cutaneous Manifestations
atrophy of the skin and subcutaneous tissues
mottled hyperpigmentation (poikiloderma)
acral sclerodermatous changes
leg ulcers

autosomal recessive

References
Bauer EA, Uitto J, Tan EML, Holbrook KA: Werner's syndrome. Evidence for preferential regional expression of a generalized mesenchymal cell defect. Arch Dermatol 1988; 124:90–101.
Beauregard S, Gilchrest BA: Syndromes of premature aging. Dermatol Clin 1987; 5:109–121.
Gilkes JJH, Sharvill DE, Wells RS: The premature ageing syndromes. Br J Dermatol 1974; 91:243–261.
Iijima S, Arinami T, Otsuka F: Possible Werner syndrome. Arch Dermatol 1992; 128:1238–1242.
Kondo S, Hozumi Y, Aso K: Werner's syndrome: no difference in *in vitro* life span of dermal fibroblasts from proximal and distal parts of the body. Acta Derm Venereol (Stockh) 1992; 72:11–14.

WHIPPLE DISEASE, INTESTINAL LIPODYSTROPHY SYNDROME

Manifestations and Major Findings
systemic bacterial infection by *Tropheryma whippelii* (Whipple bacillus)
polyarthritis
abdominal pain – exacerbated by eating
chronic diarrhea
evidence of steatorrhea
weight loss
cough

fever
lymphadenopathy
carditis/endocarditis
muscle weakness
anemia
reduced cell-mediated immunity

NEUROLOGIC ABNORMALITIES
lethargy
headache
dementia

Cutaneous Manifestations
patchy, brown pigmentation
erythema nodosum
purpura

> **References**
> **Donaldson RM:** Whipple's disease – rare malady with uncommon potential. N Engl J Med 1992; 327: 346–348.
> **Feldman M:** Southern Internal Medicine Conference: Whipple's disease. Am J Med Sci 1986; 291:56–67.
> **Relman DA, Schmidt TM, MacDermott RP, Falkow S:** Identification of the uncultured bacillus of Whipple's disease. N Engl J Med 1992; 327: 293–301.
> **Southern JF, Moscicki RA, Magro C, Dickersin GR, et al.:** Lymphedema, lymphocytic myocarditis and sarcoidlike granulomatous manifestations of Whipple's disease. J Am Med Assoc 1989; 261:1467–1470.

WHITE SPONGE NEVUS
see CANNON DISEASE

WILLIAMS SYNDROME

Manifestations and Major Findings
infantile hypercalcemia (may be transient or under-diagnosed)
cardiac abnormalities
supravalvular aortic stenosis
mental retardation (mild to severe)
hoarse voice
characteristic outgoing personality
hyperactive behavior
excessive talking (good verbal skills)
hyperacusis
dental abnormalities
joint contractures

Characteristic Facies
elfin facies in infancy
thick lips
upturned nose
depressed nasal bridge
puffy skin on malar region
epicanthal folds
blue iris with stellate pattern
large protruding ears

> **References**
> **Conway EE, Noonan J, Marion RW, Steeg CN:** Myocardial infarction leading to sudden death in the Williams syndrome: report of three cases. J Pediatr 1990; 117:593–595.
> **Kaplan P, Kirschner M, Watters G, Costa MT:** Contractures in patients with Williams syndrome. Pediatrics 1989; 84:895–899.
> **Morris CA, Demsey SA, Leonard CO, Dilts C, Blackburn BL:** Natural history of Williams syndrome: physical characteristics. J Pediatr 1988; 113:318–326.
> **Pagon RA, Bennett FC, LaVeck B, Stewart KB:** Williams Syndrome: features in late childhood and adolescence. Pediatrics 1987; 80:85–91.

WILSON DISEASE, HEPATOLENTICULAR DEGENERATION SYNDROME, CERULOPLASMIN DEFICIENCY

Manifestations and Major Findings
disturbance in copper metabolism
deposition of copper in the liver, brain, kidney, and cornea
Kayser–Fleischer rings on the cornea
azure lunulae of the nails
cirrhosis of the liver
degenerative changes of the brain
behavior disorders

autosomal recessive

> **References**
> **Danks DM:** Steely hair, mottled mice and copper metabolism. N Engl J Med 1975; 293:1147–1148.

WINCHESTER SYNDROME

Manifestations and Major Findings
short stature
joint destruction with contractures resembling rheumatoid arthritis
osteolysis of carpal and tarsal bones
severe mental retardation
may clinically resemble mucopolysaccharidosis

Characteristic Facies
coarse features
prominent forehead
large nose
depressed nasal bridge
thick lips
peripheral corneal opacities

Cutaneous Manifestations
diffuse stiffness of the skin with thickening
hyperpigmention with patchy or streaky color
hypertrichosis
gingival hypertrophy

autosomal recessive

> **References**
> Cohen AH, Hollister DW, Reed WB: The skin in the Winchester syndrome. Arch Dermatol 1975; 111:230–236.
> Winchester P, Grossman H, Lim WN, Danes BS: A new acid mucopolysaccharidosis with skeletal deformities. Am J Roentgenol 1969; 106:121–128.

WINER PORE, DILATED PORE OF WINER

Manifestations and Major Findings
large solitary pore resembling an open comedo
usually on the face
enlarged, patulous, follicular infundibulum extending down to the subcutaneous fat

> **References**
> Winer L: The dilated pore, a trichoepithelioma. J Invest Dermatol 1954; 23:181–188

WISKOTT–ALDRICH SYNDROME,
ALDRICH SYNDROME

Manifestations and Major Findings
thrombocytopenic purpura causing petechiae, epistaxis, bloody diarrhea, and intracranial bleeding
- chronic eczema (Fig. 143)
recurrent infections
– herpes
– warts
– varicella
– staphylococci
– gram-negative bacteria
– cytomegalovirus
sinopulmonary infections – onset at about 6 months of age
periodontal disease
usually fatal in childhood

IMMUNOLOGIC ABNORMALITIES
inability to form antibodies
low to absent isohemagglutinins
elevated IgA
elevated IgE
decreased IgM
normal IgG
no antibody response to polysaccharide antigens
abnormal size of lymphocyte CD43 (sialoglycoprotein)
abnormal mitogen responses to anti-CD43 and periodate

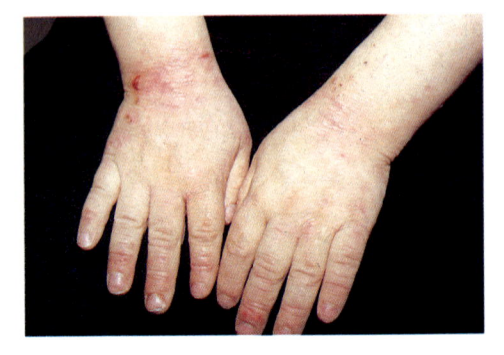

• *Figure 143 Eczematous lesions of the hands in Wiskott–Aldrich syndrome with chronic scratching.*

OTHER FINDINGS
increased risk of malignancies (lymphoma, leukemia, Hodgkin disease)
arthritic or renal autoimmune disease common
platelets decreased in number and size
prolonged bleeding time

X-linked recessive

> **References**
> Peacocke M, Siminovitch KA: Wiskott–Aldrich syndrome: new molecular and biochemical insights. J Am Acad Dermatol 1992; 27:507–519.

WITTEN AND ZAK TYPE KERATOACANTHOMA
see also KERATOACANTHOMA

Manifestations and Major Findings
combination of Ferguson–Smith type (multiple self-healing keratoacanthomas) and Grzybowski type lesions (very numerous small keratoacanthomas)

> **References**
> Street ML, White JW, Gibson LE: Multiple keratoacanthomas treated with oral retinoids. J Am Acad Dermatol 1990; 23:862–866.
> Witten VH, Zak FG: Multiple, primary, self-healing prickle-cell epithelioma of the skin. Cancer 1952; 5:539–550.

WOLFMAN SYNDROME
see CONGENITAL HYPERTRICHOSIS LANUGINOSA

WOOLF SYNDROME

Manifestations and Major Findings
piebaldism
deafness
no other features of Waardenburg syndrome

autosomal recessive

> **References**
> Bologna JL, Pawelek JM: Biology of hypopigmentation. J Am Acad Dermatol 1988; 19:217–255.
> Ortonne JP: Piebaldism, Waardenburg's syndrome, and related disorders. Dermatol Clin 1988; 6:205–216.

WORINGER–KOLOPP DISEASE,
PAGETOID RETICULOSIS, EPIDERMOTROPIC LYMPHOBLASTOMA

Manifestations and Major Findings
epidermotropic form of mycosis fungoides (cutaneous T cell lymphoma)
solitary, localized, erythematous plaque
most common on feet
asymptomatic, slowly expanding single plaque

> **References**
> Mielke V, Wolff HH, Winzer M, Sterry W: Localized and disseminated pagetoid reticulosis. Arch Dermatol 1989; 125:402–406.
> Oliver GF, Winkelmann RK: Unilesional mycosis fungoides: a distinct entity. J Am Acad Dermatol 1989; 20:63–70.
> Smoller BR, Stewart M, Warnke R: A case of Woringer–Kolopp disease with Ki-1 (CD30)+ cytotoxic/suppressor cells. Arch Dermatol 1992; 128:526–529.

WYBURN–MASON SYNDROME,
BONNET–DECHAUME–BLANC–WYBURN–MASON SYNDROME, CEREBRORETINAL ARTERIOVENOUS ANEURYSM

Manifestations and Major Findings
unilateral capillary malformation (port-wine stain) of the face
intracranial arteriovenous anomaly – predominantly around the midbrain
retinal arteriovenous malformation
exophthalmos
mental retardation
seizures

Wyburn–Mason syndrome may be associated with Sturge–Weber syndrome.

References

Brodsky MC, Hoyt WF, Higashida RT, et al.: Bonnet–Dechaume–Blanc syndrome with large facial angioma. Arch Ophthalmol 1987; 105:854–855.

Gulick AW, Taylor WB: A case of basal cell carcinoma in a patient with Wyburn–Mason syndrome. J Dermatol Surg Oncol 1978; 4:85–86.

Ward JB, Katz NNK: Combined phakomatoses: a case report of Sturge–Weber and Wyburn–Mason syndrome occurring in the same individual. Ann Ophthalmol 1983; 15:1112–1116.

X

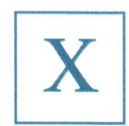

XANTHOMA DISSEMINATUM
see HISTIOCYTOSIS

XANTHOMAS
see HYPERLIPIDEMIAS

XERODERMA PIGMENTOSUM

Manifestations and Major Findings
defective repair of UV radiation damage to pyrimidine dimers in DNA
affects many cell types – epidermal, fibroblast, lymphocyte, corneal, liver
excision-defective complementation
complementation groups A, C, D, and variant groups are the most common
reduced natural killer cell activity
symptoms usually begin between 6 months and 3 years of age
shortened life expectancy

OCULAR ABNORMALITIES
ectropion
blepharitis
photophobia
keratitis
symblepharon
conjunctivitis
neoplasms of the lids, iris, and cornea (anterior compartment)
ulceration of the lids

NEUROLOGIC ABNORMALITIES
microcephaly
low intelligence
progressive dementia
cerebellar, basal ganglia, and pyramidal tract involvement
ataxia
sensorineural deafness
peripheral neuropathy
hyporeflexia

Cutaneous Manifestations
photosensitivity
- solar lentigines (Fig. 144)
- hypopigmentation (Fig. 144)

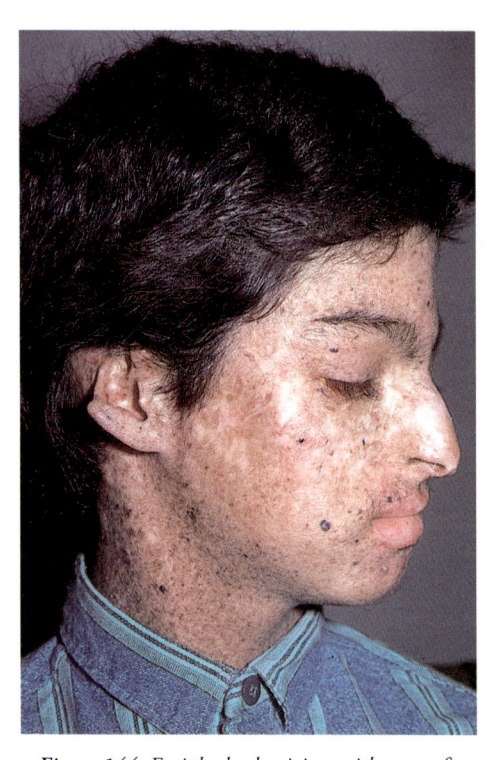

- *Figure 144 Facial solar lentigines with areas of hypopigmentation in xeroderma pigmentosum.*

premature aging
freckles
dry skin
hyperkeratoses
telangiectases
atrophy
neoplasms
- basal cell carcinomas
- squamous cell carcinomas
- lentigo maligna
- melanomas
- oral cavity neoplasms (squamous cell carcinomas)
other tumors
- keratoacanthomas
- angiomas
- fibromas
- sarcomas (angiosarcomas, fibrosarcomas)

autosomal recessive

Xeroderma Pigmentosum Complementation Groups

1. **group A**
   most severe form
   skin and central nervous system disorders
   - severe or mild
   - De Sanctis–Cacchione syndrome *see also* De Sanctis–Cacchione syndrome
   excision repair < 2% of normal
   most common in Japan
   chromosome 9

2. **group B**
   rare form
   may have Cockayne syndrome
   excision repair 3–7% of normal
   chromosome 2

3. **group C**
   common form
   usually only have skin disorders
   excision repair 10–25% of normal
   most common in USA, Europe, Egypt

4. **group D**
   common form
   skin cancer
   central nervous system disorders
   may have Cockayne syndrome
   may have trichothiodystrophy
   excision repair 25–50% of normal
   chromosome 19q

5. **group E**
   few skin cancers
   excision repair 40–50% of normal

6. **group F**
   mild skin symptoms
   excision repair 10–20% of normal

7. **group G**
   mental retardation
   neurologic abnormalities
   photosensitivity
   excision repair < 5% of normal
   chromosome 13q

8. **variant group**
   mild to severe skin disorders
   normal central nervous system function
   defect may be in postreplication repair

References
Berbis P, Beylot C, Noe C, et al.: Xeroderma pigmentosum and refractory anaemia in two first cousins. Br J Dermatol 1989; 121:767–771.
Ichihashi M, Yamamura K, Hiramoto T, Fujiwara Y: No apparent neurologic defect in a patient with xeroderma pigmentosum complementation Group D. Arch Dermatol 1988; 124:256–260.
Khatri ML, Shafi M, Mashina A: Xeroderma pigmentosum. A clinical study of 24 Libyan cases. J Am Acad Dermatol 1992; 26:75–78.
Kraemer KH, DiGiovanna JJ, Moshell AN, et al.: Prevention of skin cancer in xeroderma pigmentosum with the use of oral isotretinoin. N Engl J Med 1988; 318:1633–1637.
Kraemer KH, Lee MM, Scotto J: Xeroderma pigmentosum. Cutaneous, ocular, and neurologic abnormalities in 830 published cases. Arch Dermatol 1987; 123:241–250.
Nishigori C, Miyachi Y, Takebe H, Imamura S: A case of xeroderma pigmentosum with clinical appearance of dyschromatosis symmetrica hereditaria. Pediatr Dermatol 1986;3:410–413.
Robbins JH: Xeroderma pigmentosum. Defective DNA repair causes skin cancer and neurodegeneration. J Am Med Assoc 1988; 260:384–388.

XO SYNDROME *see* TURNER SYNDROME

XXY SYNDROME *see* KLINEFELTER SYNDROME

XYY SYNDROME

Manifestations and Major Findings
male phenotype
tall stature
occasional behavior problems (aggression)
relative weakness
poor fine-motor coordination
prominent glabella
long fingers
long ears
severe nodulocystic acne
cryptorchidism
small penis
slight mental retardation

Y

YELLOW NAIL SYNDROME,
SAMMAN SYNDROME, LYMPHEDEMA OF THE NAILS

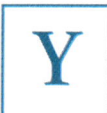

Manifestations and Major Findings
very slowly growing, discolored, yellow nails
usually involves all nails
nail thickening with increased curvature about the long axis
onycholysis
nail cuticles and lunulae are lost
usually associated with lymphedema of the extremities and/or face
recurrent pleural effusion or pulmonary abnormalities
most common in adults

Yellow nail syndrome is also associated with malignant neoplasms, D-penicillamine therapy, nephrotic syndrome, hypothyroidism, and acquired immunodeficiency syndrome.

References
DeCoste SD, Imber MJ, Baden HP: Yellow nail syndrome. J Am Acad Dermatol 1990; 22:608–611.
Govaert P, Leroy JG, Pauwels R, Vanhaesebrouck P, et al.: Perinatal manifestations of maternal yellow nail syndrome. Pediatrics 1992; 89:1016–1018.
Lodge JPA, Hunter AM, Saunders NR: Yellow nail syndrome associated with empyema. Clin Exp Dermatol 1989; 14:328–329.
Magid M, Esterly NB, Prendiville J, Fujisaki C: The yellow nail syndrome in an 8-year-old girl. Pediatr Dermatol 1987; 4:90–93.
Marks R, Ellis JP: Yellow nails: a report of six cases. Arch Dermatol 1970; 102:619–623.
Samman PD, White WF: The yellow nail syndrome. Br J Dermatol 1964; 76:153–157.
Williams HC, Buffham R, du Vivier A: Successful use of topical vitamin E solution in the treatment of nail changes in yellow nail syndrome. Arch Dermatol 1991; 127:1023–1028.

Z

ZELLWEGER SYNDROME,
CEREBROHEPATORENAL SYNDROME

Manifestations and Major Findings
absent or reduced number of peroxisomes
defects in early brain development
– large fontanels
– seizures
– severe mental retardation
– deafness
hepatomegaly
kidney cysts
extreme muscular hypotonia
speckled epiphyseal calcifications
  (especially patella)
premature death
similar to but distinct from chondrodysplasia
  punctata (rhizomelic form)

Characteristic Facies
high forehead
flat facies
shallow orbital ridges
low/broad nasal bridge
micrognathia
redundant skin folds of the neck

autosomal recessive

References
Hajra AK, Datta NS, Jackson LG, Moser AB, et al.: Prenatal diagnosis of Zellweger cerebrohepatorenal syndrome. N Engl J Med 1985; 312:445–446.
Kelley RI: Review: The cerebrohepatorenal syndrome of Zellweger, morphologic and metabolic aspects. Am J Med Genet 1983;16:503–517.
Zellweger H: The cerebro-hepato-renal syndrome. Dev Med Child Neurol 1987; 29:821–829.

ZINSSER–ENGMAN–COLE SYNDROME see DYSKERATOSIS CONGENITA

ZIPRKOWSKI–MARGOLIS SYNDROME

Manifestations and Major Findings
piebaldism-like hypomelanosis with
  hyperpigmented areas
depigmented hair
congenital deafness
heterochromia irides
most common Middle Eastern families

X-linked recessive

References
Ortonne JP: Piebaldism, Waardenburg's syndrome, and related disorders. Dermatol Clin 1988; 6: 205–216.
Ziprkowski L, Krakowski A, Adam A, Costeff H, et al.: Partial albinism and deaf mutism. Arch Dermatol 1962; 86:530–539.

ZOLLINGER–ELLISON SYNDROME

Manifestations and Major Findings
hypergastrinemia
peptic ulceration
severe diarrhea
non-β cell tumor of pancreatic islets
Zollinger–Ellison syndrome is associated with multiple endocrine neoplasia type 1.

autosomal dominant

References
Pipeleers-Marichal M, Somers G, Willems G, Foulis A, et al.: Gastrinomas in the duodenums of patients with multiple endocrine neoplasia type I and the Zollinger–Ellison syndrome. N Engl J Med 1990; 322:723–727.

ZOON BALANITIS, BALANITIS OF ZOON, BALANITIS CIRCUMSCRIPTA PLASMACELLULARIS

Manifestations and Major Findings
indolent, circumscribed, red, shiny plaque on the glans penis
plasma cell infiltrate in the dermis
affects middle-aged or elderly males

In females the condition is called vulvitis circumscripta plasmacellularis (Zoon vulvitis).

References
Ferrandiz C, Ribera M: Zoon's balanitis treated by circumcision. J Dermatol Surg Oncol 1984; 10: 622–625.
Morioka S, Nakajima S, Yaguchi H, Naito K, et al.: Vulvitis circumscripta plasmacellularis treated successfully with interferon alpha. J Am Acad Dermatol 1988; 19:947–950.
Nishimura M, Matsuda T, Muto M, Hori Y: Balantis of Zoon. Int J Dermatol 1990; 29:421–423.
Petersen CS, Thomsen K: Fusidic acid cream in the treatment of plasma cell balanitis. J Am Acad Dermatol 1992; 633–634.

APPENDIX

The following disorders are only those listed in this book and are not an exhaustive list of disorders with these features.

ACANTHOSIS NIGRICANS
- Ataxia Telangiectasia
- Bloom Syndrome
- Cardiofaciocutaneous Syndrome
- Donahue Syndrome
- Lipoatrophic Diabetes Syndrome
- Polycystic Ovary Syndrome
- Ruvalcaba–Myhre–Smith Syndrome

ACNE/ACNEIFORM ERUPTIONS
- Apert Syndrome
- Congenital Adrenal Hyperplasia
- Crohn Disease
- Cushing Syndrome
- Favre–Racouchot Syndrome
- Grover Disease
- Haber Syndrome
- Winer Pore
- XYY Syndrome

ACRAL PAPULES/ KERATOSES
- Acrokeratoelastoidosis of Costa
- Hereditary Acrokeratotic Poikiloderma
- Rothmund–Thomson Syndrome

AGING SYNDROME
- Baraitser Syndrome
- Cockayne Syndrome
- Gottron Syndrome
- Metageria
- Myotonic Dystrophy
- Progeria
- Seckel Syndrome
- Werner Syndrome
- Xeroderma Pigmentosum

ANGIOMAS
- Angiokeratomas
- Cobb Syndrome
- Cowden Disease
- Fabry Disease
- Fucosidosis
- POEMS Syndrome
- Tuberous Sclerosis
- Xeroderma Pigmentosum

ANNULAR ERYTHEMATOUS PLAQUES
- Bannwarth Syndrome
- Erythrokeratodermia Variabilis
- Gottron Syndrome
- Giroux–Barbeau Syndrome
- Glucagonoma Syndrome
- Lupus Erythematosus
- Lyme Disease
- Majocchi Granuloma
- Neonatal Lupus Erythematosus
- Oudsthoorn Disease
- Peeling Skin Syndrome
- Purpura Pigmentosa Chronica
- Rowell Syndrome
- Sarcoidosis
- Senear–Usher Syndrome
- Sneddon–Wilkinson Syndrome
- Still Disease

ATROPHY OF THE SKIN
- Aplasia Cutis Congenita
- Ataxia Telangiectasia
- Bart Syndrome
- Bazex Syndrome (Follicular)
- Beckwith–Wiedemann Syndrome
- Chondrodysplasia Punctata Syndrome
- Cushing Syndrome
- Delleman–Oorthuys Syndrome
- Ehlers–Danlos Syndrome
- Fetal Varicella Syndrome
- Focal Dermal Hypoplasia
- Hallerman–Streiff Syndrome
- Huriez Syndrome
- Jadassohn–Pellizzari Anetoderma
- Johanson–Blizzard Syndrome
- Lipoatrophic Diabetes Syndrome
- Lyme Disease
- Majocchi Disease
- Marfan Syndrome
- Metageria
- Myotonic Dystrophy
- Osteogenesis Imperfecta
- Parry–Romberg Syndrome
- Pasini and Pierini Atrophoderma
- Plummer–Vinson Syndrome
- Poikiloderma of Civatte
- Porphyria
- Progeria
- Purpura Pigmentosa Chronica
- Rombo Syndrome
- Schweninger–Buzzi Anetoderma
- Trisomy 13
- Weber–Christian Disease
- Werner Syndrome
- Xeroderma Pigmentosum

BRUISING
- Autoerythrocyte Sensitization Syndrome
- Battered Child Syndrome
- Dercum Disease
- Ehlers–Danlos Syndrome
- Gottron Syndrome
- Henoch–Schönlein Purpura
- Hermansky–Pudlak Syndrome
- Osteogenesis Imperfecta
- Von Willebrand Disease

BULLOUS/BLISTERING LESIONS
- Bart Syndrome
- Brunsting–Perry Syndrome
- Cockayne Syndrome
- Crohn Disease
- Dermatitis Herpetiformis
- Dowling–Meara Syndrome
- Epidermolysis Bullosa (all types)
- Epidermolysis Bullosa Acquisita
- Epidermolytic Hyperkeratosis
- Fogo Selvagem
- Hailey–Hailey Disease
- Hereditary Acrokeratotic Poikiloderma

Incontinentia Pigmenti
Kaposi Varicelliform Eruption
Kindler Syndrome
Lipoid Proteinosis
Mastocytosis
Mendes DaCosta Syndrome
Moynahan Syndrome
Neumann Type Pemphigus
  Vegetans
Pachyonychia Congenita
Pasini Syndrome
Polyglandular Autoimmune
  Syndrome
Porphyria
Ramsay Hunt Syndrome
Richner–Hanhart Syndrome
Staphylococcal Scalded Skin
  Syndrome
Stevens–Johnson Syndrome
Stewart–Treves Syndrome
Syphilis (Congenital)
Vohwinkel Syndrome
Weber–Cockayne Syndrome

CAFÉ AU LAIT MACULES
Bloom Syndrome
Cardiofaciocutaneous Syndrome
Ectrodactyly–Ectodermal
  Dysplasia–Clefting Syndrome
Epidermal Nevus Syndrome
Fanconi Aplastic Anemia
Johanson–Blizzard Syndrome
Maffucci Syndrome
McCune–Albright Syndrome
Morquio Syndrome
Mucosal Neuroma Syndrome
Neurofibromatosis
Niemann–Pick Disease
Proteus Syndrome
Russell–Silver Syndrome

CALCINOSIS/OSTEOMA CUTIS
Albright Hereditary
  Osteodystrophy
Hereditary Sclerosing
  Poikiloderma of Weary
Lesch–Nyhan Syndrome
Pilomatrixoma of Malherbe
Rothmund–Thomson Syndrome
Stiff Skin Syndrome

CANITIES (PREMATURE GRAYING OF HAIR)
Böök Syndrome
Branchio-Oculofacial Syndrome
Cockayne Syndrome
Cri-du-Chat Syndrome

Dyskeratosis Congenita
Fisch Syndrome
Lison Syndrome
Prolidase Deficiency
Seckel Syndrome
Waardenburg Syndrome
Werner Syndrome

CHEILITIS
Melkersson–Rosenthal Syndrome
Miescher Granulomatosis
Pachyonychia Congenita
Plummer–Vinson Syndrome

COARSE FACIAL FEATURES
Mucolipidosis II
Mucolipidosis III
Mucopolysaccharidoses
Multiple Sulfatase Deficiency
Winchester Syndrome

CONSTRICTIVE BANDS
Amniotic Band Syndrome
Multiple Pterygium Syndrome
Olmsted Syndrome
Popliteal Pterygium Syndrome
Tourniquet Syndrome
Vohwinkel Syndrome

CUTIS MARMORATA/ LIVEDO RETICULARIS
Adams–Oliver Syndrome
De Lange Syndrome
Down Syndrome
Dury–Van Bogaert Syndrome
Rett Syndrome
Rubella Syndrome
Sneddon Syndrome
Trisomy 18
Waldenström Macroglobulinemia

CUTIS VERTICIS GYRATA
Fragile X Syndrome
Pachydermoperiostosis
Rosenthal–Kloepfer Syndrome

CYSTS OF THE SKIN
Cowden Disease
Frontonasal Dysplasia Sequence
Gardner Syndrome
Pilomatrixoma of Malherbe

DENTAL ABNORMALITIES
Ankyloblepharon–Ectodermal
  Dysplasia–Clefting Syndrome
Bart Syndrome
Basal Cell Nevus Syndrome
Berlin Syndrome

Böök Syndrome
Cardiofaciocutaneous Syndrome
Cleidocranial Dysostosis
Coffin–Siris Syndrome
Congenital Hypertrichosis
  Lanuginosa
Dowling–Meara Syndrome
Down Syndrome
Ectodermal Dysplasia
Ectrodactyly–Ectodermal
  Dysplasia–Clefting Syndrome
Elejalde Syndrome
Ellis–Van Creveld Syndrome
Epidermal Nevus Syndrome
Focal Dermal Hypoplasia
Franceschetti–Jadassohn
  Syndrome
Freire–Maia Syndrome
Gardner Syndrome
Greither Syndrome
Hallerman–Streiff Syndrome
Hereditary Sclerosing
  Poikiloderma of Weary
Hypomelanosis of Ito
Incontinentia Pigmenti
Johanson–Blizzard Syndrome
KID Syndrome
Kindler Syndrome
Marinesco–Sjögren Syndrome
Monilethrix Syndrome
Moynahan Syndrome
Oculodentodigital Syndrome
Olmsted Syndrome
Orofaciodigital Syndrome
Pachyonychia Congenita
Papillon–Lefèvre Syndrome
Pili Torti Syndromes
Porphyria
Progeria
Prolidase Deficiency
Rapp–Hodgkin Ectodermal
  Dysplasia
Rothmund–Thomson Syndrome
Rubinstein–Taybi Syndrome
Sjögren–Larsson Syndrome
Syphilis (Congenital)
Trichodentoosseous Syndrome
Trichothiodystrophy
Werner Syndrome
Williams Syndrome

DIAPER DERMATITIS
Histiocytosis
Jacquet Ulcers
Leiner Disease

ECZEMATOUS/SEBORRHEIC DERMATITIS
Acrodermatitis Continua of Hallopeau
Acrodermatitis Enteropathica
Bare Lymphocyte Syndrome
Biotin Deficiency
Bruton Agammaglobulinemia
Chronic Granulomatous Disease
DiGeorge Syndrome
Down Syndrome
Dubowitz Syndrome
Ectodermal Dysplasia (Hypohidrotic)
Hartnup Disease
Hereditary Acrokeratotic Poikiloderma
Histiocytosis
Hutchinson Summer Prurigo
Hyperimmunoglobulin E Syndrome
Job Syndrome
Kaposi Varicelliform Eruption
Letterer–Siwe Disease
Mal de Meleda
Nékam Disease
Netherton Syndrome
Omenn Syndrome
Phenylketonuria
Prolidase Deficiency
Rubella Syndrome
Seckel Syndrome
Severe Combined Immunodeficiency
Sulzberger–Garbe Syndrome
Vitamin Deficiencies:
  Niacin (B_3)
  Pyridoxine (B_6)
  Riboflavin (B_2)
Wiskott–Aldrich Syndrome

EDEMA/LYMPHEDEMA
Amniotic Band Syndrome
Hansen Disease
Henoch–Schönlein Purpura
Hereditary Angioedema
Kaposi Sarcoma
Kawasaki Disease
Kwashiorkor
Melkersson–Rosenthal Syndrome
Milroy Disease
Noonan Syndrome
Papular-Purpuric 'Gloves and Socks' Syndrome
POEMS Syndrome
Prolidase Deficiency
Sézary Syndrome
Sickle Cell Disease

Staphylococcal Scalded Skin Syndrome
Stewart–Treves Syndrome
Superior Vena Cava Syndrome
Toxic Shock Syndrome
Turner Syndrome
Vitamin Deficiencies:
  Thiamine (B_1)
Yellow Nail Syndrome

ERYTHRODERMA
Biotin Deficiency
Disorders of Cornification:
  Lamellar Ichthyosis
  Lamellar Dominant Ichthyosis
  Epidermolytic Hyperkeratosis
  Harlequin Fetus
Hydantoin Syndrome
Leiner Disease
Moynahan Syndrome
Netherton Syndrome
Omenn Syndrome
Papuloerythroderma of Ofuji
Peeling Skin Syndrome
Red Man Syndrome
Sarcoidosis
Severe Combined Immunodeficiency
Sézary Syndrome
Staphylococcal Scalded Skin Syndrome
Toxic Epidermal Necrolysis
Toxic Shock Syndrome

ERYTHROKERATODERMIA
Giroux–Barbeau Syndrome
Glucagonoma Syndrome
Gottron Syndrome

FLUSHING
Carcinoid Syndrome
'Chinese Restaurant' Syndrome
Mastocytosis

GIGANTISM
Beckwith–Wiedemann Syndrome
Sotos Syndrome
Bannayan–Zonana Syndrome

GRANULOMAS/GRANULOMATOUS PROCESSES (CUTANEOUS)
Churg–Strauss Syndrome
Crohn Disease
Donovanosis
Melkersson–Rosenthal Syndrome
Miescher Granulomatosis

Parinaud Oculoglandular Syndrome
Sarcoidosis
Wegener Granulomatosis

HAIR (ALOPECIA)
Bazex Syndrome
Biotin Deficiency
CHILD Syndrome
Cronkhite–Canada Syndrome
Down Syndrome
Eosinophilia–Myalgia Syndrome
Follicular Degeneration Syndrome
Glucagonoma Syndrome
Graham Little Syndrome
Greither Syndrome
Hallerman–Streiff Syndrome
Hodgkin Disease
Hypomelanosis of Ito
Incontinentia Pigmenti
Lipoid Proteinosis
Menkes Syndrome
Moynahan Syndrome
Nevus Sebaceus of Jadassohn
Olmsted Syndrome
Pachyonychia Congenita
Parry–Romberg Syndrome
Poland Anomaly
Polycystic Ovary Syndrome
Polyglandular Autoimmune Syndrome
Porphyria
Progeria
Pseudopelade of Brocq
Rothmund–Thomson Syndrome
Severe Combined Immunodeficiency
Sézary Syndrome
Sheehan Syndrome
Sjögren Syndrome
Treacher Collins Syndrome
Ulerythema Ophryogenes
Umcombable Hair Syndrome
Vitamin Deficiencies
Vogt–Koyanagi–Harada Syndrome
Vohwinkel Syndrome

HAIR (CURLY)
Arginosuccinic Aciduria
CHAND Syndrome
Lipoatrophic Diabetes Syndrome
Menkes Syndrome
Mucopolysaccharidoses
Noonan Syndrome
Sanfilippo Syndrome
Trichodentoosseous Syndrome

HAIR (HYPERTRICHOSIS)
Coffin–Siris Syndrome
Congenital Hypertrichosis Lanuginosa
De Lange Syndrome
Donahue Syndrome
Fetal Alcohol Syndrome
Fetal Hydantoin Syndrome
Fucosidosis
G$_{M1}$ Gangliosidosis (Infantile Form)
Graves Disease
Hurler Syndrome
Klippel–Feil Syndrome
Lipoatrophic Diabetes Syndrome
Mal de Meleda
Marshall–Smith Syndrome
Michelin Tire Baby Syndrome
Mucopolysaccharidoses
Noonan Syndrome
POEMS Syndrome
Porphyria
Rubinstein–Taybi Syndrome
Sanfilippo Syndrome
Stiff Skin Syndrome
Trisomy 18
Winchester Syndrome

HAIR (HYPOTRICHOSIS)
Addison Disease
Ankyloblepharon–Ectodermal Dysplasia–Clefting Syndrome
Baraitser Syndrome
Basan Type Ectodermal Dysplasia
Bazex Syndrome
Cartilage–Hair Hypoplasia
Clouston Syndrome
Coffin–Siris Syndrome
Dubowitz Syndrome
Dyskeratosis Congenita
Ectodermal Dysplasia
Ectrodactyly–Ectodermal Dysplasia–Clefting Syndrome
Ellis–Van Creveld Syndrome
Fabry Disease
Freire-Maia Syndrome
Hallerman–Streiff Syndrome
Hansen Disease
Homocystinuria
Incontinentia Pigmenti
Johanson–Blizzard Syndrome
KID Syndrome
Klinefelter Syndrome
Loose Anagen Hair Syndrome
Marasmus
Marie Unna Hypotrichosis
Marinesco–Sjögren Syndrome

Menkes Syndrome
Metageria
Monilethrix Syndrome
Oculocerebrorenal Syndrome
Oculodentodigital Syndrome
Oculo-osteocutaneous Syndrome
Orofaciodigital Syndrome
Pachyonychia Congenita
Pierre Robin Syndrome
Pili Torti Syndromes
Progeria
Rapp–Hodgkin Ectodermal Dysplasia
Roberts Syndrome
Rombo Syndrome
Seckel Syndrome
Severe Combined Immunodeficiency
Testicular Feminization
Trichorhinophalangeal Syndrome
Trichothiodystrophy
Weaver Syndrome

HAIR SHAFT ABNORMALITIES
Arginosuccinic Aciduria
Bazex Syndrome
Björnstad Syndrome
Crandall Syndrome
Marinesco–Sjögren Syndrome
Menkes Syndrome
Monilethrix Syndrome
Netherton Syndrome
Pili Torti Syndromes
Trichothiodystrophy
Uncombable Hair Syndrome

HAIR (SILVERY BLOND)
Chédiak–Higashi Syndrome
Elejalde Syndrome
Griscelli Syndrome
Menkes Syndrome
Roberts Syndrome

HAND ABNORMALITIES
Ellis–Van Creveld Syndrome
Poland Anomaly
Popliteal Pterygium Syndrome
Potter Syndrome
Trichorhinophalangeal Syndrome

HEMANGIOMAS
Cardiofaciocutaneous Syndrome
Dandy–Walker Complex
De Lange Syndrome
Diffuse Neonatal Hemangiomatosis
Fetal Alcohol Syndrome

MULIBREY Nanism Syndrome
Trisomy 13
Trisomy 18

HIRSUTISM
Congenital Adrenal Hyperplasia
Cushing Syndrome
De Lange Syndrome
Morgagni–Stewart–Morel Syndrome
Parana Hard-Skin Syndrome
Polycystic Ovary Syndrome

HYPERHIDROSIS
Acrokeratoelastoidosis of Costa
Auriculotemporal Syndrome
Blue Rubber Bleb Nevus Syndrome
Böök Syndrome
Greither Syndrome
Mal de Meleda
Nail–Patella Syndrome
Pachydermoperiostosis
Pachyonychia Congenita
Papillon–Lefèvre Syndrome
POEMS Syndrome
Richner–Hanhart Syndrome
Unna–Thost Keratoderma
Vörner Disease

HYPERPIGMENTATION
Acropigmentation Symmetrica of Dohi
Addison Disease
Alkaptonuria
Ataxia Telangiectasia
Becker Melanosis
Bronze Baby Syndrome
Carcinoid Syndrome
Chlorpromazine Syndrome
Congenital Adrenal Hyperplasia
Cronkhite–Canada Syndrome
Cushing Syndrome
Dowling–Degos Disease
Epidermolysis Bullosa Acquisita
Fanconi Aplastic Anemia
Felty Syndrome
Fetal Hydantoin Syndrome
Fogo Selvagem
Franceschetti–Jadassohn Syndrome
G$_{M1}$ Gangliosidosis (Infantile Form)
Gaucher Disease
Gougerot–Carteaud Syndrome
Hereditary Acrokeratotic Poikiloderma
Hodgkin Disease

Incontinentia Pigmenti
Johanson–Blizzard Syndrome
Kitamura Reticulate
  Acropigmentation
Laugier–Hunziker Syndrome
LEOPARD Syndrome
McCune–Albright Syndrome
Mongolian Spot
NAME Syndrome
Neurocutaneous Melanosis
Nevus of Ito
Nevus of Ota
Niemann–Pick Disease
Parana Hard-Skin Syndrome
Parry–Romberg Syndrome
Pasini and Pierini Atrophoderma
Peutz–Jeghers Syndrome
Phakomatosis Pigmentovascularis
Piebaldism
POEMS Syndrome
Porphyria
Proteus Syndrome
Riehl Melanosis
Rubella Syndrome
Russell–Silver Syndrome
Ruvalcaba–Myhre–Smith
  Syndrome
Sickle Cell Disease
Sneddon–Wilkinson Syndrome
Tuberous Sclerosis
Vitamin Deficiencies:
  Cyanocobalamin (B_{12})
  Folic acid
Voigt Lines
Waldenström Macroglobulinemia
Whipple Disease
Winchester Syndrome
Xeroderma Pigmentosum
Ziprkowski–Margolis Syndrome

HYPOPIGMENTATION/ HYPOPIGMENTED LESIONS
Albinism
Ataxia Telangiectasia
Chédiak–Higashi Syndrome
Cross Syndrome
Epidermal Nevus Syndrome
Hansen Disease
Hermansky–Pudlak Syndrome
Homocystinuria
Hypomelanosis of Ito
Incontinentia Pigmenti
Kwashiorkor
Phenylketonuria
Piebaldism
Porphyria
Prader–Willi Syndrome

Proteus Syndrome
Russell–Silver Syndrome
Sutton Nevus
Tietz Syndrome
Tuberous Sclerosis
Waardenburg Syndrome
Woolf Syndrome
Xeroderma Pigmentosum
Ziprkowski–Margolis Syndrome

ICHTHYOSIS
Bare Lymphocyte Syndrome
Cardiofaciocutaneous Syndrome
CHILD Syndrome
Conradi–Hünermann Syndrome
Disorders of Cornification
Pili Torti Syndromes

INFECTIONS OF SKIN
Acrodermatitis Enteropathica
Agammaglobulinemia of Bruton
AIDS
Ataxia Telangiectasia
Bare Lymphocyte Syndrome
Bockhart Impetigo
Chédiak–Higashi Syndrome
Chronic Granulomatous Disease
DiGeorge Syndrome
Epidermolytic Hyperkeratosis
Griscelli Syndrome
Hyperimmunoglobulin E
  Syndrome
KID Syndrome
Leiner Disease
Madura Foot
Majocchi Granuloma
Papillon–Lefèvre Syndrome
Polyglandular Autoimmune
  Syndrome
Prolidase Deficiency
Severe Combined
  Immunodeficiency
Shwachman Syndrome
Wiskott–Aldrich Syndrome

KERATODERMAS/ HYPERKERATOSIS OF PALMS AND SOLES
Bazex Syndrome
Buschke–Fischer Disease
Cantu Syndrome
Clouston Syndrome
Cowden Disease
Darier Disease
Disorders of Cornification:
  Lamellar Dominant Ichthyosis
Dowling–Meara Syndrome

Dyskeratosis Congenita
Epidermolytic Hyperkeratosis
Franceschetti–Jadassohn
  Syndrome
Gottron Syndrome
Greither Syndrome
Haxthausen Disease
Howel–Evans Syndrome
Keratodermas
KID Syndrome
Kindler Syndrome
Mal de Meleda
Oculo-osteocutaneous syndrome
Olmsted Syndrome
Oudsthoorn Disease
Pachyonychia Congenita
Papillon–Lefèvre Syndrome
Richner–Hanhart Syndrome
Sézary Syndrome
Siemens Syndrome
Sjögren–Larsson Syndrome
Unna–Thost Syndrome
Vohwinkel Syndrome
Vörner Disease

LAXITY OF THE SKIN
Cutis Laxa
Ehlers–Danlos Syndrome
Nail–Patella Syndrome

LENTIGINES
Carney Syndrome
De Sanctis–Cacchione Syndrome
LEOPARD Syndrome
NAME Syndrome
Peutz–Jeghers Syndrome
Xeroderma Pigmentosa

LIPODYSTROPHY
Cockayne Syndrome
Donahue Syndrome
Gottron Syndrome

LIPOMAS
Bannayan–Zonana Syndrome
Basal Cell Nevus Syndrome
Cowden Disease
Dercum Disease
Gardner Syndrome
Launois–Bensaude Syndrome
Madelung Disease
Michelin Tire Baby Syndrome
Proteus Syndrome
Ruvalcaba–Myhre–Smith
  Syndrome

LIVEDO RETICULARIS
Antiphospholipid Antibody Syndrome
Churg–Strauss Syndrome
Homocystinuria

MARFANOID HABITUS
Homocystinuria
Marfan Syndrome
Mucosal Neuroma Syndrome
Pseudoxanthoma Elasticum

NAIL ABNORMALITIES
Acrodermatitis Continua of Hallopeau
Adams–Oliver Syndrome
Ankyloblepharon–Ectodermal Dysplasia–Clefting syndrome
Bart Syndrome
Bazex Syndrome
CHAND Syndrome
Clouston Syndrome
Coffin–Siris Syndrome
Cronkhite–Canada Syndrome
Darier Disease
Dyskeratosis Congenita
Ectodermal Dysplasia
Ectrodactyly–Ectodermal Dysplasia–Clefting Syndrome
Ellis–Van Creveld Syndrome
Epidermolysis Bullosa
Epidermolysis Bullosa Acquisita
Fetal Alcohol Syndrome
Focal Dermal Hypoplasia
Freire–Maia Syndrome
Glucagonoma Syndrome
Hyperimmunoglobulin E Syndrome
Hypomelanosis of Ito
Incontinentia Pigmenti
Jacquet Ulcers
KID Syndrome
Mal de Meleda
Marasmus
Marinesco–Sjögren Syndrome
Mendes Da Costa Syndrome
Monilethrix Syndrome
Morvan Syndrome
Moynahan Syndrome
Nail-Patella Syndrome
Noonan Syndrome
Olmsted Syndrome
Pachyonychia Congenita
Pili Torti Syndromes
Plummer–Vinson Syndrome
Polyglandular Autoimmune Syndrome
Popliteal Pterygium Syndrome

Progeria
Rapp–Hodgkin Ectodermal Dysplasia
Reiter Syndrome
Rothmund–Thomson Syndrome
Sézary Syndrome
Sheehan Syndrome
Stevens–Johnson Syndrome
Trichodentoosseous Syndrome
Trichorhinophalangeal Syndrome
Trichothiodystrophy
Trisomy 13
Trisomy 18
Turner Syndrome
Von Zumbusch Syndrome
Weaver Syndrome
Wilson Disease
Yellow Nail Syndrome

NEVI (INCREASED IN NUMBER OR ABNORMAL)
Baraitser Syndrome
Carney Syndrome
Cocarde Nevus
Dysplastic Nevus Syndrome
LAMB Syndrome
NAME Syndrome
Neurocutaneous Melanosis
Noonan Syndrome
Phakomatosis Pigmentovascularis
Proteus Syndrome
Spitz Nevus
Trichorhinophalangeal Syndrome
Turner Syndrome

NODULES/PLAQUES
Angiolymphoid Hyperplasia with Eosinophilia
Basal Cell Nevus Syndrome
Brooke Syndrome
Buschke–Ollendorf Syndrome
Carrion Disease
Cat-scratch Disease
Chronic Granulomatous Disease
Farber Syndrome
Hodgkin Disease
Jessner Lymphocytic Infiltrate
Kaposi Sarcoma
Keratoacanthomas
Lobo Disease
Majocchi Granuloma
Mastocytosis
Neurofibromatosis
Nevus Sebaceus of Jadassohn
Paget Disease
Porokeratosis
Rosai–Dorfman Disease
Sarcoidosis

Sister Mary Joseph Nodule
Spiegler–Fendt Pseudolymphoma
Spitz Nevus
Stewart–Treves Syndrome
Still Disease
Sweet Syndrome
Tuberous Sclerosis
Woringer–Kolopp Disease

ORAL LESIONS OR CHANGES
Bazex Syndrome
Beckwith–Wiedemann Syndrome
Behçet Syndrome
Cannon Disease
Chédiak–Higashi Syndrome
Chronic Granulomatous Disease
Cowden Disease
Crohn Disease
Darier Disease
Down Syndrome
Dyskeratosis Congenita
Ehlers–Danlos Syndrome (Type 8)
G_{M1} Gangliosidosis (Infantile Form)
Grinspan Syndrome
Hand-Foot-and-Mouth Disease
Heck Disease
Histiocytosis
Howel–Evans Syndrome
Kaposi Sarcoma
Kawasaki Disease
KID Syndrome
Kwashiorkor
Letterer–Siwe Disease
Lipoid Proteinosis
Lupus Erythematosus
MAGIC Syndrome
Mal de Meleda
Melkersson–Rosenthal Syndrome
Miescher Granulomatosis
Mucolipidosis II
Mucosal Neuroma Syndrome
Neurofibromatosis
Oculodentodigital Syndrome
Orofaciodigital Syndrome
Pachyonychia Congenita
Papillon–Lefèvre Syndrome
Papular-Purpuric 'Gloves and Socks' Syndrome
Pierre Robin Syndrome
Popliteal Pterygium Syndrome
Reiter Syndrome
Richner–Hanhart Syndrome
Ruvalcaba–Myhre–Smith Syndrome
Senear–Usher Syndrome

Sickle Cell Disease
Stevens–Johnson Syndrome
Syphilis (Congenital)
Takahara Syndrome
Toxic Epidermal Necrolysis
Tuberous Sclerosis
Unna–Thost Syndrome
Vincent Infection
Vitamin Deficiencies:
  Riboflavin (B_2)
  Pyridoxine (B_6)
  Cyanocobalamin (B_{12})
  Scurvy (C)
  Biotin (H)
  Folic acid
Von Zumbusch Syndrome
Wegener Granulomatosis
Winchester Syndrome
Wiskott–Aldrich Syndrome

PANNICULITIS
α-1-Antitrypsin Deficiency
Bazin Disease
Behçet Syndrome
Buerger Disease
Crohn Disease
Gonococcal Dermatitis Syndrome
Hansen Disease
Hemophagocytic Syndrome
Hodgkin Disease
Löfgren Syndrome
Rothmann–Makai Syndrome
Sarcoidosis
Weber–Christian Disease
Whipple Disease

PHOTOSENSITIVITY
Cockayne Syndrome
Hutchinson Summer Prurigo
Kindler Syndrome
Lupus Erythematosus
Neonatal Lupus Erythematosus
Porphyria
Prolidase Deficiency
Rothmund–Thomson Syndrome
Trichothiodystrophy
Xeroderma Pigmentosum

POIKILODERMA
Berlin Syndrome
Dyskeratosis Congenita
Hereditary Acrokeratotic
  Poikiloderma
Hereditary Sclerosing
  Poikiloderma of Weary
Kindler Syndrome
Mendes DaCosta Syndrome
Metageria

Poikiloderma of Civatte
Rothmund–Thomson Syndrome
Werner Syndrome
Xeroderma Pigmentosum

PRURITUS
Alagille Syndrome
Gottron Syndrome
Grzybowski Type
  Keratoacanthoma
Hodgkin Disease
Mastocytosis
Neurofibromatosis
Notalgia Paresthetica
Paget Disease
Papular-Purpuric 'Gloves and
  Socks' Syndrome
Papulovesicular Acrolocated
  Syndrome
Peeling Skin Syndrome
PINK Disease
Purpura Pigmentosa Chronica:
  Itching Purpura
Red Man Syndrome
Sézary Syndrome
Sulzberger–Garbe Syndrome

PSORIASIFORM DERMATITIS
Bazex Syndrome
Glucagonoma Syndrome
Mal de Meleda
Papillon–Lefèvre Syndrome
Reiter Syndrome

PURPURA/PETECHIAE
Antiphospholipid Antibody
  Syndrome
Bateman Purpura
Churg–Strauss Syndrome
Coumarin Necrosis
Gougerot–Blum Disease
Hemolytic Uremic Syndrome
Hemophagocytic Syndrome
Henoch–Schönlein Purpura
Histiocytosis
Kasabach–Merritt Syndrome
Letterer–Siwe Disease
Lupus Erythematosus
Majocchi Disease
Neonatal Lupus Erythematosus
Niemann–Pick Disease
Notalgia Paresthetica
Papular-Purpuric 'Gloves and
  Socks' Syndrome
Polyglandular Autoimmune
  Syndrome
Prolidase Deficiency
Protein C Deficiency

Purpura Pigmentosa Chronica
Rocky Mountain Spotted Fever
Schamberg Purpura
Shwachman Syndrome
Stevens–Johnson Syndrome
Toxic Shock Syndrome
Vitamin Deficiencies:
  Scurvy (C)
Waldenström Macroglobulinemia
Waterhouse–Friderichsen
  Syndrome
Whipple Disease
Wiskott–Aldrich Syndrome

PYODERMA GANGRENOSUM
Crohn Disease
Felty Syndrome
Wegener Granulomatosis

SCLERODERMA/ SCLERODERMOID CHANGES OF THE SKIN
Carcinoid Syndrome
CREST Syndrome
Eosinophilia–Myalgia Syndrome
Eosinophilic Fasciitis
Hereditary Sclerosing
  Poikiloderma of Weary
Kindler Syndrome
Metageria
Phenylketonuria
POEMS Syndrome
Porphyria
Progeria
Restrictive Dermopathy
Scleromyxedema
Sjögren Syndrome
Vitamin Deficiencies:
  Scurvy (C)
Werner Syndrome
Winchester Syndrome
Xeroderma Pigmentosum

TELANGIECTASIA
Ataxia Telangiectasia
Berlin Syndrome
Bloom Syndrome
Carcinoid Syndrome
Coats Disease
CREST Syndrome
Cushing Syndrome
Fabry Disesae
Gaucher Disease
Kaposi Sarcoma
Mastocytosis
Morquio Syndrome
Osler–Weber–Rendu Syndrome
Poikiloderma of Civatte

Pseudoxanthoma Elasticum
Purpura Pigmentosa Chronica:
 Majocchi Disease
Sjögren Syndrome
Xeroderma Pigmentosum

ULCERS OF THE SKIN
Bazin Disease
Behçet Syndrome
Buruli Ulcer
Coumarin Necrosis
Crohn Disease
Donovanosis
Hansen Disease
Heparin Necrosis
Histiocytosis
Klinefelter Syndrome
Lesch–Nyhan Syndrome
Letterer–Siwe Disease
Lipoid Proteinosis
Madura Foot
MAGIC Syndrome
Marjolin Ulcer
Meleney Ulcer
Mucha–Habermann Syndrome
Münchausen Syndrome
Prader–Willi Syndrome
Prolidase Deficiency
Severe Combined
 Immunodeficiency
Sickle Cell Disease
Trigeminal Trophic Syndrome
Werner Syndrome

URTICARIA/ANGIOEDEMA
α-1-Antitrypsin Deficiency
Churg–Strauss Syndrome
Familial Mediterranean Fever
 Syndrome
Gonococcal Dermatitis Syndrome
Hereditary Angioedema
Hypereosinophilic Syndrome
Mastocytosis
Muckle–Wells Syndrome
Porphyria
Sulzberger–Garbe Syndrome
Wegener Granulomatosis
Wells Syndrome

VASCULAR MALFORMATIONS AND/OR LESIONS
Alagille Syndrome
Bannayan–Zonana Syndrome
Beckwith–Wiedemann Syndrome
Blue Rubber Bleb Nevus
 Syndrome
Brushfield–Wyatt Syndrome
Cobb Syndrome
Epidermal Nevus Syndrome
Gorham Syndrome
Kasabach–Merritt Syndrome
Klippel–Trenaunay Syndrome
Maffucci Syndrome
Phakomatosis Pigmentovascularis
Proteus Syndrome
Riley–Smith Syndrome
Roberts Syndrome
Rubinstein–Taybi Syndrome
Sturge–Weber Syndrome
Thrombocytopenia–Absent Radii
 Syndrome
Trisomy 13
Trisomy 18
Von Hippel–Lindau Syndrome
Wyburn–Mason Syndrome

VASCULITIS
Antiphospholipid Antibody
 Syndrome
α-1-Antitrypsin Deficiency
Behçet Syndrome
Bowel Bypass Syndrome
Churg–Strauss Syndrome
Crohn Disease
Degos Disease
Familial Mediterranean Fever
Henoch–Schönlein Purpura
Kawasaki Disease
Lupus Erythematosus
Schnitzler Syndrome
Waldenström Macroglobulinemia
Wegener Granulomatosis

VITILIGO/VITILIGINOUS MACULES
Addison Disease
Alezzandrini Syndrome
Ataxia Telangiectasia
Down Syndrome
Lip-Tip Syndrome
Polyglandular Autoimmune
 Syndrome
Vogt–Koyanagi–Harada
 Syndrome
Waardenburg Syndrome

RL
100
.M35

2601

DATE DUE

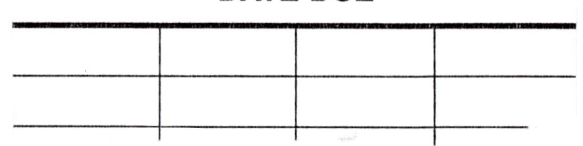

South University
709 Mall Blvd
Savannah, GA 31406